Inequalities in Health and Healthcare

Inequalities in Health and Healthcare

Editors

Jessica Sheringham
Sarah Sowden

MDPI • Basel • Beijing • Wuhan • Barcelona • Belgrade • Manchester • Tokyo • Cluj • Tianjin

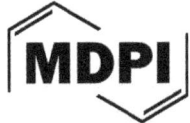

Editors
Jessica Sheringham
University College London
London
UK

Sarah Sowden
Newcastle University
Newcastle upon Tyne
UK

Editorial Office
MDPI
St. Alban-Anlage 66
4052 Basel, Switzerland

This is a reprint of articles from the Special Issue published online in the open access journal *International Journal of Environmental Research and Public Health* (ISSN 1660-4601) (available at: https://www.mdpi.com/journal/ijerph/special_issues/Inequalities_Healthcare).

For citation purposes, cite each article independently as indicated on the article page online and as indicated below:

LastName, A.A.; LastName, B.B.; LastName, C.C. Article Title. *Journal Name* **Year**, *Volume Number*, Page Range.

ISBN 978-3-0365-6978-9 (Hbk)
ISBN 978-3-0365-6979-6 (PDF)

© 2023 by the authors. Articles in this book are Open Access and distributed under the Creative Commons Attribution (CC BY) license, which allows users to download, copy and build upon published articles, as long as the author and publisher are properly credited, which ensures maximum dissemination and a wider impact of our publications.

The book as a whole is distributed by MDPI under the terms and conditions of the Creative Commons license CC BY-NC-ND.

Contents

Preface to "Inequalities in Health and Healthcare" vii

Claire Norman, Josephine M. Wildman and Sarah Sowden
COVID-19 at the Deep End: A Qualitative Interview Study of Primary Care Staff Working in the Most Deprived Areas of England during the COVID-19 Pandemic
Reprinted from: *Int. J. Environ. Res. Public Health* 2021, 18, 8689, doi:10.3390/ijerph18168689 . . . 1

Michelle Black, Amy Barnes, Mark Strong, Anna Brook, Anna Ray, Ben Holden, Clare Foster, et al.
Relationships between Child Development at School Entry and Adolescent Health—A Participatory Systematic Review
Reprinted from: *Int. J. Environ. Res. Public Health* 2021, 18, 11613, doi:10.3390/ijerph182111613 . 13

Marise S. Kaper, Jane Sixsmith, Sijmen A. Reijneveld and Andrea F. de Winter
Outcomes and Critical Factors for Successful Implementation of Organizational Health Literacy Interventions: A Scoping Review
Reprinted from: *Int. J. Environ. Res. Public Health* 2021, 18, 11906, doi:10.3390/ijerph182211906 . 49

Brenda Hayanga, Mai Stafford and Laia Bécares
Ethnic Inequalities in Healthcare Use and Care Quality among People with Multiple Long-Term Health Conditions Living in the United Kingdom: A Systematic Review and Narrative Synthesis
Reprinted from: *Int. J. Environ. Res. Public Health* 2021, 18, 12599, doi:10.3390/ijerph182312599 . 71

Louise Tanner, Sarah Sowden, Madeleine Still, Katie Thomson, Clare Bambra and Josephine Wildman
Which Non-Pharmaceutical Primary Care Interventions Reduce Inequalities in Common Mental Health Disorders? A Protocol for a Systematic Review of Quantitative and Qualitative Studies
Reprinted from: *Int. J. Environ. Res. Public Health* 2021, 18, 12978, doi:10.3390/ijerph182412978 . 95

Hannah Fairbrother, Nicholas Woodrow, Mary Crowder, Eleanor Holding, Naomi Griffin, Vanessa Er, Caroline Dodd-Reynolds, et al.
'It All Kind of Links Really': Young People's Perspectives on the Relationship between Socioeconomic Circumstances and Health
Reprinted from: *Int. J. Environ. Res. Public Health* 2022, 19, 3679, doi:10.3390/ ijerph19063679 . . 107

Elizabeth Ingram, Manuel Gomes, Sue Hogarth, Helen I. McDonald, David Osborn and Jessica Sheringham
Household Tenure and Its Associations with Multiple Long-Term Conditions amongst Working-Age Adults in East London: A Cross-Sectional Analysis Using Linked Primary Care and Local Government Records
Reprinted from: *Int. J. Environ. Res. Public Health* 2022, 19, 4155, doi:10.3390/ijerph19074155 . . . 127

Georgia Watson, Cassie Moore, Fiona Aspinal, Claudette Boa, Vusi Edeki, Andrew Hutchings, Rosalind Raine, et al.
A Protocol for a Mixed-Methods Process Evaluation of a Local Population Health Management System to Reduce Inequities in COVID-19 Vaccination Uptake
Reprinted from: *Int. J. Environ. Res. Public Health* 2022, 19, 4588, doi:10.3390/ijerph19084588 . . . 145

Liina Mansukoski, Alexandra Albert, Yassaman Vafai, Chris Cartwright, Aamnah Rahman, Jessica Sheringham, Bridget Lockyer, et al.
Development of Public Health Core Outcome Sets for Systems-Wide Promotion of Early Life Health and Wellbeing
Reprinted from: *Int. J. Environ. Res. Public Health* 2022, *19*, 7947, doi:10.3390/ijerph19137947 . . . **155**

Daniel Subel, David Blane and Jessica Sheringham
Workplace Interventions to Reduce Occupational Stress for Older Workers: A Systematic Review
Reprinted from: *Int. J. Environ. Res. Public Health* 2022, *19*, 9202, doi:10.3390/ijerph19159202 . . . **171**

Sabuj Kanti Mistry, Miranda Shaw, Freya Raffan, George Johnson, Katelyn Perren, Saito Shoko, Ben Harris-Roxas, et al.
Inequity in Access and Delivery of Virtual Care Interventions: A Scoping Review
Reprinted from: *Int. J. Environ. Res. Public Health* 2022, *19*, 9411, doi:10.3390/ijerph19159411 . . . **197**

Bartłomiej Matłosz, Agata Skrzat-Klapaczyńska, Sergii Antoniak, Tatevik Balayan, Josip Begovac, Gordana Dragovic, Denis Gusev, et al.
Chronic Kidney Disease and Nephrology Care in People Living with HIV in Central/Eastern Europe and Neighbouring Countries—Cross-Sectional Analysis from the ECEE Network
Reprinted from: *Int. J. Environ. Res. Public Health* 2022, *19*, 12554, doi:10.3390/ijerph191912554 . **209**

Jemma Keeves, Belinda Gabbe, Sarah Arnup, Christina Ekegren and Ben Beck
Serious Injury in Metropolitan and Regional Victoria: Exploring Travel to Treatment and Utilisation of Post-Discharge Health Services by Injury Type
Reprinted from: *Int. J. Environ. Res. Public Health* 2022, *19*, 14063, doi:10.3390/ijerph192114063 . **221**

Sowmiya Moorthie, Vicki Peacey, Sian Evans, Veronica Phillips, Andres Roman-Urrestarazu, Carol Brayne and Louise Lafortune
A Scoping Review of Approaches to Improving Quality of Data Relating to Health Inequalities
Reprinted from: *Int. J. Environ. Res. Public Health* 2022, *19*, 15874, doi:10.3390/ijerph192315874 . **237**

Jennifer Deane, Ruth Norris, James O'Hara, Joanne Patterson and Linda Sharp
Who Presents Where? A Population-Based Analysis of Socio-Demographic Inequalities in Head and Neck Cancer Patients' Referral Routes
Reprinted from: *Int. J. Environ. Res. Public Health* 2022, *19*, 16723, doi:10.3390/ijerph192416723 . **255**

Malcolm Moffat, Suzanne Nicholson, Joanne Darke, Melissa Brown, Stephen Minto, Sarah Sowden and Judith Rankin
A Qualitative Evaluation of a *Health Access Card* for Refugees and Asylum Seekers in a City in Northern England
Reprinted from: *Int. J. Environ. Res. Public Health* 2023, *20*, 1429, doi:10.3390/ijerph20021429 . . . **271**

Michelle S. Fitts, Jennifer Cullen, Gail Kingston, Yasmin Johnson, Elaine Wills and Karen Soldatic
Understanding the Lives of Aboriginal and Torres Strait Islander Women with Traumatic Brain Injury from Family Violence in Australia: A Qualitative Study Protocol
Reprinted from: *Int. J. Environ. Res. Public Health* 2023, *20*, 1607, doi:10.3390/ijerph20021607 . . . **287**

Edward Adinkrah, Babak Najand and Angela Young-Brinn
Race and Ethnic Differences in the Protective Effect of Parental Educational Attainment on Subsequent Perceived Tobacco Norms among US Youth
Reprinted from: *Int. J. Environ. Res. Public Health* 2023, *20*, 2517, doi:10.3390/ijerph20032517 . . . **299**

Preface to "Inequalities in Health and Healthcare"

Tackling inequalities in health and healthcare is more important than ever. The COVID-19 pandemic has already starkly illustrated the disproportional impact of the virus on those who already face disadvantage and discrimination (Bambra C et al. https://jech.bmj.com/content/74/11/964). Moreover, there is already evidence that the public health measures taken to contain the virus are likely to have longstanding differential impacts across populations.

Numerous studies have documented avoidable differences in health, within and between populations. Similarly, studies have consistently shown inequalities in access, use, experience and outcomes from many types of healthcare and public health programmes. The focus has often been on individual determinants, such as gender, age and ethnicity. Less attention has been paid to structural or contextual determinants, except for area-level socioeconomic conditions. In addition, to tackle inequalities, there is a need to move beyond measuring, in order to understand why these inequalities arise and how they can be addressed.

This Special Issue seeks to extend the parameters of inequalities research in health and healthcare beyond measuring and documenting inequalities. Reviews, observational studies, and quasi-experimental and other evaluation designs (using quantitative, qualitative or mixed methods) focusing on the following were welcomed for submission:

- understanding inequalities across health and care systems or at structural levels;
- methodological developments to understand drivers of inequalities;
- efforts to reduce inequalities, particularly in evidence-based healthcare or public health policy and practice;
- understanding and mitigating the adverse impact of the COVID-19 pandemic on inequalities.

Jessica Sheringham and Sarah Sowden
Editors

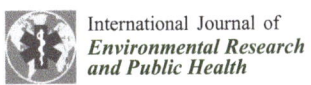

Article

COVID-19 at the Deep End: A Qualitative Interview Study of Primary Care Staff Working in the Most Deprived Areas of England during the COVID-19 Pandemic

Claire Norman *, Josephine M. Wildman and Sarah Sowden

Population Health Sciences Institute, Faculty of Medical Sciences, Newcastle University, Newcastle upon Tyne NE1 4LP, UK; josephine.wildman@newcastle.ac.uk (J.M.W.); sarah.sowden@newcastle.ac.uk (S.S.)
* Correspondence: claire.norman7@nhs.net

Abstract: COVID-19 is disproportionately impacting people in low-income communities. Primary care staff in deprived areas have unique insights into the challenges posed by the pandemic. This study explores the impact of COVID-19 from the perspective of primary care practitioners in the most deprived region of England. Deep End general practices serve communities in the region's most socioeconomically disadvantaged areas. This study used semi-structured interviews followed by thematic analysis. In total, 15 participants were interviewed (11 General Practitioners (GPs), 2 social prescribing link workers and 2 nurses) with Deep End careers ranging from 3 months to 31 years. Participants were recruited via purposive and snowball sampling. Interviews were conducted using video-conferencing software. Data were analysed using thematic content analysis through a social determinants of health lens. Our results are categorised into four themes: the immediate health risks of COVID-19 on patients and practices; factors likely to exacerbate existing deprivation; the role of social prescribing during COVID-19; wider implications for remote consulting. We add qualitative understanding to existing quantitative data, showing patients from low socioeconomic backgrounds have worse outcomes from COVID-19. Deep End practitioners have valuable insights into the impact of social distancing restrictions and remote consulting on patients' health and wellbeing. Their experiences should guide future pandemic response measures and any move to "digital first" primary care to ensure that existing inequalities are not worsened.

Keywords: COVID-19; health inequalities; general practice; primary care; social determinants of health; social prescribing; remote consulting; marginalised communities; health care inequalities; health/healthcare inequity

Citation: Norman, C.; Wildman, J.M.; Sowden, S. COVID-19 at the Deep End: A Qualitative Interview Study of Primary Care Staff Working in the Most Deprived Areas of England during the COVID-19 Pandemic. *Int. J. Environ. Res. Public Health* **2021**, *18*, 8689. https://doi.org/10.3390/ijerph18168689

Academic Editor: Myriam Khlat

Received: 2 July 2021
Accepted: 13 August 2021
Published: 17 August 2021

Publisher's Note: MDPI stays neutral with regard to jurisdictional claims in published maps and institutional affiliations.

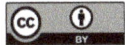

Copyright: © 2021 by the authors. Licensee MDPI, Basel, Switzerland. This article is an open access article distributed under the terms and conditions of the Creative Commons Attribution (CC BY) license (https://creativecommons.org/licenses/by/4.0/).

1. Introduction

The COVID-19 pandemic has highlighted the impact of unfair and avoidable health inequalities, with death rates in deprived areas of the UK three times those of more affluent areas [1–3]. In this article, we make known the immediate and longer-term impacts of the pandemic from the perspective of primary care staff working in areas of blanket socioeconomic deprivation.

Governments around the world have used social distancing measures to slow the transmission of the virus. Social distancing aims to reduce virus transmission between households and includes physical distancing measures and the closure of sites of transmission, including schools and non-essential businesses. These measures are also referred to as "lockdowns". Although lockdowns have been shown to be effective at suppressing the number of cases (and therefore deaths) from COVID-19 [4,5], concerns have been raised that the social distancing measures themselves are not without harm and that these harms will fall disproportionately on those living in disadvantaged circumstances [6]. These harms range from early consequences of people delaying medical assessments for COVID or non-COVID illness, to the longer-term effects of economic decline. In the UK, social distancing and lockdown policy has, at times, meant that schools have been closed to the majority of children and many services, including general practitioner (GP) surgeries, have attempted to reduce the amount of face-to-face contact they have with patients: appointments have become telephone or video by default, with 90% of consultations being via telemedicine [7]. The pandemic also necessitated the creation of "hot sites" for assessing patients with suspected COVID-19: these were often led by Primary Care Networks and staffed by local GPs [8]. Latterly, GPs have also co-ordinated community COVID-19 vaccine rollout.

North East England is the setting for this study. The North East of England has the lowest life expectancy in the country and in its most deprived areas, between the years 2010 and 2012 and the years 2016 and 2018, life expectancy has actually been decreasing [9]. The region performs the worst or second worst in the country for causes of death considered preventable: suicide and drug misuse at any age, as well as cancer, cardiovascular, respiratory, and liver diseases in those under 75. These differences can be attributed to a range of factors: high rates of poverty, poor housing, and the health and social sequelae of heavy industry and its more recent decline [10].

General Practitioners (GPs, also known as family practitioners or primary care practitioners), are the main providers of community care for acute and chronic illnesses in the UK. Everybody resident in or visiting the UK is entitled to access free medical care on the National Health Service (NHS) via their GP, although visitors may be charged for some hospital treatments or prescription medications. As one of a range of measures being implemented to address health inequalities, the North East and North Cumbria (NENC) is in the process of establishing a "Deep End" GP network of professionals working in practices in the region's most deprived areas. Deep End practices serve populations living in areas of blanket deprivation with high proportions of patients living in the 15% most deprived local areas, based on postcode data. The NENC Deep End network was inspired by the GPs at the Deep End network in Scotland: a forum for advocacy, sharing ideas and developing interventions to mitigate health inequalities [11,12]. Since the founding of the original Scottish network in 2009, Deep End GP networks have been founded in several other regions of the UK, plus Ireland, Australia and Canada.

Social prescribing is a relatively new intervention which acknowledges the impact of the social determinants of health on people's health and wellbeing. The aim is to use community organisations and other non-medical support services to address factors such as loneliness and poor housing, as an addition or alternative to offering clinical or pharmaceutical treatments to patients who may have multiple conditions or co-morbid mental and physical health problems [13]. The NHS England Long-Term Plan commits to providing social prescribing as part of its Universal Personalised Care model [14] and, typically, this is delivered by groups of GP practices via Primary Care Networks. The most common social prescribing model is for patients to be referred to a "link worker" (also known as care navigators or health trainers) who can identify the most appropriate service for their needs. Many of these link workers began working during the COVID-19 pandemic.

Deep End GPs and other primary care practitioners will have unique insights into the effect of COVID-19 on their communities, and the impact of public health measures designed to reduce viral transmission. In this qualitative study, conducted during the UK's second wave of COVID-19, we aim to explore experiences of delivering primary care in a pandemic among staff working in practices in areas of blanket deprivation in North East England.

2. Materials and Methods

Data were collected as part of a wider project on the co-design of a Deep End network for the North East and North Cumbria. There was no direct patient or public involvement in this co-design project; however, the work was informed by a multi-agency steering group of policy and practice partners and researchers from across the NENC region.

Ethical approval was granted by Newcastle University research ethics committee (ref: 4322/2020).

2.1. Participants and Recruitment

Practices included in the core Deep End NENC network were identified using the methodology applied in the Scottish Deep End project. This entails identifying the proportion of each practice population living in the 15% most deprived areas of England, based on the Index of Multiple Deprivation (2019) and NHS Digital Practice Populations by Lower layer Super Output Areas (LSOA) (January 2020). All practices were ranked, and 34 North East and North Cumbria practices were found to be amongst the 10% most deprived practices in England against this measure.

A purposive framework was used to sample within the 34 NENC Deep End practices, prioritising geographical representation from Deep End practices across the NENC region. We also aimed to speak to participants with different levels of Deep End experience. Invitations to participate were sent via email to all Deep End practices, in addition to convenience and snowball sampling of participants known to the research team and purposive sampling of staff from practices that were the only Deep End practice in their locality. All staff members in Deep End practices were invited to attend.

Participants were sent a participant information leaflet and consent was gained by electronic completion of a form or by recording verbal consent at the start of the interview.

2.2. Data Collection

Interviews were carried out between October 2020–March 2021. In the temporal context of the COVID-19 pandemic, most interviews were undertaken in the early stages of the UK second wave. Cases were once again starting to rise, and lockdown restrictions (either local or national) were being tightened. Schools were open at this time and all but two interviews were prior to the approval of any COVID-19 vaccines.

Interviews were conducted by C.N. and J.M.W. and recorded using the Zoom video conferencing platform (Zoom Client for Meetings, Version 5.7.5 (939), Zoom Video Communications, Inc., San Jose, CA, USA). A topic guide was developed by the research team and used to provide a semi-structured approach, and this guide was continuously updated in line with emerging themes and participant feedback. Interview data were stored on a secure password protected server, accessible only by the research team.

2.3. Data Analysis

Interviews were auto-transcribed using Zoom video conferencing software, with manual corrections by C.N. C.N. and J.M.W. engaged in ongoing constant comparison of the data, allowing concurrent collection and analysis. Interviews were double coded to enhance validity. Thematic content analysis was used to code the transcripts and categorise them into emerging inductive themes [15]. NVivo (version 12, QSR International (UK) Ltd., Cheshire, UK) was used for data management and to support data coding [16].

3. Results

3.1. Participants

Fifteen interviews were carried out with primary care practitioners (Table 1): eleven GPs, two social prescribing link workers (LW), one nurse practitioner (NP) and one district nurse (DN). We spoke to participants with a breadth of experience: their careers in Deep End practices ranged between 3 months and over 30 years. All participants worked in urban areas, reflective of the areas of high blanket deprivation in the region. A wide geographic coverage was achieved; all but one of the North East's Clinical Commissioning Group (CCG) areas were represented; at the time, CCGs were the organisations responsible for commissioning health services for individual geographical areas in England. A decision was taken to end recruitment as the emergence of recurrent themes suggested data saturation. We also found that the UK vaccine rollout was becoming a priority for primary care staff.

Table 1. Participant characteristics.

Characteristic	N
Gender	
Male	7
Female	8
Occupation	
General Practitioner (GP) partner	8
Salaried GP	3
Social prescribing link worker (LW)	2
Nurse practitioner (NP)	1
District nurse (DN)	1
Time spent working in the Deep End	
0–3 years	5
4–9 years	3
10–20 years	3
21–31 years	4

Our findings can be categorised into four overarching themes: (1) factors increasing the direct health risks of COVID-19 virus; (2) factors worsening pre-existing deprivation; (3) the role of social prescribing during COVID-19; (4) the benefits and costs of remote consulting.

3.2. Factors That Increased the Health Risks of COVID-19

Participants gave several reasons why COVID-19 cases and deaths might be higher in communities with high levels of deprivation. Multi-morbidity, rather than advanced age, was identified as the major risk factor for patients living in communities where *"getting to 55 would be pretty good"* (Interview 2, GP).

Concerns were raised about patients' low levels of health literacy, which reduced their understanding of health messaging around COVID symptoms. As one GP noted, even widely publicised symptoms were not triggering patients to seek testing:

> "I still find it amazing, a guy I spoke to last week, cough and breathlessness: "do you think it could be COVID?" "Oh, I don't know." "Have you had a COVID test?" "No." "Do you know how to get one?" "No, how do I do that doc?" And you just think, surely, with the last six months, the media, all the rest of it but it'd just not crossed his mind." Interview 8, GP

Some participants noted that social distancing measures were not being adhered to in their communities. A lack of understanding, rather than deliberate rule flouting, was identified as a possible cause for non-observance:

> "I did a home visit yesterday, driving up the street, and we're meant to not be socialising with anyone out of the household and I drove past about 13 people in a garden sharing a fag over the fence ... You wonder how much of it is just like, I don't want to follow it and how much is actually understanding the impact of your potential action." Interview 3, NP

Patients' ability to access to healthcare was identified as one of the most pressing challenges facing Deep End practices. One GP expressed concerns that the local "hot hub" facilities for assessing patients with suspected or confirmed COVID-19 in the community were inaccessible for those without cars.

"The local hot site, say for patients in (local area) for COVID, you have to have a car to go ... That does not help our patients" Interview 13, GP

Access issues created health risks for staff as well as patients. Lack of local testing and assessment services put pressure on GP surgeries to continue seeing symptomatic patients, potentially raising COVID case numbers among staff. Staff mentioned that their premises were smaller which made social distancing difficult.

"The rooms are a lot smaller, patients are harder to manage on the phone because there's lots of digital poverty, for example, people turn up and ask to be seen who don't have a phone ... So, I see a lot more people face-to-face here and probably as a result, I got COVID a month ago" Interview 13, GP

In addition to presenting a risk to staff health, exposure to the virus was creating staff shortages:

"We had a big outbreak of staff, having it in lockdown one, there was an entire team went off with it" Interview 5, DN

"We had 11 members of staff off last week. Just complete carnage, trying to manage" Interview 11, GP

District nursing staff felt that they were being asked to take on extra responsibilities because some GPs were, understandably, trying to reduce patient contact.

"It has been really hard to get GPs out to see anyone and a lot of the time we find as nurses that we're telling GPs what we think over the phone, and they're saying, "Okay, yeah, we'll go with that" and not seeing the patient. So, even as far as palliative care—we're having patients that haven't been seen that are dying. And it's been quite tough for the families because, you know, they would quite like to see a doctor ... it does feel a bit like we are expected to diagnose someone so that they don't have to visit." Interview 5, DN

3.3. Factors Likely to Exacerbate the Effects of Deprivation in These Areas

Although recognising the need for lockdown measures, Deep End staff found that the social distancing measures were having a huge impact on their communities. Social distancing meant that community initiatives that practices had put in place were on hold, including social groups for isolated patients and group consultations for chronic pain.

"Obviously, it's all on hold at the minute because of COVID, which is making us all feel very uncomfortable because it became a bit of a lifeline really for some of our more isolated patients" Interview 11, GP

In addition to providing clinical care, supporting patients to address the social determinants of health formed a significant part of the workload in Deep End practices. The reduction in other services such as housing and social work was proving challenging for patients.

"Housing is a recurring theme ... that's been really tricky recently, again because of COVID, it's just (they) basically aren't moving anybody. No matter what circumstances are, really they just will not move them." Interview 6, GP

Concern around child safeguarding was a common theme, with participants reporting a reduction in family contact from health visitors and social workers. School closures also meant a reduction in safeguarding oversight, which was a source of deep concern to practice staff.

"The child safeguarding situation fills me with dread ... throughout lockdown because we've been one of the services that's remained open and visible, we're being presented with a lot of this stuff which is difficult. And we're being presented with it without lots of the support that we normally have to manage it." Interview 1, GP

Although telephone contact was happening, this was not felt to be adequate.

"Health visitors are not doing a lot of face-to-face visits . . . there's always the risk that we're missing things because they're not being seen face-to-face—it's just been telephone." Interview 2, GP

The long-term effects of the pandemic were also a significant concern: communities that were already struggling economically may not be able to recover.

"The legacy of this, the unemployment, the deprivation, that's just going to get worse for patients because as with all of these things, our communities will be the hardest hit going forward. They're not going to recover. They're not going to bounce back . . . in the way that other areas may be able to. And so, yeah, it kinda depresses me really 'cos I just think this is just going to make things worse . . . That's my concern from COVID, is just it's just going to push these communities further down." Interview 11, GP

3.4. Social Prescribing during COVID-19

A lot of social prescribing services in the North East of England were commissioned just before or during the COVID-19 pandemic. Their roles were constantly changing.

"For the most part we started in the pandemic. So, a lot of it was initially just COVID response stuff. Yeah, you know. Food parcels, medication deliveries, that kind of thing and like check in calls really for vulnerable patients. So initially we were getting sent a list of COVID patients or 80 plus (year old patients) for example and pretty much cold calling them. You know, we phoned on behalf of the GP practice. "Is there anything you need in this lockdown?" that kind of thing. But we've moved away from that." Interview 14, Link worker

Lockdown periods saw an increase in referrals, particularly for mental health difficulties.

"There's a huge amount people getting referred for support with losses and also just anxiety, generally coping with the lockdown, problems with isolation, no contact with families and I think people felt were moving beyond that in the autumn of last year and then to go into another lockdown. I think a lot of people really dipped during the winter with their mental health." Interview 15, LW

Increased demand plus a reduction in other services due to the pandemic meant that waiting lists were often long, particularly for talking therapies. The social prescriber was seen as a stop gap for patients who were needing extra support *"We're doing a lot of more long-term handholding at the moment"* said one link worker (Interview 14, LW).

However, *"bearing in mind, we're not trained counsellors or therapists"* (Interview 14, LW), social prescribing link workers in the Deep End were proving a valuable resource for patients with non-clinical needs during the pandemic. One GP observed:

"They've done a lot of very intense work with quite complex and risky people. So they've contained a lot of that complexity and risk, which I hadn't really appreciate that they'd be doing." Interview 1, GP

However, the link workers themselves found that the provision of adapted services to refer patients to was very variable.

"(North East (NE) town) seems to have a lot more going on if you like, a lot more of their groups seem to have adapted to the pandemic, so they're offering remote sessions or virtual sessions instead. Whereas in (another NE town) a lot of things seem to have just ceased" Interview 14, LW

They also found that many referring practitioners and patients had great expectations of what the service could offer, which often did not reflect reality.

"You know there's a lot of sort of magic wand expectations, and you know the GP saying "right, you're really lonely or isolated. You stuck at home. I'm gonna refer you social prescribing because they can help." . . . We got to be able to do this, but those aren't

options at the moment, so we need to look at something else. And I think a lot of the time that could be quite disappointing. Because they're like, "well, you know my GP said that you could help me and, you know, get me out and about and things like that."" Interview 14, LW

3.5. Benefits and Costs of Remote Provision

Modifications to the way of working brought some positives and some participants felt that the pandemic acted as a catalyst for change.

"COVID's been a shot in the arm to make changes that we, you know, have been considering for a while anyway, like changes to our access system" Interview 1, GP

One participant felt strongly that the increased use of technology was a positive and that the pandemic had just brought forward an inevitable move away from face-to-face consulting.

"Everybody's doing telephone consultation. You don't need to push anymore. Video. Yeah, everybody's trying to do video consultation, and certainly once they know how to do it. So, I don't want to go back to the old days." Interview 10, GP

Text messaging was felt to be particularly useful, especially for reaching patients who were sometimes difficult to contact.

The social prescribing link workers found remote working meant they could support more people, because they were not spending so much time travelling; however, this came at the cost of fully assessing their circumstances.

"I mean, you are not travelling, so you've got more time....So just concentrate on having that contact with people because you're literally picking up the phone and you know you're not having to drive to them, but I think it's really hard to get a picture of people's situations over the phone." Interview 15, LW

While there was enthusiasm for the potential benefits of increased use of technology, this was tempered by an understanding of the risks of digital exclusion. Although participants understood that reducing physical contact was important during the pandemic, there was concern that the move to "remote by default" consulting may persist. Participants were keen to make sure that any change to consulting methods was not disadvantaging those who already struggled to access healthcare.

"If nothing else, making sure that what, anything we introduce doesn't disadvantage those already disadvantaged." Interview 8, GP

The drive for increased remote provision was felt to be a political decision, made without adequate knowledge of the challenges that deprived communities faced.

"In terms of the technology that Matt Hancock seems to think is the way forward and just because him and all his peers, you know, have access to all the technology and it's very convenient for them to consult with their GP via zoom, that is not how it is for the people where I work." Interview 11, GP

Online solutions were not felt to be accessible for many patients in the Deep End.

"It's so hard with COVID, because I could say if there was more ... befriending schemes and things, but at the moment, it's all kind of zoom based and none of our patients could really do that ... I don't think many of them have smartphones or laptops." Interview 5, DN

Digital poverty and lack of Information Technology (IT) literacy were often mentioned as concerns in the move to remote consulting. Participants reported that older patients in the communities often did not have internet-enabled devices at all and younger patients may have had devices, but Wi-Fi or data access was variable. Video consulting technology was available but rarely used.

"I think IT literacy, access to technology, equipment, Wi-Fi, that's been a challenge for us because video consults are often not an option. Even sometimes people who don't even have phones or are unable to take photos, that's made it difficult in terms of COVID and remote consulting." Interview 7, GP

While some initiatives have attempted to move online, this was felt to be problematic.

"If you do things via Zoom you're then immediately removing a group of the population who can't be involved." Interview 8, GP

Social prescribing link workers found that, although some services had moved online, there was mixed enthusiasm for this.

"We've gone to a digital offer but then that's only accessible to so many people, so as much as we can encourage people to become like digitally active like, not everyone wants to. People want that face-to-face contact." Interview 15, Link worker

Remote solutions were also problematic for patients with language barriers:

"I find it really hard with people via an interpreter, trying sometimes to assess what's going on...as opposed to when you just see them face-to-face, it's a lot easier." Interview 13, GP

Potentially most seriously, some felt the reduction in face-to-face contact was going to irreparably damage the relationship between primary care and the community.

"I think barriers are going up because people don't have the technology. I think barriers are going up because people like to see their GP you know, and I suspect that's even more so in deprived areas ... I think for some people we are a bit of the centre of that community and I think, you know, you put barriers up in that we're saying to them all "well you probably shouldn't be going to the surgery, we'll try and do this over the phone or I'll send something..." you know it's not good." Interview 11, GP

4. Discussion

This paper adds important context to the quantitative data on excess morbidity and mortality in deprived populations during the COVID-19 pandemic. We identify mechanisms through which socioeconomic deprivation exposes both patients and healthcare providers to an increased risk of COVID-19. We also add to the literature on the harms associated with some public health measures by highlighting the role of primary care in addressing the social determinants of health and the ways in which the pandemic is likely to worsen existing deprivation. We also highlight the work done by district nursing and social prescribing link workers during the pandemic. Finally, we contribute to the conversation around the move to remote consulting in primary care by identifying the potential risks that the drive to digital-first care poses to the provision of primary care in areas of deprivation.

Reasons for higher morbidity and mortality rates in deprived communities are multifactorial. People in deprived communities are more likely to be exposed to the virus, through overcrowded housing in built-up urban areas and through work in low-paid key worker roles [17]. As noted by the practitioners in our research, pre-existing vulnerability to the disease may be higher, due to increased rates of underlying health conditions such as smoking-related respiratory disease and hypertension [1]. The QCovid risk prediction model considers deprivation alongside other risk factors, such as ethnicity, body mass index and underlying health problems [18]. We welcome the UK government's decision to use the model to identify high-risk patients for shielding and vaccination: not only should this reduce COVID-19 morbidity and mortality in deprived areas, but it has set a precedent for publicly acknowledging the negative health impacts of deprivation. Low health literacy and ever-changing guidelines may lead to underestimation of the risks of the disease [19] which was also reflected in our findings: improving health literacy among the general population should be an urgent health and education priority.

We add that the location of COVID-19 assessment centres may make them inaccessible to low-income households without cars: this should also be considered for test centres and vaccination hubs. Without access to these sites, patients are more likely to visit their usual GP surgery and potentially increase transmission among staff and other patients. Risks to staff health are particularly important given that GP surgeries in deprived areas are likely to have fewer GPs per population, and that those who work there are more likely to be older [20] and, therefore, more vulnerable to becoming seriously unwell with COVID-19. Our participants also raise concerns that smaller premises made social distancing more challenging, potentially contributing to rates of COVID-19 transmission within the surgery. We highlight the need for healthcare spaces to have the space and ventilation required to minimise spread of diseases similar to COVID-19.

We add to the literature on the negative consequences of social distancing and remote working, highlighting the challenges that GPs faced as one of the few visible public services that remained functioning near-normally throughout the pandemic. Our findings highlight the vital role general practice plays in supporting patients with their social needs, but also the need for specific enhanced support in this area. Already vulnerable and socially isolated patients became increasingly so, with the cessation of many support services or organisations, or a move to online technologies that were not accessible for Deep End patients. However, social prescribing link workers were praised for their work, telephoning vulnerable people and navigating their non-medical needs. Concerns around child safeguarding were not unfounded, with a significant reduction in the number of children referred for Child Protection Medical Examinations during the period of the first lockdown [21,22]. A recent report highlighting Child Welfare Inequality shows the unequal distribution of safeguarding interventions across the socioeconomic spectrum and the need for enhanced safeguarding support in deprived communities during and after the pandemic [23]. As we increasingly move to remote and digital services, the value of home visiting and face-to-face encounters for picking up on signs of struggling families, or neglect and abuse, must not be forgotten.

Social prescribing is often seen as a panacea for many of the NHS's problems: supporting complex patients while increasing the amount of GP and nurse time for more traditional medical problems. Our link worker participants describe the challenges of starting new roles during a pandemic and the uncertainty and limited availability of onward and ancillary services, plus the expectation from professionals and patients that they were going to be able to wave a "magic wand". Their experiences of trying to carve out the role is similar to that described by Frostick and Bertotti [24], but likely made even more challenging by the nature of working with complex patients in the Deep End setting [25]. Primary care staff and commissioners should be clear with what they expect social prescribing to achieve in their local area and provide appropriate levels of oversight and supervision.

Our participants' experience of remote consulting matched some of those of Flemish GPs in the early part of the pandemic: fears around missed diagnoses and providing suboptimal care [26]. We add a Deep End perspective to the comprehensive review of Murphy et al., of the move to remote consulting in UK general practice [7]. Digital poverty and lack of IT literacy are major concerns for primary care staff in deprived communities and should be considered as a priority when taking forward the NHS long-term plan for a digital-first primary care [27]. Improving IT literacy among older or vulnerable populations should be considered a necessity to make sure that no-one is excluded as healthcare moves into the digital sphere; collaboration between adult education and health services may be required. Access to internet-enabled devices and affordable mobile data or Wi-Fi will also be vital.

Practitioners in these areas are aware that their surgery can often be a centre of the community. Whether this is an appropriate role for general practice, or possibly a symptom of the general decline of social capital, our participants worry that a move to remote consulting will damage this relationship. These concerns are reflected in research into the portrayal of remote consulting in the media during the pandemic, which showed a decline in popularity and acceptance between the first and second waves of COVID-19 in 2020 [28]. A recent systematic review found that telephone consulting was favoured by certain groups: women, younger people, very old people and non-immigrants. Similarly, online consulting was weakly associated with younger, more affluent and educated populations [29]. It is vital that the concerns of practitioners in areas of deprivation are reflected in changes to consulting so that the nature of community medicine is not irreversibly altered.

Our district nurse participant describes her discomfort at being asked to act beyond her usual role. This contrasted with the experiences of our GP participants who felt that the reduction in the number of home visits was patient-led. Although inter-practice variability is likely, we suspect that the district nursing views had not been directly sought. Little has been written in the peer-reviewed literature about the experiences of community nurses during the pandemic, but the Royal College of Nurses surveyed its District and Community Nursing members and found similar themes to those raised by our participant [30]. Bowers et al. raise similar concerns, particularly around palliative care, adding that the work of community teams has often been overlooked amid widespread media coverage of those working in hospital [31]. Although a reduction in GP home visits was felt to be necessary to reduce virus transmission, it is important that relationships are not damaged between doctors and their district nursing colleagues, or patients and their relatives. There may also be implications for patient care and diagnosis if nurses and other allied health professionals are not adequately supported. Macdonald et al. argue that home visits for vulnerable and end-of-life patients must remain a priority for GPs as they are the experts in continuity and overseeing complexity [32]. These experiences are unlikely to be specific to deprived communities, but they highlight the need for multidisciplinary pandemic response planning.

4.1. Strengths and Limitations

Most interviews were carried out by C.N., a GP registrar who worked in a Deep End practice during the first wave. This had a positive impact on accessing participants and was felt that this resulted in interviews that were more candid, as demonstrated in the richness of the data. There was also increased understanding of clinical terminology and local systems. A topic guide was used to avoid shared conceptual blindness and reduce the risk of biasing the agenda with C.N.'s personal experience or opinions [33].

Conducting interviews via video proved acceptable and convenient, as well as COVID-safe [34]. Participant recruitment was likely adversely affected due to the increasing clinical burden on primary care staff during the second wave of COVID-19 in late 2020 and early 2021, particularly during the vaccine rollout.

4.2. Implications for Practice and Research

Our findings are relevant to policymakers in both Primary Care and Public Health: it is vital that any public health intervention is ethically implemented, with consideration given to the most vulnerable in society [35]. Care should be taken not to increase existing inequality. They are also relevant to local authorities and adult education teams who contribute to the wider social determinants of health and the growing need for IT literacy.

Although we are pleased to have included the views of nursing staff and social prescribing link workers, future research should include other primary care practitioners, such a health visitors and midwives. Qualitative research with people who live in areas with high rates of COVID-19 infections and deaths would provide even more insight into the potential reasons behind the variation along socioeconomic lines. Further data should be collected on the benefits of social prescribing for patients and other NHS staff during the COVID-19 pandemic.

5. Conclusions

Deprived communities are facing the brunt of the COVID-19 pandemic. Through the eyes of primary care staff in these communities, we have shown that this goes beyond the impact of the disease itself, with social distancing measures and remote consulting exacerbating many existing inequalities. Deep End primary care practitioners are well-placed to advocate for their patients and their views are crucial in ensuring that future Public Health measures and major systems changes are implemented in ways that reduce rather than maintain or even increase existing inequalities in health and healthcare.

Author Contributions: Conceptualization, J.M.W., S.S. and C.N.; methodology, J.M.W., S.S. and C.N.; investigation, C.N. and J.M.W.; formal analysis, C.N., J.M.W., S.S.; writing—original draft preparation, C.N.; writing—review and editing, J.M.W. and S.S.; supervision, J.M.W. and S.S. All authors have read and agreed to the published version of the manuscript.

Funding: This research work is supported by the National Institute of Health Research (NIHR) Applied Research Collaboration (ARC) for the North East and North Cumbria (NENC). J.M.W. is a Research Fellow within the National Institute Health Research (NIHR) Applied Research Collaboration for the North East and North Cumbria. S.S. is supported by Health Education England (HEE) and the NIHR through an Integrated Clinical Academic Lecturer Fellowship (Ref CA-CL-2018-04-ST2-010) and RCF funding, NHS North of England Care System Support (NECS). C.N. is employed by Health Education England (HEE) as a GP registrar and Academic Extended Integrated Training Post Holder. The views expressed are those of the authors and not necessarily those of the NHS, the NIHR, or the Department of Health and Social Care.

Institutional Review Board Statement: Ethical approval was granted by Newcastle University research ethics committee (ref: 4322/2020).

Informed Consent Statement: Informed consent was obtained from all subjects involved in the study, including consent to publish.

Data Availability Statement: The data presented in this study are available on request from the corresponding author. The data are not publicly available due to containing potentially identifiable information about participants' places of work.

Acknowledgments: We would like to thank participants, the NENC Deep End Steering group and the Deep End network. We also thank Clare Bambra and the NENC ARC Inequalities and Marginalised Communities theme for prioritising this important workstream.

Conflicts of Interest: The authors declare no conflict of interest.

References

1. Bambra, C.; Riordan, R.; Ford, J.; Matthews, F. The COVID-19 pandemic and health inequalities. *J. Epidemiol. Community Health* **2020**, *74*, 964–968. [CrossRef]
2. Whitehead, M.; Taylor-Robinson, D.; Barr, B. Poverty, health, and covid-19. *BMJ* **2021**, *372*, n376. [CrossRef]
3. Office for National Statistics. Deaths due to COVID-19 by Local Area and Deprivation. Table 3: Number of Deaths and Age-Standardised Rates, by Sex, Deprivation Deciles in England, Deaths Registered between March and December 2020. Available online: https://www.ons.gov.uk/peoplepopulationandcommunity/birthsdeathsandmarriages/deaths/datasets/deathsduetocovid19bylocalareaanddeprivation (accessed on 22 January 2021).
4. Verma, B.K.; Verma, M.; Verma, V.K.; Abdullah, R.B.; Nath, D.C.; Khan, H.T.A.; Verma, A.; Vishwakarma, R.K.; Verma, V. Global lockdown: An effective safeguard in responding to the threat of COVID-19. *J. Eval. Clin. Pract.* **2020**, *26*, 1592–1598. [CrossRef]
5. Vinceti, M.; Filippini, T.; Rothman, K.J.; Ferrari, F.; Goffi, A.; Maffeis, G.; Orsini, N. Lockdown timing and efficacy in controlling COVID-19 using mobile phone tracking. *EClinicalMedicine* **2020**, *25*, 100457. [CrossRef]
6. Anderson, G.; Frank, J.W.; Naylor, C.D.; Wodchis, W.; Feng, P. Using socioeconomics to counter health disparities arising from the covid-19 pandemic. *BMJ* **2020**, *369*, m2149. [CrossRef] [PubMed]
7. Murphy, M.; Scott, L.J.; Salisbury, C.; Turner, A.; Scott, A.; Denholm, R.; Iyer, G.; Lewis, R.; MacLeod, J.; Horwood, J. The implementation of remote consulting in UK primary care following the COVID-19 pandemic: A mixed-methods longitudinal study. *Br. J. Gen. Pract.* **2021**, *71*, e166–e177. [CrossRef] [PubMed]
8. Thornton, J. Covid-19: How coronavirus will change the face of general practice forever. *BMJ* **2020**, *368*, m1279. [CrossRef] [PubMed]
9. Marmot, M.A.J.; Boyce, T.; Goldblatt, P.; Morrisson, J. *Health Equity in England: The Marmot Review 10 Years on*; Institute of Health Equity: London, UK, 2020.
10. Corris, V.; Dormer, E.; Brown, A.; Whitty, P.; Collingwood, P.; Bambra, C.; Newton, J.L. Health inequalities are worsening in the North East of England. *Br. Med Bull.* **2020**, *134*, 63–72. [CrossRef]

11. Watt, G.; Brown, G.; Budd, J.; Cawston, P.; Craig, M.; Jamieson, R.; Langridge, S.; Lyon, A.; Mercer, S.; Morton, C.; et al. General Practitioners at the Deep End: The experience and views of general practitioners working in the most severely deprived areas of Scotland. *Occas. Pap. R. Coll. Gen. Pract.* **2012**, *89*, 1–40.
12. Mercer, S.W.; Patterson, J.; Robson, J.P.; Smith, S.M.; Walton, E.; Watt, G. The inverse care law and the potential of primary care in deprived areas. *Lancet* **2021**, *397*, 775–776. [CrossRef]
13. Drinkwater, C.; Wildman, J.; Moffatt, S. Social prescribing. *BMJ* **2019**, *364*, l1285. [CrossRef]
14. NHS England. *Universal Personalised Care*; NHS England: London, UK, 2019.
15. Braun, V.; Clarke, V. Using thematic analysis in psychology. *Qual. Res. Psychol.* **2006**, *3*, 77–101. [CrossRef]
16. Bazeley, P.; Jackson, K. *Qualitative Data Analysis with NVivo*, 2nd ed.; SAGE Publications Ltd.: London, UK, 2013.
17. Patel, J.A.; Nielsen, F.B.H.; Badiani, A.A.; Assi, S.; Unadkat, V.A.; Patel, B.; Ravindrane, R.; Wardle, H. Poverty, inequality and COVID-19: The forgotten vulnerable. *Public Health* **2020**, *183*, 110–111. [CrossRef] [PubMed]
18. Clift, A.K.; Coupland, C.A.C.; Keogh, R.H.; Diaz-Ordaz, K.; Williamson, E.; Harrison, E.M.; Hayward, A.; Hemingway, H.; Horby, P.; Mehta, N.; et al. Living risk prediction algorithm (QCOVID) for risk of hospital admission and mortality from coronavirus 19 in adults: National derivation and validation cohort study. *BMJ* **2020**, *371*, m3731. [CrossRef] [PubMed]
19. Paakkari, L.; Okan, O. COVID-19: Health literacy is an underestimated problem. *Lancet Public Health* **2020**, *5*, e249–e250. [CrossRef]
20. Blane, D.N.; McLean, G.; Watt, G. Distribution of GPs in Scotland by age, gender and deprivation. *Scott. Med. J.* **2015**, *60*, 214–219. [CrossRef] [PubMed]
21. Bhopal, S.; Buckland, A.; McCrone, R.; Villis, A.I.; Owens, S. Who has been missed? Dramatic decrease in numbers of children seen for child protection assessments during the pandemic. *Arch. Dis. Child.* **2021**, *106*, e6. [CrossRef] [PubMed]
22. Garstang, J.; Debelle, G.; Anand, I.; Armstrong, J.; Botcher, E.; Chaplin, H.; Hallett, N.; Morgans, C.; Price, M.; Tan, E.E.H.; et al. Effect of COVID-19 lockdown on child protection medical assessments: A retrospective observational study in Birmingham, UK. *BMJ Open* **2020**, *10*, e042867. [CrossRef] [PubMed]
23. Byswaters, P.; Featherstone, B. *The Child Welfare Inequalities Project: Final Report 2020*; University of Huddersfield: Huddersfield, UK, 2020.
24. Frostick, C.; Bertotti, M. The frontline of social prescribing—How do we ensure Link Workers can work safely and effectively within primary care? *Chronic Illn.* **2019**. [CrossRef]
25. O'Brien, R.; Wyke, S.; Watt, G.G.C.M.; Guthrie, B.; Mercer, S.W. The 'Everyday Work' of Living with Multimorbidity in Socioeconomically Deprived Areas of Scotland. *J. Comorbidity* **2014**, *4*, 1–10. [CrossRef]
26. Verhoeven, V.; Tsakitzidis, G.; Philips, H.; Van Royen, P. Impact of the COVID-19 pandemic on the core functions of primary care: Will the cure be worse than the disease? A qualitative interview study in Flemish GPs. *BMJ Open* **2020**, *10*, e039674. [CrossRef]
27. NHS. The NHS Long Term Plan. Available online: https://www.longtermplan.nhs.uk/publication/nhs-long-term-plan/ (accessed on 9 February 2021).
28. Mroz, G.; Papoutsi, C.; Rushforth, A.; Greenhalgh, T. Changing media depictions of remote consulting in COVID-19: Analysis of UK newspapers. *Br. J. Gen. Pract.* **2021**, *71*, e1–e9. [CrossRef] [PubMed]
29. Parker, R.F.; Figures, E.L.; Paddison, C.A.; Matheson, J.I.; Blane, D.N.; Ford, J.A. Inequalities in general practice remote consultations: A systematic review. *BJGP Open* **2021**, *5*, BJGPO.2021.0040. [CrossRef] [PubMed]
30. Royal College of Nursing. *RCN DCN Forum Covid-19 Survey Results*; RCN: London, UK, 2020.
31. Bowers, B.; Pollock, K.; Oldman, C.; Barclay, S. End-of-life care during COVID-19: Opportunities and challenges for community nursing. *Br. J. Community Nurs.* **2020**, *26*, 44–46. [CrossRef]
32. Macdonald, G.; Vernon, G.; McNab, D.; Murdoch, J. Home visits for vulnerable older people: Journeys to the 'Far End'. *Br. J. Gen. Pract.* **2020**, *70*, 479–480. [CrossRef] [PubMed]
33. Chew-Graham, C.A.; May, C.R.; Perry, M.S. Qualitative research and the problem of judgement: Lessons from interviewing fellow professionals. *Fam. Pract.* **2002**, *19*, 285–289. [CrossRef]
34. Archibald, M.M.; Ambagtsheer, R.C.; Casey, M.G.; Lawless, M. Using zoom videoconferencing for qualitative data collection: Perceptions and experiences of researchers and participants. *Int. J. Qual. Methods* **2019**, *18*. [CrossRef]
35. Kass, N.E. An ethics framework for public health. *Am. J. Public Health* **2001**, *91*, 1776–1782. [CrossRef] [PubMed]

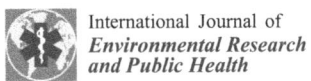

Review

Relationships between Child Development at School Entry and Adolescent Health—A Participatory Systematic Review

Michelle Black [1,*], Amy Barnes [1], Mark Strong [1], Anna Brook [1], Anna Ray [2], Ben Holden [1], Clare Foster [1] and David Taylor-Robinson [3]

[1] School of Health and Related Research, The University of Sheffield, Regent Court, 30 Regent Street, Sheffield S1 4DA, UK; a.barnes@sheffield.ac.uk (A.B.); m.strong@sheffield.ac.uk (M.S.); anna.brook@sheffield.ac.uk (A.B.); b.holden@sheffield.ac.uk (B.H.); clare.foster@sheffield.ac.uk (C.F.)
[2] Department of Health Sciences, University of York, Seebohm Rowntree Building, Heslington, York YO10 5DD, UK; annamarie.ray@nhs.net
[3] Public Health, Policy and Systems, Institute of Population Health, University of Liverpool, Liverpool L69 3GL, UK; David.Taylor-Robinson@liverpool.ac.uk
* Correspondence: michelle.black@sheffield.ac.uk

Abstract: The relationship between child development and adolescent health, and how this may be modified by socio-economic conditions, is poorly understood. This limits cross-sector interventions to address adolescent health inequality. This review summarises evidence on the associations between child development at school starting age and subsequent health in adolescence and identifies factors affecting associations. We undertook a participatory systematic review, searching electronic databases (MEDLINE, PsycINFO, ASSIA and ERIC) for articles published between November 1990 and November 2020. Observational, intervention and review studies reporting a measure of child development and subsequent health outcomes, specifically weight and mental health, were included. Studies were individually and collectively assessed for quality using a comparative rating system of stronger, weaker, inconsistent or limited evidence. Associations between child development and adolescent health outcomes were assessed and reported by four domains of child development (socio-emotional, cognitive, language and communication, and physical development). A conceptual diagram, produced with stakeholders at the outset of the study, acted as a framework for narrative synthesis of factors that modify or mediate associations. Thirty-four studies were included. Analysis indicated stronger evidence of associations between measures of socio-emotional development and subsequent mental health and weight outcomes; in particular, positive associations between early externalising behaviours and later internalising and externalising, and negative associations between emotional wellbeing and later internalising and unhealthy weight. For all other domains of child development, although associations with subsequent health were positive, the evidence was either weaker, inconsistent or limited. There was limited evidence on factors that altered associations. Positive socio-emotional development at school starting age appears particularly important for subsequent mental health and weight in adolescence. More collaborative research across health and education is needed on other domains of development and on the mechanisms that link development and later health, and on how any relationship is modified by socio-economic context.

Keywords: child development; childhood education; school; adolescent health; health inequality; adolescent mental health; adolescent weight

1. Introduction

Inequalities in many child health outcomes are increasing in the UK and the health of those living in its most disadvantaged areas are amongst the worst in the developed world [1]. Some of the roots of health inequality are thought to be in early childhood with socio-economically driven inequalities in child development persisting across the life course, negatively impacting people's future health, wellbeing and life chances, and perpetuating health inequalities into adulthood [2]. Evidence that the early years, or the first "1000 days", is a critical period of development [3,4] (together with health economics research in this field [5]) has meant that the early years have become a prime area for public policy and public health investment in many high-income countries including the UK [6].

All of the countries of the UK provide early childhood programmes, which aim to improve outcomes for children by supporting optimal health and development through access to services such as early education and care, between the ages of 0–4 years or pre-school [7]. There is evidence that programmes which support child development in readiness for school can improve cognitive and non-cognitive skills [8]. There is also evidence that positive cognitive development on starting school is associated with academic achievement by age 13 years [9] and positive socio-emotional development by age 10 years [10]. Non-cognitive skills, such as social skills and self-regulation on starting school, are also associated with later academic success and psychosocial outcomes in subsequent years of childhood and early adolescence [11]. There is less evidence for whether and how child development, or interventions to support child development, are related to subsequent health in childhood. For example, there is limited evidence on the effect of early child development programmes (such as attending pre-school, accessing health services and parenting programmes) on adolescent health, with one systematic review finding little to no effect of early childhood programmes on later child health, although with some evidence for obesity reduction, greater social competence, improved mental health and crime prevention [12]. A review of Sure Start (a UK early years programme from 1999 to 2017, for families with children under the age of four years and targeted in more disadvantaged areas) found that access to Sure Start was associated with fewer childhood hospitalisations for infections and injury [13]. Potential mechanisms proposed for this association were: the provision of information to parents and changing parents behaviour, leading to a safer and more nurturing home, and to reducing externalising behaviour in children, leading to less fights or dangerous activities [13].

To better understand whether and how child development at school starting age is associated with subsequent health in childhood requires a clear understanding of what is meant by "child development", reliable measures of child development, and also the development and testing of conceptual frameworks or theories regarding the relationships between child development and later adolescent health. In terms of defining what we mean by child development, this is contested academic and policy terrain and, as such, is difficult to define. For some, child development is understood through a narrow focus on cognitive education, whereas for others it is about broader life skills, including confidence and social competencies [14]. In English health and education policy, child development has tended to be defined in the former, relatively narrow manner, with, for example, child development at school starting age understood through a specific composite measure of a child's personal, social and emotional, physical, cognitive, and communication and language development, termed "school readiness" [15]. Internationally, school readiness, when considered more broadly, has been seen as a viable strategy to reduce inequalities in learning and development gaps at the start of formal education [16]. However, how it is defined and used in England has been criticised as reductionist, with school readiness used as a performance and accountability measure, resulting in a narrowing of the curriculum, marginalisation of children who fail to achieve required levels of development through grouping by ability, and subjugation of teachers and schools to meet targets [17]. Moving beyond targets to understanding child development more broadly, as an ongoing developmental process in a social context [18], is important if we are to develop interventions to support equitable health and development. Therefore, we consider "child development" in this review as any measure of child development which encapsulates a process of change in what a child is capable or able of doing, or in how they are feeling. There is no existing framework for characterising different aspects or measures of child development. Therefore, in this review we use four over-arching domains of child development: socio-emotional development, cognitive development, language and communication, and physical development. These domains broadly encompass the areas of learning within the early years curriculum in England [15]. We see these categories as potentially useful despite the described shortcomings of England's composite measure, "school readiness". Conceptualising child development in this way provides a platform for learning about the relationships between specific domains of child development (using a range of child development measures) and subsequent health.

Understanding whether and how child development and adolescent health outcomes are related presents opportunities for interventions to improve health and reduce health inequalities at an important time in the life-course, adolescence. There is evidence that health in adolescence is on the causal pathway to socio-economic status (SES) in adulthood by enabling "selection" into education [19]. Therefore, focusing on health in this period is critical to enable children to optimise their subsequent educational outcomes for wellbeing and employment opportunities. Informing interventions requires evidence not just on associations between child development and adolescent health but also on the effect of socio-economic circumstances on any associations found. In our protocol we outlined pathways by which socio-economically driven health inequalities may manifest (family stress, material living circumstances and parental health behaviours) and also possible direct pathways (social and cognitive) between child development and subsequent health. This provides a conceptual framework for the review. To inform interventions on any of these pathways there is a need to identify factors which may explain, and the socio-economic circumstances which may modify, the associations between child development and adolescent health. This requires a public health lens and, as far as we are aware, no review has analysed the evidence on relationships between different dimensions of child development and adolescent health outcomes or assessed the factors which may shape the relationships.

In summary, there is evidence that aspects of child development at school starting age are associated with later academic success, but less is known about whether and how particular dimensions of child development influence health outcomes in adolescence. This gap in understanding limits cross-sector interventions to improve adolescent health and reduce health inequality. This review addresses this gap by undertaking a participatory systematic review to: (1) synthesise evidence on the relationship between child development at school starting age (3–7 years) and subsequent health in adolescence (8–15 years) and (2) identify factors that shape the relationship.

2. Materials and Methods

2.1. Protocol Registration

The study protocol was registered with PROSPERO (CRD42020210011) and published [20]. The review is reported according to the Preferred Reporting Items for Reporting Systematic Reviews and Meta-Analyses (PRISMA) 2020 Statement [21,22]; the checklist available in additional file 1. Any deviations from protocol are stated and explained in the relevant sections.

2.2. Review Questions

- What are the associations between measures of child development recorded at school starting age (3–7 years) and subsequent health in adolescence (8–15 years)?
- What are the effect modifiers (socio-economic factors) of this relationship? (This will identify factors which alter the strength of the observed associations.)
- What are the mediators of this relationship? (This will identify factors or set of factors (pathways) which explain the observed associations.)

2.3. Definition of Terms

Child development is defined as a developmental process incorporating measures of development that record changes within a child's cognitive or physical development, or language and communication, or socio-emotional development.

2.4. Study Design

The design for this study was a participatory systematic review, involving engagement with national and local stakeholders across health and education sectors.

Stakeholder Engagement to Design the Conceptual Diagram

The lead reviewer held discussions with stakeholders to develop a conceptual model of the relationship under study. This process is described in full in the study protocol [20]. Their views, together with a scoping review of the evidence, led to an initial conceptual diagram (available in additional file 2). This diagram highlights the main pathways by which socio-economically driven health inequalities manifest; family stress, material living circumstances and parental health behaviours [23]; and also illustrates possible direct pathways (knowledge/literacy and social/cognitive) between child development and education and subsequent health. The diagram acted as a framework for the review, providing initial categories for extracting and analysing evidence from published studies.

2.5. Eligibility

Studies needed to include children, some or all of whom were aged between 3 and 15 years, in high-income country settings defined as a member country of the Organisation for Economic and Co-operation and Development (OECD). Exposures were characteristics of child development at school starting age (3–7 years), defined as: cognitive or physical development, or communication and language, or socio-emotional development. Primary outcomes were health and wellbeing outcomes, reported between the ages of 8 and 15 years: specifically, weight, mental health and proxy measures such as dietary habits and behaviour and measures of wellbeing. Secondary outcomes were academic outcomes of academic tests and proxy measures such as executive function during the outcome age of interest. Secondary outcomes were only included if they were found in a study with a primary outcome of interest. Executive function was included as a secondary outcome of interest because it allows for the regulation, control and management of learning, and thus appears an important link between child development and academic outcomes. In addition, executive function is a good predictor of academic achievement [24]. Studies that provided data on associations between the exposures and outcomes in the age period of interest, and additionally those that provided evidence on mechanisms, were required. The population and context, exposure, outcomes and study designs are described in full in the published protocol [20] and summarised in relation to inclusion and exclusion criteria in Table 1.

Table 1. Summary of eligibility criteria.

	Inclusion	Exclusion
Population and context	Studies must include children, some or all of whom are aged between 3 and 15 years, across socio-economic strata in high-income country settings, defined as OECD membership.	Studies of children from non-OECD countries. Studies which focus solely on a particular subset of children with a particular health or development need.

Table 1. *Cont.*

	Inclusion	Exclusion
Exposure	A measure of child development at school starting age (3–7 years), defined as: cognitive or physical or linguistic or socio-emotional development at school starting age, measured by any of the following: - School readiness, as measured by scales such as the Bracken Basic Concepts Scale Revised (BBCS-R) [25]. - Cognitive development as measured by, for example, non-reading intelligence tests, vocabulary tests, mathematics tests or parent/teacher ratings. - Language and literacy (as measured by academic achievement test scores such as pre-reading/reading, vocabulary, oral comprehension, phonological awareness, pre-writing/writing or verbal skills. - Emotional well-being and social competence (as measured by behavioural assessments of social interaction, problem behaviours, social skills and competencies, child-parent relationship/child-teacher relationship). - Physical development. Studies that explore socio-economic factors which affect associations between child development at school starting age and these outcomes. Studies that explore mechanisms or pathways between child development at school starting age and these outcomes.	Studies reporting neither data nor mechanism between exposure and outcome will be excluded.
Outcome	Primary Outcome(s) The review will incorporate evidence health and wellbeing outcomes, reported between the ages of 8 and 15 years, specifically: - Weight (BMI). - Mental Health (as measured by standard questionnaires or clinically). - Socio-emotional behaviour. - Proxy measures such as dietary habits and behaviour and measures of wellbeing will be included. Secondary Outcome(s) - Performance at the end of primary school (age 10–11), measured by standardized tests. - Proxy measures such as executive function.	Studies reporting neither data nor mechanism between exposure and outcome will be excluded.
Study design and sources	Observational studies (ecological, case-control, cohort (prospective and retrospective)) RCTs, Quasi-experimental, Review level studies including theory papers.	Cross-sectional studies, conference abstracts, books, dissertations, or opinion pieces.

2.6. Search Strategy

We searched four electronic databases for articles published from November 1990 to November 2020: MEDLINE (OVID), PsycINFO (OVID), ASSIA (ProQuest) and ERIC (EBSCO). We also searched the reference lists from all included articles for additional eligible articles. Further relevant literature was identified through stakeholder discussions. Grey literature searching was undertaken by searching relevant organisations' websites.

The search strategy was informed by a scoping review of the literature and focused on terms relating to child development, school readiness and adolescent health. The search strategy is available in additional file 3.

2.7. Study Selection and Data Extraction

Retrieved citations were uploaded to EndNote and duplicates removed. Titles and abstracts were screened by five reviewers against the inclusion and exclusion criteria. A 10% sample of papers was independently checked by two reviewers and inter-rater reliability was 86%. Any disagreements were resolved by discussion between the reviewers, so that a consensus was reached. The full texts of papers were read in the second stage of the screening process, by five reviewers, to produce a final list of papers for full text review. The final list of papers included was exported to excel to be assessed for the data extraction process. The lead reviewer extracted data for those articles that met the inclusion criteria in full. Reasons for exclusion were recorded and a list of excluded papers, together with the reason, is available in additional file 4. Data extraction was undertaken solely by the lead reviewer using a bespoke form (additional file 5), which had been trialled on a sample of different sources, and a sample of 10% was second checked. The following data were extracted: author and year, study design, analysis method, country and setting, participants, exposure measure and age, exposure measurement instrument, outcome measure and age, outcome measurement instrument, association and effect size, mechanism (studied and proposed), and factors which moderate the association, strengths and weaknesses.

2.8. Quality Assessment

Our protocol stipulated the use of Liverpool Quality Assessment Tool (LQAT) [26]. However, it was found that LQAT was insufficiently detailed for this review. Therefore, in a deviation from protocol we adapted a tool appropriate for the study designs used in previous systematic reviews [27,28]. The methodological quality of each observational study was assessed for risk of bias and clarity of study description to assign studies to one of three categories of methodological quality: high, moderate or low, using the template in additional file 6. Specifically, studies were assessed against 12 criteria within the following categories: study population, study attrition, data collection and data analysis with each pertaining to validity, precision or informativeness. In line with the recommendations of Cochrane [29], studies were not scored, and instead a narrative indication of quality (using +, − and ? against each criteria) was made based on all criteria, with criteria pertaining to validity and precision carrying a greater weight in guiding overall quality. Quality assessments were undertaken by the main author and a 10% sample independently assessed by a member of the review team. In all cases the overall assessments of quality made by the reviewers were consistent.

In addition to assessing the quality of each individual paper, the overall strength of evidence for papers grouped by outcome and domain was assessed, e.g., mental health outcomes and the socio-emotional domain of child development. Within these groupings the overall findings were graded as providing either: stronger evidence (generally consistent findings in higher quality studies); weaker evidence (generally consistent findings in one higher quality study, or in multiple lower quality studies); inconsistent evidence (inconsistent findings across multiple studies); or very limited evidence (a single study). This method draws on techniques used by Hoogendoom [27] and Baxter [30,31].

2.9. Data Synthesis

As per the protocol, we undertook a narrative synthesis using the SwIM guidelines [32] (additional file 7) to guide reporting. This was in anticipation of heterogeneity in the variety of exposures, analysis methods and outcomes in the studies. Each study was assessed and associations between exposures and outcomes recorded as either "positive", "negative" or "no association". Studies were grouped by outcome and, within this, organised by exposure domain and tabulated to illustrate both the associations and assigned quality. The groupings for the outcome measure were undertaken by allocating the measure into either mental health, obesity or academic outcomes. The grouping for exposure measures was an inductive process involving an interpretation of the way child development had been understood and measured in each included paper, and then classifying and allocating these into a particular domain of child development; namely, a socio-emotional domain, cognitive domain, language and communication domain, physical domain or multiple domains. This was a subjective process because, as indicated in the introduction, there is no existing framework for understanding child development and characterising measures of child development.

An overall rating on the strength of the evidence for each grouping (studies allocated within each domain of child development for each outcome: weight, mental health, academic) was derived as described in the quality assessment section. The results for factors which mediate or moderate associations between child development and subsequent health in adolescence (review question 2) was synthesised in relation to the conceptual diagram (additional file 2) of the relationship (produced with stakeholders at the outset of the review). Factors were classed as either mediators (those that explain associations) or moderators (those that alter the strength of associations) and assigned to a pathway (grouping of factors): family stress, knowledge/literacy, social/cognitive, material living and parent health behaviours. The overall ratings on the strength of the evidence for each domain and outcome, and stakeholder discussions, were used to inform a final diagram of the relationship between child development and adolescent health.

3. Results

3.1. Literature Results

Following the screening of 10,657 retrieved citations, 34 articles were included in the review. See Figure 1 for PRISMA diagram illustrating the study selection process. Fifty-two studies were excluded on full text review; the list of studies excluded, with the reason, is available in additional file 4.

3.2. Study Design and Setting

Of the 34 included studies there were 32 prospective longitudinal studies [33–64], one retrospective longitudinal study [65] and one meta-analysis [66]. Detailed descriptions of the included studies are available in additional file 8. Of the 34 studies, 14 were set in the United States [35,36,39,43,45,47,49–51,56–59,64], seven in Canada [38,46,52–55,63], five in Australia [34,41,44,48,62], three in the UK [40,42,61], three in The Netherlands [33,37,65], one in Denmark [60] and one in which the countries included in the analysis were not explicitly stated [66].

3.3. Sample Size and Participant Characteristcs

The total number of children in included studies in the review was 69,152 (48% female, in those where sex was reported). Participants were recruited from pre-birth (through mother's pregnancy) to age 12 years, with the majority recruited between the ages of 4–6 years, at pre-school or kindergarten. Across the studies recruitment took place between 1986 and 2009. The majority of the children were enrolled in existing longitudinal studies, were mainly Caucasian and from a mix of socioeconomic backgrounds. Six studies focused on socioeconomic disadvantage; three were of children from socio-economically disadvantaged families recruited from child care centres [50] or Head Start programmes (early years services to support low-income children and families in the US) [39,58], two studies oversampled for greater socioeconomic risk [51,61] and one oversampled for non-marital status [47]. A further two studies had children from majority low income [42] and low to middle income families [49]. There were three studies in which children from socioeconomic disadvantage were less well represented [34,38,52]. Children were assessed either in their own homes, pre-school or school apart from in two studies where lab-based assessments were made [46,51] and two where routinely collected healthcare data was used [61,65].

3.4. Studies Identified across Different Domains of Child Development (Exposures) and Adolescent Outcomes

Studies were found that focused on all domains of child development, namely: socio-emotional development, cognitive development, language and communication, and physical development. Table 2 illustrates the number of studies within each domain and the related adolescent outcome measure(s). Table 3 provides a summary of the main study characteristics and describes the exposures by domain of child development, outcomes and how they were measured. The main domain of child development studied in included papers was socio-emotional development with 24 studies [33–35,37–39,42,44–48,50,53,54,56–60,62,64–66]. Exposures included behaviours such as internalizing and externalizing behaviours, social competence, emotion knowledge, emotional wellbeing, emotional reactivity and peer relations. Exposures within the socio-emotional domain were generally measured using the relevant sections of standardized instruments such as the Child Behaviour Checklist (CBCL), the Social Behaviour Questionnaire (SBQ) or the Strengths and Difficulties Questionnaire (SDQ), with a mixture of child report, teacher report and parent report across the studies.

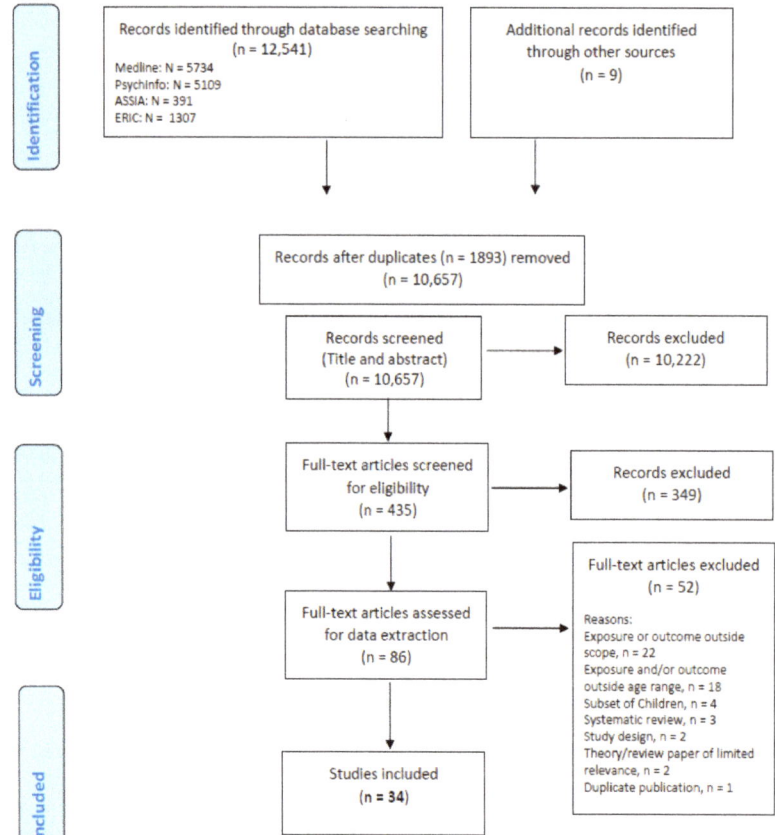

Figure 1. PRISMA flowchart of study selection process.

Four studies [40,51,52,63] had an aspect of cognition as the exposure of interest, namely: mathematics skills, executive control, foundational cognitive ability, verbal ability/literacy and Intelligence Quotient (IQ). Executive control refers to a set of cognitive processes necessary for cognitive control of behaviour and was measured by observing tasks. Verbal ability was measured using literacy tests, mathematics skills by number knowledge tests or standardized assessments relating to the relevant country's curriculum, and foundational cognitive ability and IQ by standardized instruments.

Two studies [36,43] had language and communication as the main exposures and a further study [52] included language as one of multiple exposures. Exposures included receptive and expressive vocabulary. These were measured using the relevant sections of standardised assessments such as the Peabody Picture Vocabulary Test.

Two studies [49,55] incorporated exposures in the physical domain of child development. Exposures included fundamental movement skills (balance, agility, hand-eye co-ordination) and participation in structured and unstructured physical activity. These were measured by either parent report or assessment of skills by assessors in the child's home.

Two studies [41,61] measured across all domains of child development and education. One study assessed the component parts of teacher-rated school readiness in relation to the country's early development instrument and one focused on child development in all domains in a health visitor check as a composite measure. In the main, studies analysed the effect of the exposure at a certain time point on an outcome at one later time point. However, two studies repeated measures at subsequent ages to assign children to a trajectory for the exposure of interest [38,58] and four studies repeated measures to study trends over time [43,48,57,64].

Table 2. Studies by child development domain and adolescent outcome.

Number of Studies by Exposure Domain		Outcome Measures		
		Primary		Secondary
Domain:	Total studies	Mental Health	Weight	Academic
Socio-emotional	24 *	18	5	3
Cognitive	4 *	3	1	1
Communication and Language	2	2	1 ^	-
Physical	2	1	1	-
Composite/All domains measured	2 *	2	1	-
	34	26	9	4

* Includes one study which measured several outcomes. ^ From a study centrally coded to a different domain due to multiple exposures studied.

3.5. Quality Assessment

Thirty-three of the 34 included studies were assessed using the methodological assessment tool for observational studies, available in additional file 6. One study, a meta-analysis, was assessed using AMSTAR (A MeaSurement Tool to Assess systematic Reviews). Results of the quality assessment process for all included studies is available in additional file 9. Ten were rated as low, 16 moderate and eight high in methodological quality. High implies a low risk of bias, moderate implies a moderate risk of bias and low quality implies a high risk of bias.

As outlined in quality assessment section of the methods, confidence in cumulative evidence was assessed within each grouping of papers, grouped by outcome and domain. This is referred to throughout the synthesis of the findings.

Table 3. Summary of study characteristics.

Author (Citation)	Study Design	Country	Participants (% Females)	Exposure (Development Characteristic) and Age	Exposure Measurement Instrument	Outcome and Age	Outcome Measurement Instrument
Ashford et al. [33]	Longitudinal	Holland	294 (49.2)	Behaviour internalising and externalising—age 4	Child Behaviour Checklist (CBCL)—parent and teacher rated.	Internalising behaviours—age 11	CBCL—parent and teacher report.
Berthelsen et al. [34]	Longitudinal	Australia	4819 (49.1)	Child behaviour at age 4–5 and early ecological risk factors SEP, MMH, parenting anger, parenting warmth, parenting consistency	Child behaviour risk index measured as the sum of scores: sleep (emotional and dysregulation (both parent report) and inattention/hyperactivity symptoms (mother rated).	Executive Function (age 14–15)	A composite score from three computerised tasks for assessing cognition (visual attention, visual working memory and spatial problem solving).
Bornstein et al. [35]	Longitudinal	US east coast	118 (42.0)	Social competence at age 4	Social competence as a construct, of: the peer acceptance subscale of the Pictorial Scale of Perceived Competence and Social Acceptance Preschool Form, the Friendship Interview, and the socialization domain of the Vineland Adaptive Behavior Scales (VABS).	Internalising and externalising behaviours at age 10 and 14	At age 10 years—the CBCL and Teacher Report Form At age 14 years—the CBCL and Youth Self-Report
Bornstein et al. [36]	Longitudinal	US east coast	Two studies Study 2 extracted—139 (39.6)	Language—communication skills—at age 4	Two verbal subtests of the Wechsler Preschool and Primary Scale of Intelligence—Revised and the VABS.	Internalising and externalising behaviours at age 10 and 14	At age 10 years—the CBCL and Teacher Report Form At age 14 years—the CBCL and Youth Self-Report
Derks et al. [37]	Cohort	The Netherlands	One study of three extracted: Generation R study, 3794 (50.4)	Aggressive behaviour—at ages 5–7, 10 and 14	CBCL—mother rated	BMI and body composition (fat mass and fat free mass)—at ages 6 and 10	BMI—the Dutch national reference in the Growth Analyser program. FM and FFM—dual-energy X-ray absorptiometry scanner

Table 3. *Cont.*

Author (Citation)	Study Design	Country	Participants (% Females)	Exposure (Development Characteristic) and Age	Exposure Measurement Instrument	Outcome and Age	Outcome Measurement Instrument
Duchesne et al. [38]	Longitudinal	Canada	2000 (49.9)	Behaviour—hyperactivity, inattention, aggressiveness and prosociality—age 6 Maternal warmth and maternal control also studied	Social Behaviour Questionnaire (SBQ)—teacher rated	Trajectory of anxiety at age 11–12	Rated annually from kindergarten to Grade 6 using the Anxiety Scale from the SBQ—teacher report Children put into trajectory of anxiety
Fine et al. [39]	Longitudinal	US	154 (50.0)	Emotional knowledge, internalising and externalising behaviours age 7	Emotion knowledge—composite score from two tasks: (Emotional labelling & Emotion situation knowledge) Internalising and externalising behaviours—CBCL (teacher report)	Internalising behaviours age 11	Child self-report aggregate of the following measures: Depression—Children's Depression Inventory (CDI) Anxiety—The State-Trait Anxiety Inventory Loneliness. The Loneliness Scale Negative emotions—Differential emotions scale
Glaser et al. [40]	Longitudinal	UK	5250 (50.7)	IQ age 8	Wechsler Intelligence Scale for Children	Depression symptoms—age 11, 13, 14 and 17	Self-reported depressive symptoms were measured with the 13-item Short Mood and Feelings Questionnaire (SMFQ) Moderator: Pubertal stage at 11, 13 and 14 years was measured using a five-point rating scale

Table 3. Cont.

Author (Citation)	Study Design	Country	Participants (% Females)	Exposure (Development Characteristic) and Age	Exposure Measurement Instrument	Outcome and Age	Outcome Measurement Instrument
Gregory et al. [41]	Longitudinal	Australia	3906 (49)	School readiness across 5 domains (physical, social, emotional, language and cognitive, communication and general knowledge)—age 5	Australian version of the Early Development Instrument—teacher rated. Children scored as vulnerable, at risk or on-track	Age 11: four aspects of student wellbeing (life satisfaction, optimism, sadness and worries)	Middle Years Development Instrument—child self-report
Hay et al. [42]	Longitudinal	UK	134 (53)	Co-operation (one form of prosocial behaviour) at age 4	Tester's rating of cooperativeness during the cognitive test (Tester's Rating of Children's Behaviour) and an observational measure of cooperation with the mother during the Etch-A-Sketch task	Internalising and externalising behaviour problems—at age 11	SDQ and CAPA (Child and Adolescent Psychiatric Assessment)
Hooper et al. [43]	Longitudinal	US	74 (52.7)	Language—receptive and expressive language, receptive vocab and working memory—age 5 and 7–8 (kindergarten and second grade)	Receptive and expressive language -The Clinical Evaluation of Language Fundamentals. Receptive vocab (Peabody test) and Working memory (Competing Language Processing Task)	Behaviour problems—externalising problems (conduct and hyperactivity)—kindergarten, first, second, and third grade	Teachers completed assessments of the children's behaviour using a standardized scale of behaviour—Conner's Teacher Rating Scale-Revised

Table 3. Cont.

Author (Citation)	Study Design	Country	Participants (% Females)	Exposure (Development Characteristic) and Age	Exposure Measurement Instrument	Outcome and Age	Outcome Measurement Instrument
Howard et al. [44]	Cohort	Australia	4983 (49)	Self-regulation—age 4–5 and 6–7	Self-regulation problems were indexed by combining parent-, teacher-, and interviewer-report ratings of children's self-regulatory behaviours	Academic and weight, mental health, substance use, crime, self-harm and suicidal ideation—age 15	Academic achievement—children's total scores on the Year 9 National Assessment Program—Literacy and Numeracy Mental health problems were measured in a private face-to-face interview with the parent/carer who knew the adolescent best Overweight and obesity—BMI
Howes et al. [45]	Longitudinal	US	307 (49.5)	Preschool social—emotional climate, Peer play, Behaviour problems, Teacher-child relationship quality—age 4	Preschool social—emotional climate—average of children's scores on measures in class. Peer play-peer play scale Behaviour problems—classroom behaviour inventory (CBI) Teacher-child relationship quality—The Pianta Student Teacher Relationship Scale	Social competence—Behaviour with peers at age 8	Teacher reports using the Cassidy and Asher Teacher Assessment of Social behaviour Questionnaire
Jaspers et al. [65]	Longitudinal (retrospective)	Holland	2139 (50.9)	Behavioural features at age 4—"sleeping, eating, and enuresis problems" and "emotional and behaviour problems"	Assessed by Preventative Child Healthcare professionals.	Behavioural and emotional problems at age 10 to 12	CBCL—parent completed

Table 3. *Cont.*

Author (Citation)	Study Design	Country	Participants (% Females)	Exposure (Development Characteristic) and Age	Exposure Measurement Instrument	Outcome and Age	Outcome Measurement Instrument
Lecompte et al. [46]	Longitudinal	Canada	68 (48.5)	Emotional wellbeing—Child-parent attachment at age 3–4	Lab based separation reunion procedure	Anxiety and depressive symptoms and self-esteem (age 11–12)	Dominic Interactive Questionnaire-computerised self-report measure of common mental health disorders in childhood. Self-esteem-self-perception profile for children—self-report
Lee et al. [47]	Longitudinal	US	762 (46.3)	Behaviour internalising and externalising—age 5	CBCL—primary caregiver completed	Behaviour internalising and externalising—age 9	CBCL—primary caregiver completed
Louise at al. [48]	Longitudinal	Western Australia	2900 (not stated)	Behaviour—aggressive—age 5, 8, 10 and 14	CBCL, youth self-report at age 14 and teacher report at age 10 and 14	Weight at age 5, 8, 10 and 14	Weight—Wedderburn digital chair scale Height was measured using a Holtain Stadiometer. BMI was calculated as weight (kg)/height^2 (m^2)
McKenzie et al. [49]	Longitudinal	USA	207 (49.7)	Fundamental movement skills—Balance, agility, eye-hand coordination—age 4,5 and 6	Movement skill tests in the child's home	Physical Activity—age 12	Trained assessors administered the 7-day Physical Activity Recall (PAR) in the child's home on two occasions, approximately 6 months apart
Meagher et al. [50]	Longitudinal	USA	56 (55.4)	Socio-emotional behaviours observed in pre-school—age 4	Externalising and internalising symptoms from the CBCL—teacher report Observed negative effect by research assistants	Depression symptoms—age 8	Child depression inventory—self-report

Table 3. Cont.

Author (Citation)	Study Design	Country	Participants (% Females)	Exposure (Development Characteristic) and Age	Exposure Measurement Instrument	Outcome and Age	Outcome Measurement Instrument
Nelson et al. [51]	Longitudinal	US	280 (47.9)	Executive control and Foundational Cognitive Abilities at age 5	EC-9-tasks administered to each child during individual sessions in the laboratory (working memory, inhibitory control, and flexible shifting) FCA—via the Woodcock-Johnson-III Brief Intellectual Assessment	Depression and Anxiety symptoms—Age 9–10.	Child Depression Inventory—child self-report Anxiety symptoms—Revised Child Manifest Anxiety Scale—child self-report Externalising symptoms—parents completed the ODD and ADHD-Hyperactivity subscales of the Conners 3rd Edition Parent Ratings Scale
Pedersen et al. [53]	Longitudinal	Canada	551 (45.4)	Behaviour—anxiety/social withdrawal and disruptive behaviour—age 6	Social Behaviour Questionnaire (SBQ)—mother and teacher rated	Peer rejection & Friendedness (at age 8 to 11) Depressive symptoms Loneliness Delinquency—at age 13	Peer rejection—peer nominations. Friendedness—Children were also asked to nominate up to four best friends Depressive symptoms—CDI—child report Loneliness-self-report measure developed by Asher et al. 1984 Delinquency—Self-Reported Delinquency Questionnaire (SRDQ)
Piche et al. [54]	Longitudinal	Canada	966 (47.0)	Self-regulatory skills: classroom engagement and behavioural regulation (emotional distress, physical aggression, impulsivity)—age 6	Classroom engagement (teacher rated) and Behavioural regulation using the SBQ (teacher rated)	Child Sports Participation and BMI—Age 10	Parents reported on their child's weekly involvement in structured sports outside of school during the past school year BMI was derived from direct height and weight measures made by trained, independent examiners

Table 3. Cont.

Author (Citation)	Study Design	Country	Participants (% Females)	Exposure (Development Characteristic) and Age	Exposure Measurement Instrument	Outcome and Age	Outcome Measurement Instrument
Piche et al. [55]	Longitudinal	Canada	1516 (51.9)	Participation in structured and unstructured physical activity—age 7	Parents reported on their children's participation in structured and unstructured physical activity	Age 8 Depressive symptoms	Depression symptoms assessed through the Social Behaviour Questionnaire
Rudasill et al. [56]	Longitudinal	USA	1156 (48.8)	Child temperament (negative emotionality at age 4½ and emotional reactivity at age 7–12) (Student-teacher relationship-teacher perception and child perception tested as mediators)	Negative emotionality: Mothers completed eight subscales from the Children's Behaviour Questionnaire Emotional reactivity: Children's emotional responses to events and environmental stimuli were rated by mothers using a measure designed for use in the NICHD SECCYD	Depressive symptoms in sixth grade (age 11–12)	Mother report of their children's depressive symptoms was measured in 6th grade with the Diagnostic and Statistical Manual of Mental Disorders oriented Affective Problems subscale of the Child Behaviour Checklist
Rudolph et al. [57]	Longitudinal	USA	433 (55.0)	Peer Victimization (static and dynamic) (Age 7–12, 2nd to 5th grade)	Children and teachers completed a revised version of the Social Experiences Questionnaire to assess children's exposure to peer victimization.	Depression symptoms and Aggressive behaviour—Age 11–12 (5th grade)	Depression symptoms—Short Mood and Feelings Questionnaire (Child report) Aggressive behaviour—Children's Social Behaviour Scale (teacher report)
Sandstrom et al. [66]	Meta-analysis	Any	8836 (51.5)	The mean age at the first BI assessment was 3.61 years	BI: defined as shyness, fear, and avoidance when faced with new stimuli	The mean age at the anxiety assessment was 10.39 years	Anxiety and specific anxiety types searched

Table 3. *Cont.*

Author (Citation)	Study Design	Country	Participants (% Females)	Exposure (Development Characteristic) and Age	Exposure Measurement Instrument	Outcome and Age	Outcome Measurement Instrument
Sasser et al. [58]	Longitudinal	USA	356 (54.0)	Intervention targeting social-emotional functioning and language-emergent literacy skills in the first year of pre-school. Executive function measured before and after preschool and each year to third grade (age 8)	Executive function assessment by trained examiners. Children assigned to either low, moderate or high executive function trajectory	Third grade academic outcomes	Reading fluency, language-arts and mathematics (all teacher rated), children self-evaluation of reading ability
Shapero et al. [59]	Longitudinal	USA	958 (48.0)	Emotional—emotional reactivity at age 8. (Household income and household chaos also studied. Household Chaos and Household income also studied.)	Emotional reactivity—mother report—10-item questionnaire about their perceptions of how their child expresses emotions in response to events	Emotional and behavioural problems—age 15	Adolescent Emotional and Behavioural Problems—Youth Self-Report.
Slemming et al. [60]	Longitudinal	Denmark	1336 (49.0)	Behaviour: anxious–fearful, hyperactive–distractible, and hostile–aggressive—age 3–4	Preschool behaviour questionnaire (PBQ)—parent report	Internalising problems—age 10–12	Emotional difficulties were measured at age 10–12 years with the parent-administered strength and difficulties questionnaire (SDQ)

Table 3. *Cont.*

Author (Citation)	Study Design	Country	Participants (% Females)	Exposure (Development Characteristic) and Age	Exposure Measurement Instrument	Outcome and Age	Outcome Measurement Instrument
Straatmannet al. [61]	Longitudinal	UK	10262 (not stated)	Five central domains of a health check in England: (1) personal, social and emotional development, (2) communication and language, (3) physical health, (4) learning and cognitive development and (5) physical development and self-care)—at age 3	Health visitor assessment at routine health check	Language, weight, socioemotional behaviour—age 11	Language—British Ability Scale Second Edition (BAS II) Verbal Similarities test Weight was derived from the body mass index (BMI), using the age and sex- International Obesity Task Force cut-offs Socio-emotional behaviour—SDQ—mother report
Sutin et al. [62]	Longitudinal	Australia	4153 (71.6)	Temperament—sociability, persistence, negative reactivity. Age 4–5	Parents completed a 12-item measure of temperament based on the Childhood Temperament Questionnaire	Weight and weight attitudes and behaviour—age 14–15	Weight—BMI and waist circumference at all ages Weight attitudes and behaviour. At ages 14–15 years, study children self-reported on several aspects of their attitudes and behaviours.
Weeks et al. [63]	Longitudinal	Canada	4405 (50.0)	Verbal ability (age 4–5) and Math skills—age 7–11	Verbal Ability: Peabody Picture Vocabulary Test-Revised (PPVT-R) Math skills—Mathematics Computation Test (MCT)	Internalising symptoms of anxiety and depression—age 12–13 and 14–15	Questionnaire that included 7 items from the Ontario Child Health Study (OCHS-R), assessing symptoms of anxiety and depression—self-report.
Yan et al. [64]	Longitudinal	USA	695 (49.1)	Emotional Wellbeing—child parent relationship—Age 6	Both fathers and mothers rated their relationships (conflict and closeness) with the child at Grade 1, 3, 4 and 5—Child-Parent Relationship Scale	Loneliness at grades 1, 3 and 5 (age 10–11)	Loneliness and Social Dissatisfaction Questionnaire—child self-report

3.6. Narrative Synthesis

There was a range of exposures and outcomes reported across the included literature. Studies were organised by outcomes and grouped as follows:

- "Mental health related symptoms"—this incorporated: internalising symptoms (general, depression, anxiety, loneliness and self-esteem), externalising (general and 'delinquency'), socio-emotional behaviour problems, social competence, wellbeing, self-harm and suicidal ideation.
- "Weight, diet and physical activity"—this incorporated: BMI, overweight/obese, sports participation, unhealthy weight attitudes, and healthy dietary habits.
- For secondary outcomes, the group included executive function and outcomes from academic tests.

Within these above groupings, studies were subsequently organised by exposure and by each domain of child development as follows:

- Domain: Social and emotional development. This was further subdivided to aid analysis, as follows:
    - Internalising—internally focused behaviour such as inhibition and withdrawal.
    - Externalising—externally focused behaviour such as aggression, attention problems, hyperactivity and "delinquent" behaviour.
    - Emotional—internal factors such as social competence, emotion knowledge, pro-social, co-operative and self-regulation skills. External factors such as peer relations, parent-child relationships, teacher-child relationships, socio-emotional climate of school/pre-school setting.
    - Temperament—negative emotionality, emotional reactivity and persistence.
- Domain: Language and communication. This comprised the ability to listen, understand and speak. Exposures included: receptive and expressive vocabulary. Receptive relates to understanding of words and expressive relates to the ability to use words for expression.
- Domain: Cognitive development. This comprised mathematics skills, executive control, foundational cognitive ability, verbal ability/literacy and Intelligence Quotient (IQ)
- Domain: Physical development. This involved fundamental movement skills (balance, agility, hand-eye co-ordination) and participation in structured and unstructured physical activity
- Multiple domains.

A summary of the evidence on associations between exposures (domains of child development) and outcomes is presented in Figure 2. Each annotation does not always represent a study in its entirety as many studies analysed multiple exposures and outcomes.

3.7. Primary Outcomes

3.7.1. Mental Health

Summary of Associations between Child Development and Mental Health

Positive development on starting school is associated with subsequent positive mental health. There is stronger evidence for associations between the socio-emotional domain of child development and later mental health, weaker evidence for the cognitive domain, inconsistent evidence for language and communication and limited evidence for physical development.

Summary of Associations between Socio-Emotional Development and Mental Health

Eighteen studies analysed associations between a socio-emotional exposure of child development and later mental health [33,35,38,39,42,44–47,50,53,56,57,59,60,64–66]. All associations highlighted that positive socio-emotional development is good for subsequent mental health, apart from five studies where no associations were found for some exposures and outcomes studied [39,42,50,60,65]. The evidence is stronger for exposures of externalising behaviour and emotional wellbeing at school entry, weaker for exposures of internalising behaviour and limited for exposures relating to temperament.

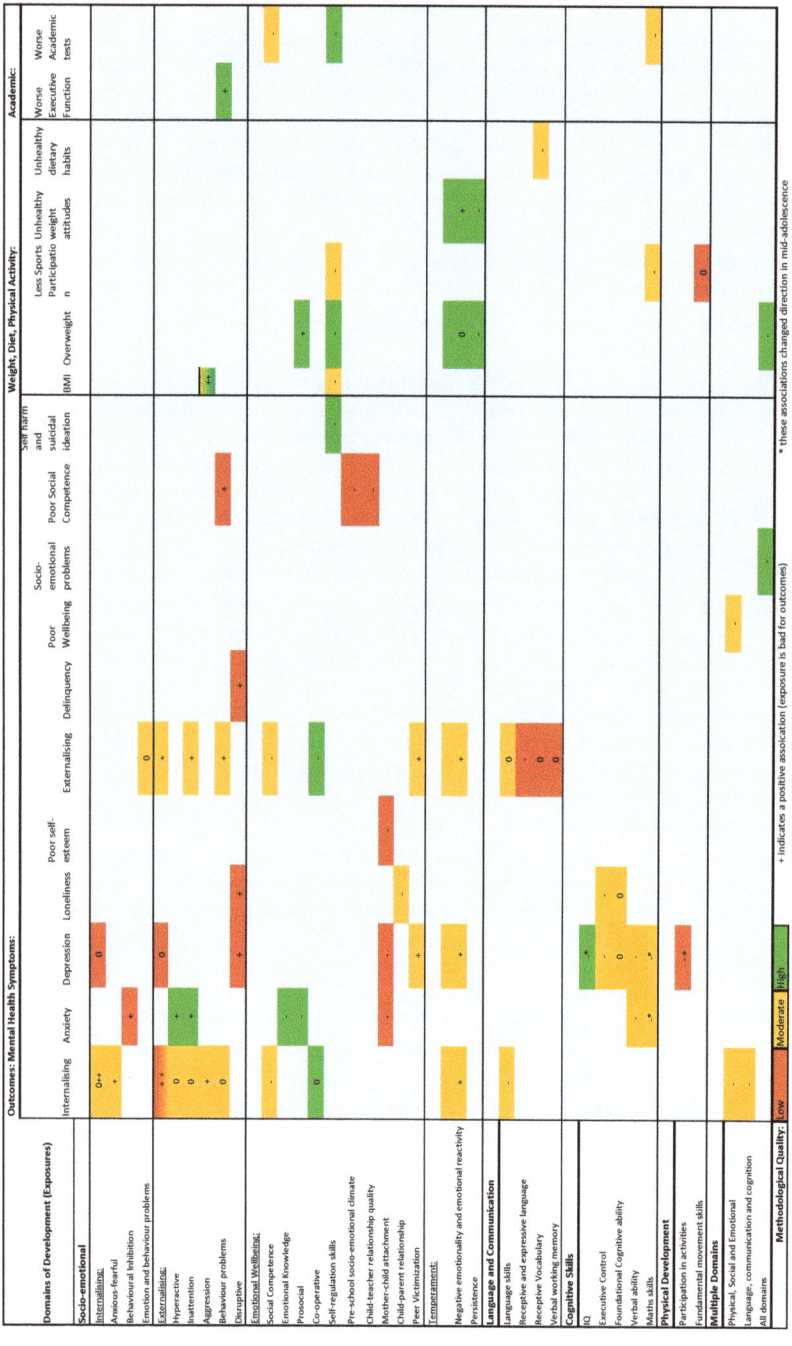

Figure 2. Evidence of associations between domains of "child development" (exposures) and outcomes of mental health symptoms, weight and academic.

Exposure of Internalising Behaviours at School Entry and Subsequent Mental Health

Eight studies analysed the relationship between early internalising behaviour and later mental health [33,39,47,50,53,60,65,66], highlighting weaker evidence for positive associations with internalising outcomes and limited evidence for positive associations with externalising outcomes. Of these, six studies analysed the association between early internalising and later internalising behaviours, with two studies of moderate quality showing positive associations [33,47], one high quality study where no association was found [39], and one low quality study, of 56 children, where no association was found with depression symptoms [50]. Specifically, anxious-fearful behaviour is associated with later emotional difficulties as reported by parents [60] in a study of moderate quality. Behavioural inhibition is associated with anxiety but this evidence was from a lower quality review [66]. Evidence on the relationship between early internalising and later externalising behaviours was scant; only limited evidence was provided, with two studies not studying that relationship specifically [47,53] and one study where no association was found between early emotional and behaviour problems and later externalising [65].

Exposure of Externalising Behaviours at School Entry and Subsequent Mental Health

Nine studies were found on the relationship between externalising behaviours and later mental health [33,38,39,45,47,50,53,60,65], highlighting stronger evidence for positive associations with both internalising and externalising outcomes. Of these, seven studies analysed the associations between early externalising and later internalising, with six studies showing positive associations and one study where no association was found. There was evidence of positive associations between general externalising behaviour problems [33,39] and later internalising symptoms, and specifically aggression [60] was associated with later internalising symptoms. However, although two studies showed no association between hyperactive behaviour [60] or inattention [65] and later general internalising symptoms, one high quality study of 2000 children did evidence an association between these behaviours and later anxiety symptoms [38]. One study, of lower quality, evidenced that disruptiveness was associated with later depression symptoms and loneliness [53].

Similar to internalising symptoms, whereby the continuity of association was found for early and later symptoms, the same is true for externalising symptoms, whereby early problems are associated with externalising at a later age. However, the evidence is stronger with two studies of moderate quality evidencing associations between general externalising [47], inattention and behaviour problems [65] and later general externalising symptoms, with a further study evidencing a relationship between poorer social competence with peers in mid-childhood and earlier behaviour problems [45]. Specifically, disruptiveness was associated with delinquency in one low quality study [53].

Exposures of Emotional Wellbeing at School Entry and Subsequent Mental Health

Nine studies were found on the associations between a child's emotional wellbeing and later mental health [35,38,39,42,44–46,57,64] with stronger evidence found for the association with internalising outcomes and weaker evidence for externalising outcomes. A child's emotional wellbeing, in terms of social competence, emotional knowledge (the ability to identify and label emotions), self-regulation and prosociality (behaviour intended to benefit others), appears beneficial to later health in adolescence. Negative associations were found between early social competence and internalising and externalising problems [35]. In two high quality studies, associations were found for emotional knowledge [39] and prosocial skills [38] and later anxiety, with increasing emotional knowledge and prosocial skills both associated with less anxiety symptoms. A child's ability to co-operate, a particular prosocial skill, highlighted mixed results in one study [42], with increasing co-operation associated with less externalising but no association found with internalising problems. Self-regulation problems, in terms of ability to control behaviours, attention, thinking, social interaction and emotions, were subsequently associated, in adolescence, with an increase in the risk of self-harm ideation and behaviour, suicidal ideation, school truancy, mental health problems, smoking and alcohol use, and violent and property crime [44]. When self-regulation problems reduced, from age 4–5 to 6–7, the association between these adolescent outcomes and earlier self-regulation problems was no longer found [44].

In relation to the child's emotional wellbeing in the context of relationships or setting specific (external factors), studies were found on: mother–child attachment, relationship with parents, teachers, and peers (victimisation), and the socio-emotional climate in a pre-school setting, and all proved important for positive mental health in adolescence. A small study of 68 children, rated low quality, evidenced that disorganised maternal attachment at pre-school age was associated with greater depression and anxiety symptoms and lower self-esteem in early adolescence [46]. A positive relationship with parents, in terms of closeness, was associated with less loneliness, particularly for father–daughter relationships [64]. In one low quality study, a good quality relationship with teachers and a positive socio-emotional climate in a pre-school setting were both associated with improved social competence in mid-childhood [45]. With regard to relations with peers, one study evidenced that early and increasing peer victimisation was associated with depression symptoms and aggression [57].

Exposures of Temperament at School Entry and Subsequent Mental Health

Two studies were found on the association between temperament and later mental health highlighting limited evidence of a negative association, with higher levels of certain traits associated with worse outcomes. These studies investigated child temperament, in terms of negative emotionality and emotional reactivity (the former refers to the propensity to react with negative emotions and the latter relates to the intensity of emotion) [56,59] and both were of moderate quality. One showed an association between negative emotionality, emotional reactivity and depression symptoms [56] and one between emotional reactivity and internalising and externalising symptoms [59].

Summary of Associations between Language and Communication, Cognitive Development, Physical Development, and Multiple Domains and Mental Health

Eight studies analysed the associations between exposures relating to either language and communication, cognitive development, physical development or multiple domains of child development and later mental health. All associations highlighted that positive development across all of the domains of child development are good for subsequent mental health. There was weaker evidence for the effect of cognitive skills and the positive effect of cognitive development appears to alter with age. The evidence for associations between language and communication and later mental health outcomes was inconsistent in relation to internalising and externalising outcomes. There was limited evidence for both physical development and measures incorporating multiple domains.

Exposures within the Language and Communication Domain and Subsequent Mental Health

The results for the effect of language and communication skills on later mental health symptoms was inconsistent with two studies investigating these associations [36,43]. One study of 129 children evidenced that language skills at pre-school age predict internalising but not externalising behaviour problems in adolescence. Conversely, one low quality study of 74 children did find an association between good language skills (receptive and expressive language) and less externalising problems, namely, conduct problems but not hyperactivity.

Exposures within the Cognitive Domain and Subsequent Mental Health

Three studies analysed the effect of cognitive skills on later mental health symptoms, [40,51,63] with weaker evidence found. One study found that deficits in executive control predicted depression and anxiety symptoms and clinical level of depression [51]. The same study showed that foundational cognitive ability did not predict these outcomes. One high quality study showed an association between cognition, measured as IQ, and depression symptoms with an increased IQ in early childhood associated with less depression symptoms at age 11 [40]. However, by age 13–14 the association reversed. The loss of protective effect of cognition was also found in relation to the effect of cognitive skill (measured as mathematics skills and verbal ability) on internalising symptoms, whereby a protective effect seen at age 12-13 was reversed or had no associated effect at age 14–15 [63].

Exposures within Physical Development Domain and Subsequent Mental Health

There was limited evidence for the effect of physical development on later mental health related symptoms. One lower quality study, in which time between exposure and outcome was one year, found that structured physical activity was associated with less depression symptoms in boys, whereas unstructured physical activity was associated with more depression in girls [55].

Exposures Incorporating Multiple Domains and Subsequent Mental Health

Two studies provided evidence across multiple domains [41,61]. One study evidenced that all components of school readiness (as part of a model of early years data), measured by UK health visitors before starting school, predicted socio-emotional behaviour problems in early adolescence [61]. An Australian study which investigated the relationships between all domains of school readiness and wellbeing at the end of primary school found that all domains were negatively associated with internalising symptoms, whereas only physical and socio-emotional development were positively associated with overall wellbeing [41].

3.7.2. Weight, Diet and Physical Activity Outcomes

Summary of Associations between Child Development and Weight

Positive development on starting school is associated with subsequent healthy weight related outcomes. There is stronger evidence for the socio-emotional domain of child development, and limited evidence for language and communication, cognitive and physical domains of child development.

Summary of Associations between Socio-Emotional Development and Weight

Five studies analysed the associations between a socio-emotional measure of child development and later weight diet or physical activity outcomes [37,44,48,54,62]. All associations highlighted that positive socio-emotional development is good for subsequent weight-related outcomes, apart from one study where mixed associations were found for exposures of certain temperamental traits and later weight related outcomes. The evidence is stronger for exposures within the emotional wellbeing domain, specifically self-regulation skills, with weaker evidence found for exposures of externalising behaviour and no evidence found for internalising behaviour.

Exposures of Externalising, Emotional Wellbeing and Temperament and Subsequent Weight

In relation to externalising, specifically aggressive behaviour, one higher quality study found a positive association with higher BMI [37] and one of moderate quality found an association with higher rate of change in BMI but in girls only [48]. In relation to self-regulation, one higher quality study [44] evidenced that early problems in self-regulation (ability to control attention, behaviour and emotion at age 4–5) were associated with being overweight or obese in adolescence but that a change in self-regulation (less problems) at a later age (age 6–7) had no effect on the association. Another study highlighted that increasing self-regulation skills (measured as class room engagement) were associated with lower BMI and increased sports participation [54]. Additionally, this study evidenced that emotional distress (a measure of self-regulation) was associated with less sports participation. In relation to temperament, one higher quality study [62] looked at the associations between the traits of persistence sociability and negative reactivity, and later BMI and weight attitudes and behaviours, and found that persistence decreased the risk of obesity and overweight, sociability increased the risk of overweight but not obesity, and negative reactivity was not associated with either. In relation to weight attitudes and behaviours, all three traits were associated with restrained eating habits in adolescence, with lower persistence and higher negative reactivity or sociability associated with restrained eating and use of unhealthy weight management strategies.

Summary of Associations between Domains of: Language and Communication, Cognitive, Physical Development, Multiple Domains and Weight

There was limited evidence on associations between the domains of language and communication, cognitive skills, and physical development, and later weight-related outcomes. One study, which looked at evidence on a range of school readiness skills and later wellbeing measures, evidenced that receptive vocabulary was associated with healthier dietary habits [52], with increasing receptive vocabulary predicting reduced sweet snack intake and increased dairy intake. The same study [52] evidenced that increasing mathematics skills predicted increasing involvement in physical activity, providing limited evidence for an association between cognitive skills and later weight-related outcomes. There was limited evidence on the association between physical development and weight-related outcomes, with one lower quality study finding no association between fundamental movement skills and later involvement in physical activity [49]. One study evidenced that all components of school readiness (as part of a model of early years data), as measured by UK health visitors before starting school, predicted overweight and obesity in early adolescence [61].

3.8. Secondary Outcomes

3.8.1. Academic Tests and Executive Function

Summary of Associations between Child Development and Academic Outcomes

Four studies analysed associations between a domain of child development and later academic outcomes: three in relation to socio-emotional development and one in relation to cognitive development. All associations highlighted that positive development is good for subsequent academic outcomes. The evidence is stronger for exposures within the socio-emotional domain, specifically self-regulation skills and less behaviour problems, with weaker evidence found for exposures within the cognitive domain of child development. There were no studies found looking at the association between language and communication or physical development and academic outcomes.

Exposures within the Socio-Emotional and Cognition Domains and Subsequent Academic Outcomes

There were two studies found on associations between socio-emotional development and the secondary academic outcomes, both of higher quality [34,44]. One studied the effect of behaviour risk (a composite of poor sleep, emotions and inattention) on adolescent executive function and found that poorer behaviour is associated with lower executive function [34]. Another study highlighted that self-regulation problems are associated with reduced scores on numeracy and literacy tests in adolescence [44]. An additional study [58] investigated the effect of an intervention targeting socio-emotional functioning and language emergent literacy skills in pre-school, through comparing the impact of executive function trajectories on academic test results of children in the intervention group compared to those who were not. This study showed that socio-emotional and language programmes improved executive function and academic outcomes for children with the lowest executive function trajectory. There was limited evidence on associations between early cognitive skills and later academic outcomes, with one study showing a positive association between kindergarten mathematics skills and later academic outcomes [52].

3.9. Factors Affecting Relationships

Summary of findings on factors affecting associations (mediation and moderation)

Limited evidence was found on factors affecting associations. Some evidence, however, was found on factors affecting associations between socio-emotional development and subsequent mental health and academic outcomes. The factors are discussed in relation to the pathways identified in the initial conceptual model devised with stakeholders. Factors were found in relation to family stress, knowledge/literacy and social/cognitive pathways. No factors were found that pertained to the material living or parent health behaviour pathways. All of the findings within this section fall into the category of limited evidence as all of the factors described were found in single studies only.

3.9.1. Mediators

Six studies included data on mediating variables: five related to studies focusing on mental health outcomes [35,36,46,53,56] and one relating to academic outcomes [34]. None of the studies that focused on weight as an outcome included data on mediation. Factors mediating associations between socio-emotional development and mental health were self-esteem, type of internalising or externalising in mid-childhood, and relationships with teachers and friends. Factors mediating associations between socio-emotional development and academic outcomes were approaches to learning and attentional regulation.

3.9.2. Moderators

Seven studies included data on variables to test for moderation effects on associations between exposure and outcome: five in relation to mental health [38,40,47,59,64], one in relation to weight [62] and one in relation to academic outcomes [58]. Factors moderating associations between socio-emotional development and mental health were household chaos and parenting. Household chaos had a negative effect, and aspects of parenting had a positive effect on the associations between the socio-emotional domain of child development and mental health outcomes. A factor found to moderate the association between socio-emotional development and academic outcomes was trajectory of executive function.

3.9.3. Factors Pertaining to the Family Stress Pathway—Moderating Associations between Child Development and Mental Health

This pathway incorporates factors related to stress in the home, which can affect parenting ability, parenting style and consequently child health and development. Household chaos and aspects of parenting were identified as moderators of the relationship between the socio-emotional domain of child development and later mental health symptoms. Household chaos was found to disproportionately affect children with higher emotional reactivity resulting in greater internalising problems [59]. This effect was not found for household income; that is, level of emotional reactivity made no difference to the impact of income on adolescent emotional and behaviour problems. This implies that the impact of low income on adolescent mental health is pervasive and not amenable to individual interventions promoting self-regulation (in terms of emotional response to events) but that interventions of this type might support how children respond to household chaos. Three studies analysed the moderating role of aspects of parenting on the relationships between socio-emotional measures and later mental health related symptoms [38,47,64], with all finding positive effects of aspects of child/parent relationships on adolescent outcomes. Two studies found a protective effect of relationships with fathers on continuity of behaviour problems. One found a protective effect for fathers' positive engagement on the continuity of earlier to later internalising and externalising behaviour problems, and for those in the greatest poverty, fathers' positive engagement was associated with a reduction in the continuity of internalising problems from age 5 to 9 years [47]. The authors hypothesize that this is due to development of secure attachment and the development of emotional and behavioural regulation skills. Another looked at the moderating role of parent–child closeness on the continuity of loneliness from age 6–11 years and found that as parent–child closeness increased, loneliness reduced and this relationship was particularly strong for girls and their fathers [64]. Another study looked at the moderating role of maternal parenting practices, warmth and discipline, on the relationship between behavioural characteristics of; inattention, hyperactivity, aggressiveness and low prosociality and trajectory of anxiety in children between the ages of 6 and 12 years [38]. It found that a lack of maternal warmth increased the association between hyperactivity and anxiety. It also found that high level of maternal discipline (rules and controlling child's behaviour) increased the probability of belonging to the high anxiety group.

3.9.4. Factors Pertaining to the Knowledge/Literacy Pathway—Moderating and Mediating Associations between Child Development and Academic Outcomes

This pathway relates to the way knowledge and literacy can lead to behaviours that can be positive for wellbeing [67]. Two studies analysed factors within this category, both on the relationship between the socio-emotional domain and later academic outcomes. One highlighted a moderating role of executive function on the relationship between an intervention to improve socio-emotional and language emergent skills and later academic outcomes, and found that the effect of the intervention was higher in children with low executive function in the intervention group resulting in better academic outcomes compared to controls [58]. Another highlighted attentional regulation and approaches to learning as mediators, partially explaining the relationship between child behaviour (composite of sleep, emotional dysregulation and inattention/hyperactivity) and later executive functioning.

3.9.5. Factors Pertaining to the Social/Cognitive Pathway—Mediating Associations between Child Development and Mental Health

This pathway relates to the influence of individual experiences, the actions of others and environmental factors that provide the social context for learning to influence health behaviours [68]. Five studies analysed mediators pertaining to this pathway and all in relation to mental health related symptoms: four in relation to the socio-emotional domain [35,46,53,56] and one from the language and communication domain [36]. In relation to the socio-emotional domain of child development and later mental health there is limited evidence that self-esteem, type of internalising or externalising in mid-childhood, and relationships with teachers and friends all play a role in explaining the relationship. One study evidenced the role of self-esteem, which partially mediated the relationship between emotional wellbeing (measured as parental attachment) and depression but not anxiety [46]. Two studies highlighted the role of relationships: one with peers [53] and one with teachers [56]. In relation to peers, peer rejection and number of friends in mid-childhood mediated the relationship between disruptiveness at age 6 and depression at age 13 years, with peer rejection also mediating the relationship between disruptiveness and loneliness. Relationships with teachers (closeness and conflict) also appear important, with one study analysing the effect of child–teacher relationships on the relationship between negative emotionality at age 4, emotional reactivity at age 7 and depression symptoms at age 11–12 years [56]. This study found that teacher-child conflict mediated the relationship between emotional reactivity and depression symptoms, with children higher in emotional reactivity having more depression symptoms, and this was partially explained by conflict with teachers (teacher reported).

3.9.6. Factors Pertaining to Child Characteristics—Moderating Associations between Child Development and Weight and Mental Health

Sex moderated the association between socio-emotional domain of child development and weight outcomes, with worse outcomes for girls. Age moderated the association between the cognitive domain of child development and subsequent mental health, with a protective role of positive cognitive development on mental health in early adolescence reversing in mid-adolescence.

Two studies analysed the effect of age on the relationship between cognition and later depression symptoms, and found that age reversed the protective effect of cognition on early adolescent (age 11) mental health by age 13–15 years [40,63] but that this reversed again at age 17 for females [40]. This study also found that pubertal status mimicked the relationship by age but that this was stronger for females. The loss of the health protective effect of cognition may be due to exam pressures at certain time points or, for females, biological hormonal changes. Sex was the only factor studied in relation to weight. One study evidenced that girls with higher aggression cores throughout childhood had a higher rate of change in their BMI [48]. Another study highlighted that girls higher in sociability in early childhood had a greater fear of weight gain at age 14–15 years [62].

3.10. Conceptual Model/Diagram Development

A summary of findings and revised conceptual model was discussed with stakeholders and a final diagram of the relationships, as informed by this systematic review, was discussed and agreed—see Figure 3. Factors which were not found in the review but were deemed important by stakeholders are highlighted on the diagram. These included neighbourhood factors, such as community engagement and community environment, which stakeholders felt could create conditions conducive for optimal health and development. Political and system factors were also identified, such as short political cycles not giving policy sufficient time to embed and effect change, and regulators focusing narrowly on academic outcomes rather than broader social and emotional wellbeing, which dictates the focus of a school. The stakeholder group identified these factors as potential moderators of the relationships between child development and health.

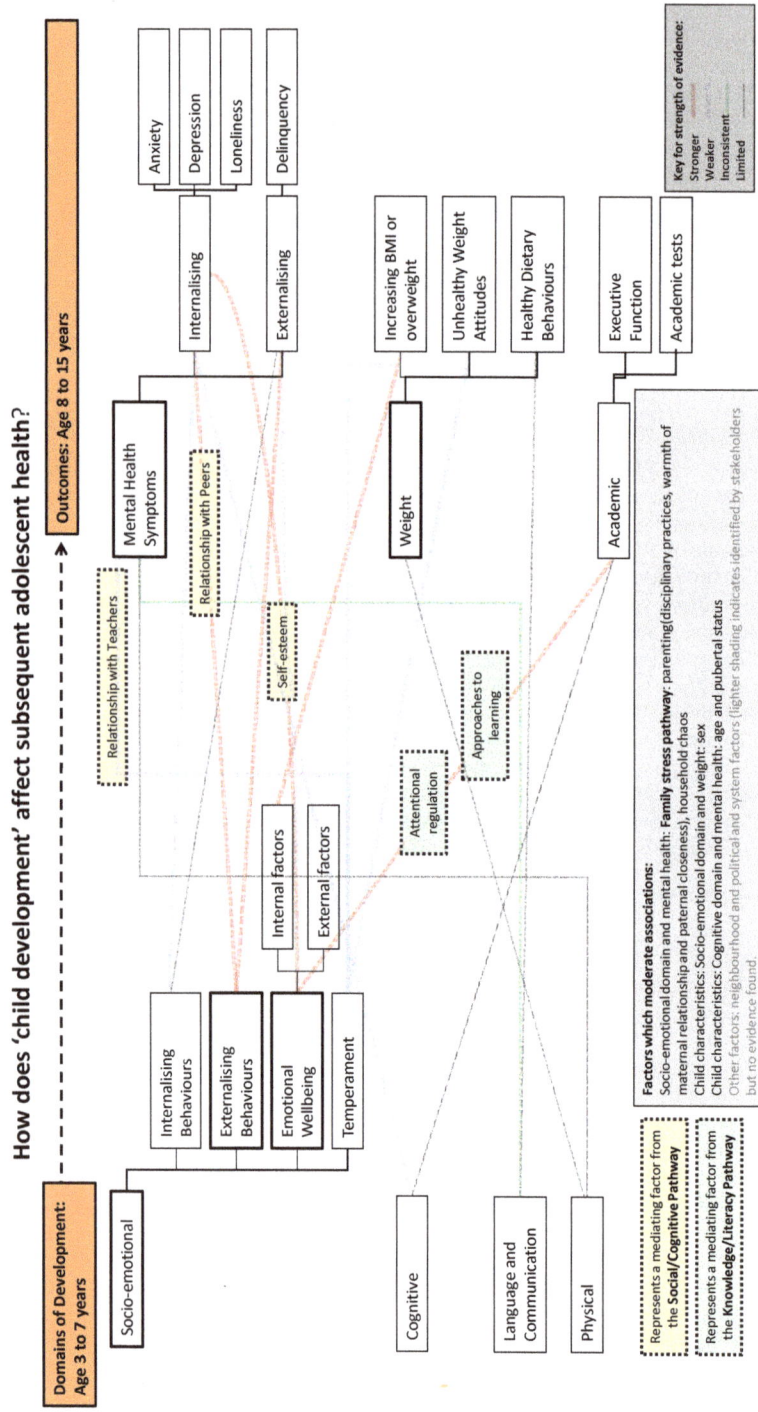

Figure 3. Diagram of the relationship between domains of child development and adolescent outcomes.

4. Discussion

This review asked the questions: what are the associations between child development and adolescent health, and what factors explain or alter the associations. The review clearly shows that positive development on starting school is good for later health outcomes, but that the evidence is stronger for relationships between some domains of child development than others, with gaps in the evidence base across domains. In relation to mental health outcomes, there is stronger evidence for associations between socio-emotional development and later mental health, weaker evidence for associations with cognitive development, inconsistent evidence for language and communication, and limited evidence for physical development. In relation to adolescent weight, there is stronger evidence for associations with children's socio-emotional development and limited evidence of relationships with language and communication, cognitive development or physical development. In relation to secondary (academic) outcomes, there is stronger evidence for associations with socio-emotional development, limited evidence for an association with cognitive development and no evidence found for an association with language and communication or physical development. In relation to what factors explain or moderate the associations, the evidence identified in this review is largely limited to factors shaping the relationship between socio-emotional development and mental health and academic outcomes with factors pertaining to the pathways of family stress, knowledge/literacy and social/cognitive.

Our findings build upon the existing limited evidence that attendance at pre-school (a proxy for good child development) is associated with positive mental wellbeing and healthy weight in adolescence [12], and provides detail on which domains of child development are associated with these positive health outcomes. Supporting the existing literature, we found positive relationships between both cognitive and socio-emotional development (such as self-regulation and social competence) on mental health and academic outcomes in early adolescence [9–11], with stronger evidence found for socio-emotional development. Additionally, we identified evidence of a negative relationship between socio-emotional wellbeing and unhealthy weight. The review provided a test of our conceptual model and we found that the evidence base was lacking for some of the proposed pathways between child development and later health.

Undertaking this review highlighted a complexity in classifying the rich and broad literature that exists on child development. In consequence, the review had to embed an inductive process of interpretation of how included studies had understood and measured child development. Using a classification system of four domains of child development to aid analysis of a very broad concept enabled us to categorise a multitude of measures of child development within this system. This complexity and the need for interpretation is perhaps unsurprising given that the field of child development spans the disciplines of psychology, sociology education, biology, genetics and public health. That a classification system for understanding child development does not exist is in itself a finding of our review. Our classification of four domains of child development adds to the literature, providing a framework for other researchers to use and to critique.

Our findings show that conceptualising child development into domains of development matters because different aspects of development seem to have different impacts on later health outcomes. Understanding this can help to inform public health interventions in childhood. For example, in our review, we found that socio-emotional development when children start school has the most evidence for subsequent impact on adolescent health, in terms of mental health and healthy weight, and as such could be a focus for intervention. The findings in relation to mental health are to be expected, with much literature highlighting the continuity of early problems with socio-emotional functioning and later onset of mental health conditions [69]. The evidence is stronger for early externalising behaviours and their impact on both internalising and externalising behaviours in adolescence, and this is supported by wider literature [70,71]. A finding of this review is that there is more evidence that behaviours such as aggression and hyperactivity pose a risk to future mental health than anxious/withdrawn behaviour, particularly for externalising outcomes. This finding should be interpreted cautiously because it may be that early internalising behaviours, compared to externalising, are more likely to resolve by early adolescence [72], or it may be that internalising is harder to identify, whereas externalising behaviours are more obvious and easier for parents and teachers to report, which could lead to less associations being observed for internalising behaviours and consequently less associations found [39,70]. The finding that emotional wellbeing was more closely associated with later internalising may be because emotional stability promotes regulation and mood stability leading to less internalising [73], but other studies have found that emotional wellbeing (in terms of regulation skills) is associated quite strongly with both internalising and externalising, but particularly so for internalising after the early years [74].

The findings in relation to stronger evidence on the associations between socio-emotional development and weight add to a growing field of evidence exploring this relationship, with evidence of co-development and temporal associations in mid-childhood [75], evidence of obesity having a detrimental impact on socio-emotional behaviour [76], and evidence on associations between social competence and weight with social competence reducing the odds of later overweight [77]. From this review, emotional wellbeing and, in particular, self-regulation skills, appear to be important factors to study in this complex relationship between socio-emotional development and weight. However, other developmental pathways in the development of obesity, such as physical activity and cultural and social factors, are important to consider alongside self-regulation development [44].

More evidence is needed on how adolescent health outcomes are shaped by other domains of child development, particularly the impact of language and communication, and cognitive and physical development at school starting age. Evidence on these domains are important for engaging health and education sectors to work together because education and health services share a common goal for optimal developmental potential of children [78]. This evidence would help the development of a shared understanding and provide a platform from which to develop the context and settings that may work best for optimal health and development of children, regardless of their stage of development when starting school. Including executive function as an exposure and outcome in this review allowed for inclusion of any evidence on the bi-directional relationship between executive function and health [79]. The analysis of secondary outcomes of academic tests and executive function highlight the importance of socio-emotional development on these outcomes (health improves executive function). Conversely, the protective effect of cognitive skills (measured as executive control) on adolescent mental health highlights that executive function improves health. However, age appears to be an important factor in this latter relationship, with the protective effects of cognition on mental health being reversed or no associations found in mid-adolescence [40,63], and this warrants further research.

Understanding the impact of domains of child development on later health has important policy implications in relation to reducing inequalities, and in relation to a policy extension beyond the first 1000 days. In relation to reducing inequalities, our review highlights a strong relationship between socio-emotional development and later health. Applying a public health lens to "child development" helps to understand exactly what it is that pre-school provision or early years centres may need to focus on if we are to improve adolescent health and wellbeing. Re-invigoration of early childhood programmes such as Sure Start, with a renewed focus on socio-emotional development, may be one area of policy improvement, particularly if we are to focus on their longer-term potential to reduce inequalities [80].

In addition, arguably a policy shift is required, which extends beyond the first 1000 days, to understand and support optimal development throughout childhood and into adolescence [81], to address the consequences of inequalities in child development as children age and because adolescence is a significant period of development and an important period in the life course [82]. If we are to maximise the opportunities conferred by education as a platform to improve public health and reduce health inequalities [83], policy that incorporates a life course approach to healthy development is needed, and this requires cross-sector collaboration.

Fostering collaboration to inform policy on reducing child and adolescent health inequalities beyond the first 1000 days requires more research on how development and education translates into health throughout childhood, and on the effect of socio-economic circumstances on this relationship. Findings in relation to the factors that explain or alter associations between child development and subsequent health were limited in this review, with all findings pertaining to single studies. The most evidence was within the social-cognitive pathway with self-esteem, relations with peers and teachers all providing some explanation for the relationship between socio-emotional development and subsequent mental health outcomes, and this can inform interventions for optimal health and development through the primary school years. Surprisingly, in relation to the original conceptual diagram designed with stakeholders, there was no literature found on material living circumstances, parent health behaviours, community factors, and political and system factors. To some extent this was because the studies controlled for the effect of income, housing, parental education and parent health behaviours. However, this presents a problem because we need to know more about how these elements of socio-economic circumstance affect the associations under study in this review. For example, we know that children from more deprived backgrounds experience poorer health and development than their more affluent peers [7]. If we are to pragmatically intervene to improve the health and development trajectory of children in more deprived circumstances, and reduce the attainment and health gap, we need to understand exactly how poverty, household circumstances and home environments affect learning and the co-development of education and health. This requires the design of public health research that respects agency but more clearly theorizes children within their social and economic context [84], so as to encapsulate socio-political cultural and familial environments because, in many ways, this is what "defines" child development in practice, over and above genetic make-up.

In addition to collaborating to produce more evidence on individual, home or school-level interventions to mitigate against poor development, interventions at system level are required to tackle prevention earlier so that children reach a good stage of development, and to reduce inequalities in development measures upon starting school. This requires evidence in relation to macro-determinants such as political and system factors, e.g., addressing poverty, the role of regulators in generating a target-driven culture that focuses attention on academic achievement, a political system not conducive to cross-departmental perspectives or action, and a system which stifles innovation and creativity. Larger studies, such as natural experiments or evaluations of existing policies, are needed that perhaps compare areas with different working systems or policies to identify any particular cultures or practices that are conducive to promoting positive trajectories for the health and development of children. The participatory element of this research identified some of these macro-determinants, identifying a gap between research and practice. This finding highlights the need to bring research and practice closer together [85] through listening to views and experiences of those working in service roles, at the system level and/or with children. It is hoped that this method can help to inform future research by highlighting what is evidenced in the literature, but also bringing to light views from lived experience, which may not be captured in any published evidence but could steer future research.

The strengths of this review are in its systematic design aiming to incorporate all relevant studies to answer the research question and in its engagement with a stakeholder group to steer the review and engage research with practice. The involvement of a sample of stakeholders raises the potential for biases to be introduced by selection of stakeholders with particular views, opinions or experiences. The use of replicable and transparent systematic review methods helps to minimise this risk. The research question was broad. This limited the search strategy in incorporating all possible terms to address the breadth of the research question and this may mean that some evidence was not found. Another limitation is that the secondary outcomes were only included where they were found in papers that also encompassed the primary outcome. This likely means that the associations found are underestimated. Including any paper with the secondary outcomes would have led to an unmanageable number of papers and, given that the focus of the review was health outcomes, it steered the decision on only including secondary outcomes where relevant in understanding any temporal dynamics to the relationship under study. The grouping of child development measures, used for data synthesis, could be seen as both a strength and a weakness: a strength in that it allowed for the classification of a range of child development measures into developmental domains, and a limitation in that it was a subjective process and, as such, is open to critique.

5. Conclusions

Positive socio-emotional development at school starting age appears particularly important for subsequent mental health and weight in adolescence. There are gaps in the evidence about what factors affect the relationships between child development and subsequent health, in particular, the effect of socio-economic factors. More collaborative research across health and education is needed to develop and define appropriate measures of child development across key domains of child development, and also on the relationships and mechanisms between domains of development, particularly cognitive, language and communication, and physical development, and later health, in the context of socio-economic inequality. This requires the design of public health research that respects agency but more clearly theorizes children within their social and economic context [84], so as to encapsulate socio-political, cultural and familial environments. Research designed using longitudinal cohorts could be one way forward here and be considered in future work on this topic. This theoretically informed research and knowledge is imperative to inform interventions to address health inequalities in mid-childhood and adolescence.

Supplementary Materials: The following are available online at https://www.mdpi.com/article/10.3390/ijerph182111613/s1, Additional file 1: PRISMA Checklist, Additional file 2: Conceptual diagram, Additional file 3: Search Strategy, Additional file 4: Excluded papers, Additional file 5: Data extraction form, Additional file 6: Quality assessment form, Additional file 7: SWIM Checklist, Additional file 8: Table of study characteristics, Additional file 9: Results of quality assessment process.

Author Contributions: M.B. identified the topic and led the study design process with contributions from A.B. (Amy Barnes), M.S. and D.T.-R.; M.B., A.B. (Anna Brook), A.R., B.H. and C.F. screened the search results; M.B. extracted data and undertook the quality assessments, with input from A.B. (Amy Barnes), A.B. (Anna Brook), B.H. and C.F.; M.B. drafted the manuscript with input from all authors. All authors have read and agreed to the published version of the manuscript.

Funding: This research was funded by the National Institute for Health Research (NIHR Doctoral Fellowship, Mrs Michelle Black, NIHR300689). The views expressed are those of the authors and not necessarily those of the NHS, the National Institute for Health Research or the Department of Health and Social Care. DTR is funded by the MRC on a Clinician Scientist Fellowship (MR/P008577/1).

Institutional Review Board Statement: Not applicable.

Informed Consent Statement: Not applicable.

Data Availability Statement: Lists of included and excluded articles are available in the published article and the associated supplementary files.

Acknowledgments: We would like to thank Susan Baxter, Andrew Booth and Mark Clowes for their helpful comments on the methods for the review. We are also very grateful to the stakeholders who contributed to the discussion in designing the conceptual model.

Conflicts of Interest: The authors declare no conflict of interest.

References

1. Royal College of Paediatrics and Child Health. *State of Child. Health 2020*; RCPCH London, 2020.
2. Strategic Review of Health Inequalities in England post-2010. *Fair Society, Healthier Lives: The Marmot Review*. 2010. Available online: https://www.instituteofhealthequity.org/resources-reports/fair-society-healthy-lives-the-marmot-review/fair-society-healthy-lives-full-report-pdf.pdf (accessed on 3 November 2021).
3. Centre on the Developing Child. *The Foundations of Lifelong Health Are Built in Early Childhood*. 2010. Available online: https://developingchild.harvard.edu/resources/the-foundations-of-lifelong-health-are-built-in-early-childhood/ (accessed on 3 November 2021).
4. Fox, S.E.; Levitt, P.; Nelson, C.A. How the Timing and Quality of Early Experiences Influence the Development of Brain Architecture. *Child. Dev.* **2010**, *81*, 28–40. [CrossRef]
5. Heckman, J.J. Skill Formation and the Economics of Investing in Disadvantaged Children. *Science* **2006**, *312*, 1900–1902. [CrossRef] [PubMed]
6. Darling, J.C.; Bamidis, P.D.; Burberry, J.; Rudolf, M.C.J. The First Thousand Days: Early, integrated and evidence-based approaches to improving child health: Coming to a population near you? *Arch. Dis. Child.* **2020**, *105*, 837. [CrossRef]
7. Black, M.; Barnes, A.; Baxter, S.; Beynon, C.; Clowes, M.; Dallat, M.; Davies, A.R.; Furber, A.; Goyder, E.; Jeffery, C.; et al. Learning across the UK: A review of public health systems and policy approaches to early child development since political devolution. *J. Public Health* **2019**, *42*, 777–780. [CrossRef] [PubMed]
8. Britto, P.R.; Lye, S.J.; Proulx, K.; Yousafzai, A.K.; Matthews, S.G.; Vaivada, T.; Perez-Escamilla, R.; Rao, N.; Ip, P.; Fernald, L.C.H.; et al. Nurturing care: Promoting early childhood development. *Lancet* **2017**, *389*, 91–102. [CrossRef]
9. Pan, Q.; Trang, K.T.; Love, H.R.; Templin, J. School Readiness Profiles and Growth in Academic Achievement. *Front. Educ.* **2019**, *4*. [CrossRef]
10. Sabol, T.J.; Pianta, R.C. Patterns of school readiness forecast achievement and socioemotional development at the end of elementary school. *Child. Dev.* **2012**, *83*, 282–299. [CrossRef]
11. Smithers, L.G.; Sawyer Alyssa, C.P.; Chittleborough, C.R.; Davies, N.M.; Davey Smith, G.; Lynch, J.W. A systematic review and meta-analysis of effects of early life non-cognitive skills on academic, psychosocial, cognitive and health outcomes. *Nat. Hum. Behav.* **2018**, *2*, 867–880. [CrossRef]
12. D'Onise, K.; Lynch, J.W.; Sawyer, M.G.; McDermott, R.A. Can preschool improve child health outcomes? A systematic review. *Soc. Sci. Med.* **2010**, *70*, 1423–1440. [CrossRef]
13. Cattan, S.; Conti, G.; Farquharson, C.; Ginja, R. The Health Effects of Sure Start. London, UK, 2019.
14. PACEY. *What Does "School Ready" Really Mean?—A Research Report from Professional Association for Childcare and Early Years*; Professional Association for Childcare and Early Years: London, UK, 2013.
15. Department for Education. *Statutory Framework for the Early Years Foundation Stage Setting the Standards for Learning, Development and Care for Children from Birth to Five*; London, UK, 2014. Available online: https://www.gov.uk/government/publications/early-years-foundation-stage-framework--2 (accessed on 24 October 2021).
16. United Nations Children's Fund. *School Readiness: A Conceptual Framework*; New York, NY, USA, 2012. Available online: https://sites.unicef.org/earlychildhood/files/Child2Child_ConceptualFramework_FINAL(1).pdf (accessed on 24 October 2021).
17. Bradbury, A.; Roberts-Holmes, G. *The Datafication of Primary and Early Years Education: Playing with Numbers*; Routlege: Abingdon, UK; New York, NY, USA, 2017.
18. Zajacova, A.; Lawrence, E.M. The relationship between education and health: Reducing disparities through a contextual approach. *Annu. Rev. Public Health* **2018**, *39*, 273–289. [CrossRef]
19. Lynch, J.; von Hippel, P. An Education Gradient in Health, a Health Gradient in Education, or a Confounded Gradient in Both? *Soc. Sci. Med.* **2016**, *154*. [CrossRef] [PubMed]
20. Black, M.; Barnes, A.; Strong, M.; Taylor-Robinson, D. Impact of child development at primary school entry on adolescent health—protocol for a participatory systematic review. *Syst. Rev.* **2021**, *10*, 142. [CrossRef]
21. Moher, D.; Liberati, A.; Tetzlaff, J.; Altman, D.G.; The, P.G. Preferred Reporting Items for Systematic Reviews and Meta-Analyses: The PRISMA Statement. *PLoS Med.* **2009**, *6*, e1000097. [CrossRef]
22. Page, M.J.; McKenzie, J.E.; Bossuyt, P.M.; Boutron, I.; Hoffmann, T.C.; Mulrow, C.D.; Shamseer, L.; Tetzlaff, J.M.; Akl, E.A.; Brennan, S.E.; et al. The PRISMA 2020 statement: An updated guideline for reporting systematic reviews. *BMJ* **2021**, *372*, n71. [CrossRef]
23. Pearce, A.; Dundas, R.; Whitehead, M.; Taylor-Robinson, D. Pathways to inequalities in child health. *Arch. Dis. Child.* **2019**, *104*, 998–1003. [CrossRef] [PubMed]
24. Cortés Pascual, A.; Moyano Muñoz, N.; Quílez Robres, A. The Relationship Between Executive Functions and Academic Performance in Primary Education: Review and Meta-Analysis. *Front. Psychol.* **2019**, *10*. [CrossRef]
25. Bracken, B.A. *Basic Concept Scale Revised*; The Psychological Corporation: San Antonio, TX, USA, 1998.
26. Pope, D. *Introduction to Systematic Reviews (Lecture)*; University of Liverpool: Liverpool, UK, 2015.
27. Hoogendoorn, W.E.; van Poppel, M.N.; Bongers, P.M.; Koes, B.W.; Bouter, L.M. Physical load during work and leisure time as risk factors for back pain. *Scand. J. Work. Environ. Health* **1999**, *25*, 387–403. [CrossRef] [PubMed]

28. te Velde, S.J.; van Nassau, F.; Uijtdewilligen, L.; van Stralen, M.M.; Cardon, G.; De Craemer, M.; Manios, Y.; Brug, J.; Chinapaw, M.J.; ToyBox-Study Group. Energy balance-related behaviours associated with overweight and obesity in preschool children: A systematic review of prospective studies. *Obes. Rev.* **2012**, *13* (Suppl. S1), 56–74. [CrossRef]
29. Sterne, J.A.C.; Hernán, M.A.; McAleenan, A.; Reeves, B.C.; Higgins, J.P.T. Chapter 25: Assessing risk of bias in a non-randomized study. In *Cochrane Handbook for Systematic Reviews of Interventions Version 6.2*; Higgins, J., Thomas, J., Chandler, J., Cumpston, M., Li, T., Page, M., Welch, V., Eds.; 2021; Available online: https://training.cochrane.org/handbook/current/chapter-25 (accessed on 24 October 2021).
30. Baxter, S.K.; Blank, L.; Woods, H.B.; Payne, N.; Rimmer, M.; Goyder, E. Using logic model methods in systematic review synthesis: Describing complex pathways in referral management interventions. *BMC Med. Res. Methodol.* **2014**, *14*, 62. [CrossRef]
31. Baxter, S.; Johnson, M.; Chambers, D.; Sutton, A.; Goyder, E.; Booth, A. The effects of integrated care: A systematic review of UK and international evidence. *BMC Health Serv. Res.* **2018**, *18*, 350. [CrossRef] [PubMed]
32. Campbell, M.; McKenzie, J.E.; Sowden, A.; Katikireddi, S.V.; Brennan, S.E.; Ellis, S.; Hartmann-Boyce, J.; Ryan, R.; Shepperd, S.; Thomas, J.; et al. Synthesis without meta-analysis (SWiM) in systematic reviews: Reporting guideline. *BMJ* **2020**, *368*, l6890. [CrossRef] [PubMed]
33. Ashford, J.; Smit, F.; van Lier, P.A.; Cuijpers, P.; Koot, H.M. Early risk indicators of internalizing problems in late childhood: A 9-year longitudinal study. *J. Child. Psychol. Psychiatry* **2008**, *49*, 774–780. [CrossRef] [PubMed]
34. Berthelsen, D.; Hayes, N.; White, S.L.J.; Williams, K.E. Executive Function in Adolescence: Associations with Child and Family Risk Factors and Self-Regulation in Early Childhood. *Front. Psychol.* **2017**, *8*, 903. [CrossRef] [PubMed]
35. Bornstein, M.H.; Hahn, C.-S.; Haynes, O. Social competence, externalizing, and internalizing behavioral adjustment from early childhood through early adolescence: Developmental cascades. *Dev. Psychopathol.* **2010**, *22*, 717–735. [CrossRef]
36. Bornstein, M.H.; Hahn, C.-S.; Suwalsky, J.T. Language and internalizing and externalizing behavioral adjustment: Developmental pathways from childhood to adolescence. *Dev. Psychopathol.* **2013**, *25*, 857–878. [CrossRef]
37. Derks, I.P.M.; Bolhuis, K.; Yalcin, Z.; Gaillard, R.; Hillegers, M.H.J.; Larsson, H.; Lundstrom, S.; Lichtenstein, P.; van Beijsterveldt, C.E.M.; Bartels, M.; et al. Testing Bidirectional Associations Between Childhood Aggression and BMI: Results from Three Cohorts. *Obesity* **2019**, *27*, 822–829. [CrossRef]
38. Duchesne, S.; Larose, S.; Vitaro, F.; Tremblay, R.E. Trajectories of anxiety in a population sample of children: Clarifying the role of children's behavioral characteristics and maternal parenting. *Dev. Psychopathol.* **2010**, *22*, 361–373. [CrossRef]
39. Fine, S.E.; Izard, C.E.; Mostow, A.J.; Trentacosta, C.J.; Ackerman, B.P. First grade emotion knowledge as a predictor of fifth grade self-reported internalizing behaviors in children from economically disadvantaged families. *Dev. Psychopathol.* **2003**, *15*, 331–342. [CrossRef]
40. Glaser, B.; Gunnell, D.; Timpson, N.J.; Joinson, C.; Zammit, S.; Smith, G.D.; Lewis, G. Age- and puberty-dependent association between IQ score in early childhood and depressive symptoms in adolescence. *Psychol. Med.* **2011**, *41*, 333–343. [CrossRef]
41. Gregory, T.; Dal Grande, E.; Brushe, M.; Engelhardt, D.; Luddy, S.; Guhn, M.; Gadermann, A.; Schonert-Reichl, K.A.; Brinkman, S. Associations between School Readiness and Student Wellbeing: A Six-Year Follow Up Study. *Child. Indic. Res.* **2021**, *14*, 369–390. [CrossRef]
42. Hay, D.F.; Pawlby, S. Prosocial development in relation to children's and mothers' psychological problems. *Child. Dev.* **2003**, *74*, 1314–1327. [CrossRef] [PubMed]
43. Hooper, S.R.; Roberts, J.E.; Zeisel, S.A.; Poe, M. Core Language Predictors of Behavioral Functioning in Early Elementary School Children: Concurrent and Longitudinal Findings. *Behav. Disord.* **2003**, *29*, 10–24. [CrossRef]
44. Howard, S.J.; Williams, K.E. Early Self-Regulation, Early Self-Regulatory Change, and Their Longitudinal Relations to Adolescents' Academic, Health, and Mental Well-Being Outcomes. *J. Dev. Behav. Pediatrics* **2018**, *39*, 489–496. [CrossRef]
45. Howes, C. Social-emotional classroom climate in child care, child-teacher relationships and children's second grade peer relations. *Soc. Dev.* **2000**, *9*, 191–204. [CrossRef]
46. Lecompte, V.; Moss, E.; Cyr, C.; Pascuzzo, K. Preschool attachment, self-esteem and the development of preadolescent anxiety and depressive symptoms. *Attach. Hum. Dev.* **2014**, *16*, 242–260. [CrossRef] [PubMed]
47. Lee, J.-k.; Schoppe-Sullivan, S.J. Resident fathers' positive engagement, family poverty, and change in child behavior problems. *Fam. Relat. Interdiscip. J. Appl. Fam. Stud.* **2017**, *66*, 484–496. [CrossRef]
48. Louise, S.; Warrington, N.; McCaskie, P.; Oddy, W.; Zubrick, S.; Hands, B.; Mori, T.; Briollais, L.; Silburn, S.; Palmer, L.; et al. Associations between aggressive behaviour scores and cardiovascular risk factors in childhood. *Pediatric Obes.* **2012**, *7*, 319–328. [CrossRef]
49. McKenzie, T.L.; Sallis, J.F.; Broyles, S.L.; Zive, M.M.; Nader, P.R.; Berry, C.C.; Brennan, J.J. Childhood movement skills: Predictors of physical activity in Anglo American and Mexican American adolescents? *Res. Q Exerc. Sport* **2002**, *73*, 238–244. [CrossRef]
50. Meagher, S.M.; Arnold, D.H.; Doctoroff, G.L.; Dobbs, J.; Fisher, P.H. Social-Emotional Problems in Early Childhood and the Development of Depressive Symptoms in School-Age Children. *Early Educ. Dev.* **2009**, *20*, 1–24. [CrossRef]
51. Nelson, T.D.; Kidwell, K.M.; Nelson, J.M.; Tomaso, C.C.; Hankey, M.; Espy, K.A. Preschool executive control and internalizing symptoms in elementary school. *J. Abnorm. Child. Psychol.* **2018**, *46*, 1509–1520. [CrossRef]
52. Pagani, L.S.; Caroline, F. Children's School Readiness: Implications for Eliminating Future Disparities in Health and Education. *Health Educ. Behav.* **2014**, *41*, 25–33. [CrossRef]

53. Pedersen, S.; Vitaro, F.; Barker, E.D.; Borge, A.I. The Timing of Middle-Childhood Peer Rejection and Friendship: Linking Early Behavior to Early-Adolescent Adjustment. *Child. Dev.* **2007**, *78*, 1037–1051. [CrossRef]
54. Piché, G.; Fitzpatrick, C.; Pagani, L.S. Kindergarten Self-Regulation as a Predictor of Body Mass Index and Sports Participation in Fourth Grade Students. *Mind Brain Educ.* **2012**, *6*, 19–26. [CrossRef]
55. Piché, G.; Huỳnh, C.; Villatte, A. Physical activity and child depressive symptoms: Findings from the QLSCD. *Can. J. Behav. Sci. Rev. Can. Des Sci. Du Comport.* **2019**, *51*, 114–121. [CrossRef]
56. Rudasill, K.M.; Pössel, P.; Winkeljohn, B.S.; Niehaus, K. Stephanie Winkeljohn; Niehaus, Kate. Teacher support mediates concurrent and longitudinal associations between temperament and mild depressive symptoms in sixth grade. *Early Child. Dev. Care* **2014**, *184*, 803–818. [CrossRef]
57. Rudolph, K.D.; Troop-Gordon, W.; Hessel, E.T.; Schmidt, J.D. A Latent Growth Curve Analysis of Early and Increasing Peer Victimization as Predictors of Mental Health across Elementary School. *J. Clin. Child. Adolesc. Psychol.* **2011**, *40*, 111–122. [CrossRef]
58. Sasser, T.R.; Bierman, K.L.; Heinrichs, B.; Nix, R.L. Preschool Intervention Can Promote Sustained Growth in the Executive-Function Skills of Children Exhibiting Early Deficits. *Psychol. Sci.* **2017**, *28*, 1719–1730. [CrossRef]
59. Shapero, B.G.; Steinberg, L. Emotional reactivity and exposure to household stress in childhood predict psychological problems in adolescence. *J. Youth Adolesc.* **2013**, *42*, 1573–1582. [CrossRef] [PubMed]
60. Slemming, K.; Sørensen, M.J.; Thomsen, P.H.; Obel, C.; Henriksen, T.B.; Linnet, K.M. The association between preschool behavioural problems and internalizing difficulties at age 10-12 years. *Eur. Child. Adolesc. Psychiatry* **2010**, *19*, 787–795. [CrossRef] [PubMed]
61. Straatmann, V.S.; Pearce, A.; Hope, S.; Barr, B.; Whitehead, M.; Law, C.; Taylor-Robinson, D. How well can poor child health and development be predicted by data collected in early childhood? *J. Epidemiol. Community Health* **2018**, *72*, 1132–1140. [CrossRef] [PubMed]
62. Sutin, A.R.; A Kerr, J.; Terracciano, A. Temperament and body weight from ages 4 to 15 years. *Int. J. Obes.* **2017**, *41*, 1056–1061. [CrossRef]
63. Weeks, M.; Wild, T.; Ploubidis, G.; Naicker, K.; Cairney, J.; North, C.; Colman, I. Childhood cognitive ability and its relationship with anxiety and depression in adolescence. *J. Affect. Disord.* **2014**, *152–154*, 139–145. [CrossRef]
64. Yan, J.; Feng, X.; Schoppe-Sullivan, S.J. Longitudinal associations between parent-child relationships in middle childhood and child-perceived loneliness. *J. Fam. Psychol.* **2018**, *32*, 841–847. [CrossRef]
65. Jaspers, M.; De Winter, A.F.; De Meer, G.; Stewart, R.E.; Verhulst, F.C.; Ormel, J.; Reijneveld, S.A. Early findings of preventive child healthcare professionals predict psychosocial problems in preadolescence: The TRAILS study. *J. Pediatrics* **2010**, *157*, 316–321.e312. [CrossRef]
66. Sandstrom, A.; Uher, R.; Pavlova, B. Prospective Association between Childhood Behavioral Inhibition and Anxiety: A Meta-Analysis. *J. Abnorm. Child. Psychol.* **2020**, *48*, 57–66. [CrossRef] [PubMed]
67. Michie, S.; Van Stralen, M.M.; West, R. The behaviour change wheel: A new method for characterising and designing behaviour change interventions. *Implement. Sci. IS* **2011**, *6*, 42. [CrossRef]
68. Bandura, A. Social Cognitive Theory. In *The International Encyclopedia of Communication*; Donsbach, W., Ed.; Blackwells: Oxford, UK, 2008. [CrossRef]
69. Thomson, K.C.; Richardson, C.G.; Gadermann, A.M.; Emerson, S.D.; Shoveller, J.; Guhn, M. Association of Childhood Social-Emotional Functioning Profiles at School Entry With Early-Onset Mental Health Conditions. *JAMA Netw.* **2019**, *2*, e186694. [CrossRef] [PubMed]
70. Arslan, İ.B.; Lucassen, N.; van Lier, P.A.C.; de Haan, A.D.; Prinzie, P. Early childhood internalizing problems, externalizing problems and their co-occurrence and (mal)adaptive functioning in emerging adulthood: A 16-year follow-up study. *Soc. Psychiatry Psychiatr. Epidemiol.* **2021**, *56*, 193–206. [CrossRef]
71. Willner, C.J.; Gatzke-Kopp, L.M.; Bray, B.C. The dynamics of internalizing and externalizing comorbidity across the early school years. *Dev. Psychopathol.* **2016**, *28*, 1033–1052. [CrossRef] [PubMed]
72. Stringaris, A.; Lewis, G.; Maughan, B. Developmental pathways from childhood conduct problems to early adult depression: Findings from the ALSPAC cohort. *Br. J. Psychiatry* **2014**, *205*, 17–23. [CrossRef]
73. Arbel, R.; Mason, T.B.; Dunton, G.F. Transactional links between children daily emotions and internalizing symptoms: A six-wave ecological momentary assessment study. *J. Child. Psychol. Psychiatry* **2021**, *06*, 17. [CrossRef]
74. Eisenberg, N.; Spinrad, T.L.; Eggum, N.D. Emotion-related self-regulation and its relation to children's maladjustment. *Annu. Rev. Clin. Psychol.* **2010**, *6*, 495–525. [CrossRef]
75. Patalay, P.; Hardman, C.A. Comorbidity, Codevelopment, and Temporal Associations Between Body Mass Index and Internalizing Symptoms From Early Childhood to Adolescence. *JAMA Psychiatry* **2019**, *76*, 721–729. [CrossRef] [PubMed]
76. Pearce, A.; Scalzi, D.; Lynch, J.; Smithers, L.G. Do thin, overweight and obese children have poorer development than their healthy-weight peers at the start of school? Findings from a South Australian data linkage study. *Early Child. Res. Q.* **2016**, *35*, 85–94. [CrossRef]
77. Jackson, S.L.; Cunningham, S.A. Social Competence and Obesity in Elementary School. *Am. J. Public Health* **2015**, *105*, 153–158. [CrossRef] [PubMed]

78. Taylor, C.L.; Christensen, D.; Jose, K.; Zubrick, S.R. Universal child health and early education service use from birth through Kindergarten and developmental vulnerability in the Preparatory Year (age 5 years) in Tasmania, Australia. *Aust. J. Soc. Issues* **2021**, *00*, 1–25. [CrossRef]
79. Allan, J.L.; McMinn, D.; Daly, M. A Bidirectional Relationship between Executive Function and Health Behavior: Evidence, Implications, and Future Directions. *Front. Neurosci* **2016**, *10*, 386. [CrossRef] [PubMed]
80. Cattan, S.; Conti, G.; Farquharson, C.; Ginja, G.; Pecher, M. *The Health Impacts of Sure Start*; The Institute for Fiscal Studies, 2021. Available online: https://ifs.org.uk/publications/14139 (accessed on 24 October 2021).
81. Bundy, D.A.P.; de Silva, N.; Horton, S.; Patton, G.C.; Schultz, L.; Jamison, D.T. Child and Adolescent Health and Development: Realizing Neglected Potential. In *Child and Adolescent Health and Development*, 3rd ed.; Bundy, D.A.P., de Silva, N., Horton, S., Jamison, D.T., Patton, G.C., Eds.; World Bank: Washington, DC, USA, 2017; Volume 8.
82. Viner, R.M.; Allen, N.B.; Patton, G.C. Puberty, Developmental Processes and Health Interventions. In *Child and Adolescent Health and Development*, 3rd ed.; Bundy, D.A.P., de Silva, N., Horton, S., Jamison, D.T., Patton, G.C., Eds.; World Bank: Washinton, DC, USA, 2017.
83. Hahn, R.A.; Truman, B.I. Education Improves Public Health and Promotes Health Equity. *Int. J. Health Serv.* **2015**, *45*, 657–678. [CrossRef] [PubMed]
84. Burke, N.J.; Joseph, G.; Pasick, R.J.; Barker, J.C. Theorizing social context: Rethinking behavioral theory. *Health Educ. Behav.* **2009**, *36*, 55s–70s. [CrossRef] [PubMed]
85. McAteer, J.; Di Ruggiero, E.; Fraser, A.; Frank, J.W. Bridging the academic and practice/policy gap in public health: Perspectives from Scotland and Canada. *J. Public Health* **2018**, *41*, 632–637. [CrossRef] [PubMed]

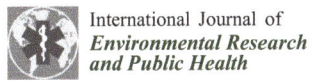

Review

Outcomes and Critical Factors for Successful Implementation of Organizational Health Literacy Interventions: A Scoping Review

Marise S. Kaper [1,2,*], Jane Sixsmith [3], Sijmen A. Reijneveld [1] and Andrea F. de Winter [1]

1. Department of Health Sciences, University Medical Center Groningen, University of Groningen, Hanzeplein 1, P.O. Box 30.001, FA10, 9713 RB Groningen, The Netherlands; s.a.reijneveld@umcg.nl (S.A.R.); a.f.de.winter@umcg.nl (A.F.d.W.)
2. Center for Dentistry and Oral Hygiene, University Medical Center Groningen, University of Groningen, Antonius Deusinglaan 1, 9713 AV Groningen, The Netherlands
3. Health Promotion Research Centre, National University of Ireland Galway, University Road, H91 TK33 Galway, Ireland; jane.sixsmith@nuigalway.ie
* Correspondence: m.s.kaper@umcg.nl

Abstract: Organizational health literacy (OHL)-interventions can reduce inequality and demands in health care encountered by patients. However, an overview of their impact and critical factors for organization-wide implementation is lacking. The aim of this scoping review is to summarize the evidence on: (1) the outcomes of OHL-interventions at patient, professional and organizational levels; and (2) the factors and strategies that affect implementation and outcomes of OHL-interventions. We reviewed empirical studies following the five-stage framework of Arksey and O'Malley. The databases Scopus, PubMed, PsychInfo and CINAHL were searched from 1 January 2010 to 31 December 2019, focusing on OHL-interventions using terms related to "health literacy", "health care organization" and "intervention characteristics". After a full-text review, we selected 24 descriptive stu-dies. Of these, 23 studies reported health literacy problems in relation to OHL-assessment tools. Nine out of thirteen studies reported that the use of interventions resulted in positive changes on OHL-domains regarding comprehensible communication, professionals' competencies and practices, and strategic organizational changes. Organization-wide OHL-interventions resulted in some improvement of patient outcomes but evidence was scarce. Critical factors for organization-wide implementation of OHL-interventions were leadership support, top-down and bottom-up approaches, a change champion, and staff commitment. Organization-wide interventions lead to more positive change on OHL-domains, but evidence regarding OHL-outcomes needs strengthening.

Keywords: health literacy; organization and administration; health care settings; organizational innovation; culture; program development

Citation: Kaper, M.S.; Sixsmith, J.; Reijneveld, S.A.; de Winter, A.F. Outcomes and Critical Factors for Successful Implementation of Organizational Health Literacy Interventions: A Scoping Review. *Int. J. Environ. Res. Public Health* **2021**, *18*, 11906. https://doi.org/10.3390/ijerph182211906

Academic Editors: Jessica Sheringham and Sarah Sowden

Received: 3 October 2021
Accepted: 10 November 2021
Published: 12 November 2021

Publisher's Note: MDPI stays neutral with regard to jurisdictional claims in published maps and institutional affiliations.

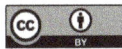

Copyright: © 2021 by the authors. Licensee MDPI, Basel, Switzerland. This article is an open access article distributed under the terms and conditions of the Creative Commons Attribution (CC BY) license (https://creativecommons.org/licenses/by/4.0/).

1. Introduction

Almost one in every two people in Europe encounter problems handling health issues because of limited health literacy skills [1]. These problems are more prominent among people of a higher age and lower educational level [1]. Health literacy is defined as 'the degree to which people are able to access, understand, appraise and communicate information to engage with the demands of different health contexts' [2]. As Rudd et al. consistently point out [3–5], a health literacy gap is emerging between the abilities of patients and the demands placed by increasingly complex health services. This gap can contribute to a range of negative consequences for people with limited health literacy [1,6], who find it difficult to access and navigate health care organizations, communicate with health professionals, understand information, and engage in decision making and self-management [3,6–10]. These consequences can have a profound impact on patients, affecting their safety, quality of care, and health outcomes [1,6]. In order to reduce and prevent these problems, it has been recommended to reduce the complex demands in health care organizations [5,11–13].

Health care organizations can reduce these demands and "make it easier for people to navigate, understand, and use information and services to take care of their health" [13,14], which is the definition of the concept of organizational health literacy (OHL). Contextualising health literacy to health care organizations involves the design of accessible and easy to use health services, including health promotion and ill health prevention, fostering equality and a responsive health system, supporting people to navigate that system, and engaging them in making informed health related decisions [15–17]. Palumbo [15] conducted a literature review with a preventive medicine orientation, and distinguished five themes from the identified OHL literature: (1) understanding OHL as a preventive health policy issue and promoting the integration of health literacy into organizations po-licies and daily activities; (2) contextualizing OHL in a patient-centred care perspective, building on a combination of formal (top-down) and informal (bottom-up) approaches to improve the accessibility of health services and engagement of patients; (3) raising awareness and strengthening commitment for achieving OHL, (4) preparing a health literate workforce using tailored training and capacity building, and (5) measuring efforts and outcomes related to OHL by using a systematic approach. Measurement should focus on the ability of health organizations to engage patients in a co-creation relationship, the quality of communication, supportive services and technologies.

Reducing the organizational demands for people with limited health literacy requires a combination of approaches targeted at the level of patients, professionals and the organization [13,18], denoted as organizational health literacy (OHL)-interventions. At the patient level, interventions can improve oral, written, and digital communication, and accessibility of services and physical navigation, as well as involve patients more actively in improving health information and services. At the professional level, OHL-interventions can improve capacity building and promotion of health literacy friendly communication practices. OHL improvement at the organizational level involves domains such as leadership and culture, organizational policies, systems processes, and structures. Over the last decade, a number of such OHL-interventions have been developed [19,20]. These interventions usually involve two phases: (1) assessment of health literacy problems from the perspectives of patients, professionals and independent observers; and (2) planning and application of interventions aimed at reducing demands in healthcare organizations.

Two reviews concluded that evidence on the planning, application, and outcomes of OHL-interventions was limited [19,20]. Until recently, these interventions focused mostly on the assessment of health literacy problems at the patient and professional levels, including physical navigation, and written-, digital-, and spoken communication, but with limited attention to an organization-wide approach [19,20]. The available studies of applied interventions reported a number of facilitators and barriers that influenced OHL-interventions, such as lack of health literacy awareness, staff commitment, and leadership support [19,20]. The evidence on outcomes indicated that implementation periods were brief and improvement of OHL-outcomes limited.

Since the publication of these reviews, new insight has been gained regarding outcomes and implementation of OHL-interventions, and on how organizational transformation may improve patient outcomes. Current research on health literate organizations focuses more on facilitating sustainable transformation to improve OHL outcomes at patient, professional and organizational levels [14]. This scoping review summarizes the evidence regarding: (1) outcomes of OHL-interventions at patient, professional and organizational levels; and (2) factors and strategies that influence implementation and outcomes of these interventions.

2. Materials and Methods

To guide this scoping review we used the five-stage framework for scoping reviews developed by Arksey and O'Malley (2005) [21]. The five stages are: (1) Identify the research questions, (2) Identify and retrieve relevant articles, (3) Select articles, (4) Chart the data, (5) Collate, summarize and report. We structured the methods section in line with these stages.

2.1. Stage 1. Identify the Research Questions

Before conducting the review, within the group of authors we defined two preliminary research objectives and discussed the concepts to guide the literature search. We aimed at a sensitive search to catch all potentially relevant studies regarding the domains of OHL interventions, and criteria to specify the interventions regarding the phases of assessment and application of OHL interventions.

2.2. Stage 2. Identify and Retrieve Relevant Articles

First, to identify and retrieve relevant articles, we set up a literature search strategy based on search terms and inclusion criteria used in two previous reviews of OHL interventions [19,20]. Second, with the help of a librarian (TvI), we refined the research objectives and search strategy, and developed a protocol, all of which we discussed among the co-authors (MK, JS, SAR, AFdW). This was to ensure that methods and search strategies were consistent and comprehensive. We applied the final search strategy to the MEDLINE/PubMed databases and then adapted it for the other databases, covering all publications up to 31 December 2019. We searched the databases PubMed, Scopus, PsychInfo and CINAHL. In the literature search we included keywords and MESH terms related to the concept of "health literacy"; we combined these with Boolean operator AND search terms related to the health care setting, and Boolean operator OR search terms involving intervention characteristics. The complete search string is provided in Table S1 as supplementary material.

To ensure inclusion of all relevant studies in the review we used reference searches of retrieved articles to complement the electronic searches. Inclusion criteria were: (1) publication between January 2010 and December 2019; (2) inclusion of an abstract written in English; (3) an OECD country as geographical setting; (4) a study setting involving a health care setting in primary or secondary care; (5) a study aimed at assessment of organizational barriers and improvement of outcomes for adults with limited health literacy; (6) a study design involving an intervention, evaluation of a program, a pilot-study or needs assessment; (7) an intervention focused on assessing problems or changing two or more domains of organizational health literacy: changes at patient level (oral, written and digital communication and health literacy levels); changes at professional level (health literacy capacities and communication practices); or changes at organizational level (leadership and culture, organizational policies, systems processes, and structures).

2.3. Stage 3. Selection of Articles

After removing duplicate articles, we reviewed the title and abstract of identified articles against the following exclusion criteria: (1) health literacy was assessed or addressed only at the individual or family level (e.g., validation of screening tools or educational interventions for patients); (2) the only focus was to investigate determinants associated with health literacy and health outcomes; (3) the aim was to develop and validate instruments to measure organizational health literacy without investigating their implementation in organizations.

One investigator (MK) did the initial screening. In cases of uncertainty, a second investigator (AFdeW) reviewed the abstract or full text of an article; together consensus was reached on inclusion or exclusion in the review. Articles identified for inclusion underwent full text screening and two investigators screened a sub-section to ensure fit to criteria and consistency.

2.4. Stage 4. Charting the Data

In three steps we extracted the data from the selected studies in Excel, sorted them in tables, and analysed them based on the study purpose. First we extracted descriptive data: author, year and country, design and evaluation method, aim, setting, sample, and OHL-intervention components. Second, we extracted data on outcomes of OHL-interventions at patient, professional and organizational levels. Third, we extracted data on whether critical factors and strategies were considered to be facilitators or barriers to implementation processes.

2.5. Stage 5. Collate, Summarize and Report

In three steps we extracted the data from the selected studies, sorted them in tables and analysed them based on key themes informed by the study purpose, to: (1) assess the outcomes of OHL-interventions, and (2) to unravel the factors and strategies affecting the implementation and outcomes of OHL-interventions. First, we tabulated the selected studies by author, year and country, research design, setting, sample, OHL domains addressed, and focus of the study, i.e., assessment or application of OHL-interventions. Second, we summarized and reported the outcomes of OHL-interventions following their assessment or application, and the level to which the outcome applied: patient, professional, and/or organization. Third, we summarized and reported factors and strategies which influenced the assessment and application of OHL-interventions, and analysed whether these were facilitators or barriers at patient, professional, and/or organizational level.

3. Results

We identified 5420 records from the literature search and one record through reference searching (we retrieved 1511 records from Pubmed; 1351 from Scopus; 1750 from Cinahl; and 808 from Psychinfo). After removing 2223 duplicates, we screened 3197 titles and abstracts and included 82 articles for full-text review. After reading the full text, we selected and excluded articles based on the criteria specified above. We included twenty-four articles in the data extraction. This results section presents: (1) description of the studies, (2) outcomes of OHL-interventions, and (3) strategies and factors that influence the implementation of OHL-interventions. Figure 1 presents the results of the literature search and study selection.

3.1. Description of Studies

The 24 selected articles involved 17 original research projects (Table 1); several studies were part of larger research projects (these were: Grabeel [22], Grabeel [23], and Tester [24]; Beauchamp [25], Goeman [26], and Jessup [27]; Mabachi [28] and Brega [29]; Vellar [30] and Mastroianni; Weaver [31] and Wray [32]). We included some articles because, although they reported on a single domain, they were connected with other articles reporting different domains of the same study. We sorted the studies according to the results of the assessment of OHL-domains, and the planning and delivery of interventions aimed at improvement of health literacy related problems. Unlike the study conducted by Cawthon et al. [33], the remaining 23 studies conducted an OHL-assessment. Thirteen of these studies focused solely on assessment of health literacy related problems [3,17,22–24,34–40]. Together with the assessment, these studies also often evaluated the feasibility of the OHL-instrument. Eleven studies reported on both the assessment and on findings regarding the planning and delivery of interventions [22,25–33,41–43]. Fourteen studies were conducted in the United States [22–24,28,29,31–34,36,38–40,43]; other studies were conducted in Australia [25–27,30,41], New Zealand & Canada [37], and several European countries including Austria [35], Italy [17], Ireland and the Netherlands [42], and Spain [3]. Study settings involved hospitals, as well as general health care settings like community and primary care practices, pharmacies and dental clinics.

The majority of the studies used a mixed-method approach (n = 16), or qualitative (n = 4) or quantitative approaches (n = 4). Multiple informants and methods were used to report on the assessment and application of OHL-interventions; these included managers, professionals, patients and observers who had taken part in surveys, interviews, focus group discussions, and observation and review of documents. The interventions targeted a variety of OHL domains using different tools and approaches. Domains most frequently addressed were the comprehensibility of written patient information materials, digital communication, oral communication, and navigation. Fewer studies targeted OHL as a strategic priority, health literacy policies, and capacity building of staff [17,25,30–32,35]. A number of studies [3,17,31,36,40,42] used or adapted the toolkit "The Health Literacy Environment of Hospitals and Health Centers. Partners for Action: Making Your Healthcare Facility Literacy-Friendly" (HLEHHC Toolkit) developed by Rudd and Anderson [44]. Other studies used, e.g., the HLUP toolkit [28,29,34] or the Agency for Healthcare Research and Quality (AHRQ) Health Literacy Assessment Tool [39,43].

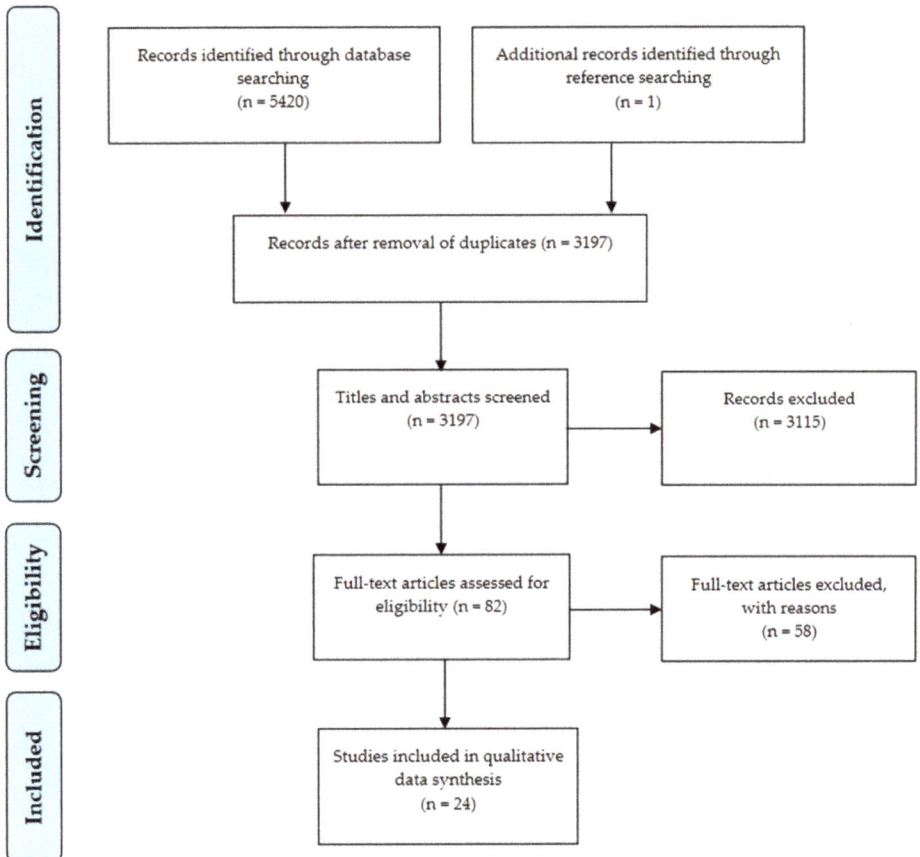

Figure 1. Flow of studies through the review.

Table 1. Descriptive results of OHL-interventions regarding research design, aim, setting, sample, and OHL-intervention.

Author, Year	Research Design	Focus	Setting	Sample	OHL-Intervention
De Walt (2011) [34]	Qualitative study: Interviews	Assessment	Primary care practices (n = 10)	Staff and health professionals (number not reported)	Assessment (using HLUP toolkit): 20 tools organized under five sections: - path to improvement - improve spoken communication - improve written communication - improve self-management and empowerment - improve supportive systems
Dietscher (2016) [35]	Mixed methods: Survey Interviews	Assessment	Hospitals (n = 9)	Coordinators (n = 9) Other hospital staff (number not reported)	Assessment (using WGKKO-I toolkit, which has 9 OHL standards) (summarized here): - policy, organizational structures and resources on OHL - staff training and promoting of HL communication - initiation of HL improvement and supportive physical environment - participation of patients in design of services and materials
Grabeel (2018) [22]	Quantitative study: Survey	Assessment	University medical centre	Nurses and other staff (n = 196)	Assessment (using HLEHHC toolkit) of: - current health literacy knowledge - interest in training
Grabeel (2018) [23]	Quantitative study: Rating of materials	Assessment	University medical centre	Sample: NA	Assessment (using HLEHHC toolkit) of printed patient education materials, comparing: - hand-scored SMOG method - computerized F-K grade level method
Tester (2019) [24]	Quantitative study: Structured interviews Observation	Assessment	University medical centre	Patients (n = 298) Observers/auditors	Assessment (using HLEHHC toolkit) of oral communication: - Patient Satisfaction Survey Interview Form (PSSIF) - Oral Exchange Rating Form (OERF)

Table 1. *Cont.*

Author, Year	Research Design	Focus	Setting	Sample	OHL-Intervention
Groene (2011) [3]	Mixed methods: Surveys Interviews Observation	Assessment	Hospitals (n = 10)	Patients (n = 313) Coordinators (n = 6)	Assessment (using HLEHHC toolkit) of three domains: - navigation: walking interviews undertaken by researcher - written communication: Flesch–Szigriszt readability formula - patients' perceptions of written and oral communication
Horowitz (2014) [36]	Mixed methods: Surveys Interviews Observation	Assessment	Community-based dental clinics (n = 26)	Dental providers (n = 60) Patients (n = 67)	Assessment (informed by HLEHHC and HLUP toolkits) on four domains: - review of accessibility, signage and navigation, including website and phone - written communication; educational materials and patient forms - provider perspective regarding health literacy friendly communication - patient perspectives regarding navigation, communication and treatment
Lambert (2014) [37]	Qualitative study: Interviews Focus group	Assessment	Primary health care services (n = 4)	Health professionals (n = 29)	Assessment on three domains: - understanding of health literacy and needs of indigenous patients - suitability of the health care environment for people with limited health literacy - opinions and strategies to address health literacy problems
Martinez-Donate (2013) [38]	Mixed methods: Interviews Surveys	Assessment	Clinics provide outreach oncology services (n = 5)	Various clinical staff (n = 41) Patients (n = 53)	Assessment (informed by Chronic Care model) on four domains: - community resources - self-management support - delivery system design - decision support

Table 1. Cont.

Author, Year	Research Design	Focus	Setting	Sample	OHL-Intervention
O'Neal (2013) [39]	Mixed methods (post-test control group): Survey Interviews Observation	Assessment	Community pharmacies (n = 8)	Staff (n = 21) Patients (n = 60) Auditors (n = 4)	Assessment (using AHRQ Health Literacy Assessment Tool) on three domains: - promotion of services and pharmacy environment - printed materials - health literacy-sensitive verbal communication. Brief training intervention on HL knowledge and HL sensitive communication
Shoemaker (2013) [43]	Mixed methods: Document review Observation Interviews	Assessment and delivery	Pharmacies (n = 8)	Coordinating staff (n = 8) Other staff (number not reported)	Assessment (using AHRQ Health Literacy Assessment Tool) on three domains: - promotion of services and pharmacy environment - printed materials - health literacy-sensitive verbal communication
Palumbo (2017) [17]	Mixed methods: Document review Interviews Survey	Assessment	Public hospitals (n = 3).	Senior managers and health professionals (n = 6) Patients (n = 9)	Assessment (using Italian version of HLEHHC toolkit) on five domains: - navigation - printed communication - oral exchange - technology - policy and protocols
Smith (2010) [40]	Mixed methods: Interviews Observation Rating of materials	Assessment	Stroke unit and a senior independent living facility.	Auditors (n = 12) Health professionals and various staff (number not reported)	Assessment (using HLEHHC toolkit) on five domains: - navigation - printed communication—Fry Readability Graph (Schrock, 2009) - oral exchange - technology - policy and protocols

Table 1. *Cont.*

Author, Year	Research Design	Focus	Setting	Sample	OHL-Intervention
Beauchamp (2017) [25]	Multi-centre mixed methods: Surveys Interviews Focus groups	Assessment and delivery	8 health service organizations	Clinicians (n = 43) Clients (n = 228)	Assessment and delivery of OHL-interventions in three phases: - assessment using HLQ questionnaire to identify local strengths needs and problems, results used by stakeholders to identify local solutions - local stakeholders prioritize action areas and co-design interventions - interventions implemented through quality improvement cycles Principles of the Ophelia approach: focused outcomes, equity driven, needs diagnosis, co-design, driven by local wisdom, sustainable, responsive, and systematically applied.
Goeman (2016) [26]	Mixed methods: Surveys Interviews	Assessment and delivery	Home nursing service setting (7 sites)	Nurses (n = 9) Clients with diabetes (n = 113)	Assessment, development and pilot of tailored diabetes self-management intervention: - education tool - online resources - teach-back training
Jessup (2018) [27]	Mixed methods: Surveys Interviews	Assessment and delivery	8 health service organizations	Staff (n = 23) Patients (n = 384)	Assessment and co-design of local OHL-interventions targeting: - patients - provider-patient interface - system-level
Cawthon (2014) [33]	Mixed methods: Observation Focus group Interviews Process recordings	Delivery	University medical centre	Nurses and staff (number not reported) Patients (n = 74,249)	Implementation of the three Brief Health Literacy Screening items into the nursing work flow: - How confident are you when filling out medical forms by yourself? - How often do you have someone help you read hospital materials? - How often do you have problems learning about your medical condition because of difficulty understanding written information?

Table 1. *Cont.*

Author, Year	Research Design	Focus	Setting	Sample	OHL-Intervention
Mabachi (2016) [28]	Qualitative study Interviews Observation	Assessment and delivery	Primary care practices (n = 12)	3 staff members per practice (total N = 36)	Implementation guided by a quality improvement framework consisting of leadership support, training, monitoring uptake of screening items, and feedback Assessment and delivery of 13 of the 20 tools in the HLUP Toolkit in one or more practices. Tools were organized under five sections: - path to improvement - improve spoken communication - improve written communication - improve self-management and empowerment - improve supportive systems
Brega (2015) [29]	Mixed method pre-post study Interviews Rating materials	Assessment and delivery	Primary care practices (n = 4)	Professionals (n = 12) 3 per practice	Assessment and delivery with HLUP toolkit 11: design Easy-to-Read Material
Kaper (2019) [42]	Mixed methods: Surveys Interviews Observation	Assessment and delivery	Hospitals (n = 4)	Staff (n = 24) Older adults (n = 40)	- Assessment (using Quickscan Health literacy toolbox [in NL] and Literacy Audit for Health Care Settings [in IRL]), on four domains: navigation, digital-, written-, and oral communication - Planning and delivery of interventions to improve navigation and digital-, written-, and oral communication
Vellar (2017) [30]	Mixed methods: Observation Interviews Survey	Assessment and delivery	Regional health service (9 hospitals)	Health professionals & various staff (exact number not reported) Patients (n = 1179)	Design of OHL-framework in three phases: 1. review of literature and clinical incidents; 2. organizational consultations; 3. piloting of HL strategiesFocus of OHL-framework: ensure effective communication, embed HL in health systems, and integrate HL into clinical incident management, education and clinical QI

Table 1. Cont.

Author, Year	Research Design	Focus	Setting	Sample	OHL-Intervention
Mastroianni (2019) [41]	Quantitative pre-post study: Rating of materials	Assessment and delivery	Regional health service (9 sites)	Sample: NA	Implementation of the PiP (Patient information Portal) process: - organization-wide approach for staff to develop plain-language patient information together with patients - supported by an interactive intranet site, a coordinator, and an HL ambassador training program
Weaver (2012) [31]	Mixed methods: Observation Interviews	Assessment	Clinics of a rural health centre (n = 3)	Various staff (n = 19) Patients (n = 16)	Assessment on six domains using an open-ended approach (informed by toolkits of: HLEHHC, Joint commission, the HLUP and AHRQ): - patient–provider interaction - patient education - printed materials - technology - inter-staff interaction - policy
Wray (2019) [32]	Qualitative study: Interviews	Delivery	Clinics of a rural health centre (n = 3)	Various staff (n = 19) Patients (n = 16)	Planning and delivery of interventions to enhance health literacy: - staff orientation to increase knowledge of HL and HL-friendly practices - formation of task force from several staff levels - development of a logic model and strategic planning of activities to enhance HL - improvement of complicated patient forms, and plain language diabetes self-care patient education materials - implementation of HL practices with staff at each level - identification of criteria for HL outcomes for program evaluation: increased HL awareness and capacities, HL practices, and sustainability in these practice

3.2. Outcomes of OHL-Interventions

In this section, we present first the outcomes of the OHL-assessments, and second the impact after the delivery of interventions (Table 2). Findings are the result of descriptive studies. Most studies (n = 23) assessed and identified OHL-related problems at the levels of patients, professionals and organizations. Patients encountered problems relating to navigation, spoken communication, and understanding and acting upon written and digital information [3,17,23,25,28–31,34,36–43], although they also reported positive experiences [3,31,36,40]. Professionals reported limited understanding of health literacy, a lack of training, and infrequent use of recommended health literacy practices, such as use of plain language and the teach-back method [3,17,24–27,30,31,34–40,42,45]. Other studies reported that professionals had a patient-centred attitude and applied health literacy practices, but on an informal basis [17,36]. However, the assessment itself often increased awareness of health literacy problems among professionals [3,30,31,34,42]. At the organizational level, OHL was rarely considered a strategic priority, and strategic plans, policies, and routine procedures were often considered insufficient to address pro-blems related to OHL [17,25,30,31,35,38,42,43]. For example, the concept of patient-centred care was not translated into a concrete plan, and procedures to improve coordination of care were lacking [3,17,37,38].

The application of organization-wide OHL-interventions resulted in some improvement of patient outcomes [25–27,30,41], and greater changes in intermediate outcomes at professional and organizational levels [25–27,30,32,33,41,42]. Despite relatively small sample sizes, two research projects reported some improvement in patient-related outcomes [25–27,30,41], such as increased health literacy skills, participation in health care, and increased self-management abilities following interventions involving peer community members. Although not evaluated by patients, independent assessors reported both improved comprehensibility related to patient information materials [30,41], and some li-mited changes in the complexity of materials [29]. Improved health outcomes were not reported. Studies which reported greater change on intermediate outcomes at professional and organizational levels [25–27,30,32,33,41,42] used an organization-wide and long-term approach to deliver OHL-interventions. After training, (health) professionals in these studies reported increased competency to address health literacy and application of recommended practices [25–27,30,32,41,42]. Intermediate outcomes at the organizational level included integration of OHL into policies and systems, redesign of services, organization-wide programs to promote staff capacity building, and promotion of health literacy strategies by professionals in written, digital, and spoken communication [25–27,30,32,41]. Limited impact was reported regarding routine organization-wide application of practices [25,32,42], navigation, and distal outcomes such as health indicators, quality of care, patient safety, and cost-effectiveness [25,28,29,32,42,43]. A few studies with only brief implementation periods struggled with defining priorities and action plans, and reported limited changes among professionals and organizations [28,29,43], although they undertook preliminary attempts to improve written communication and train staff.

3.3. Factors and Strategies Influencing the Application of OHL-Interventions

Reported facilitators of a comprehensive OHL-assessment were: patient engagement, a change champion, commitment and capacity of staff, support from leadership and researchers, and an innovation culture, see Table 3 [3,28,31,34,39,42,43]. Patient engagement was found to be crucial for identifying health literacy problems from their perspective [25,30,42]. Health professionals needed to perceive the OHL-assessment as relevant and feasible, be committed to its implementation, and have knowledge of quality improvement [3,28,34,42,43]. Clear introduction meetings were found to increase HL awareness and staff buy-in [34,39,42,43]. Support from researchers added credibility to the intervention and promoted its quality of implementation [3,28,34,42,43]. Facilitators at the orga-nizational level were: an innovation culture focused on quality improvement, leadership support, and coordination by a change champion [28,30,32,34,43].

Table 2. Outcomes of OHL Assessments and Interventions.

Stage	Outcome Level		
	Patient	Professional	Organization
OHL-Assessment	Problems with communication and navigation [3,17,23,25,28–31,34,36–43]: - Navigation: difficulties due to inconsistent terms and signage in larger buildings. - Written- and digital information too long and complex due to high reading levels. - Oral communication: difficulty with understanding information and participating in treatment. Positive experiences [3,31,36,40]: - Satisfaction on interaction with providers - Staff responsive to help with navigation, questions, and explaining information. - Information easy to read and accessible.	OHL problems identified among staff [3,17,24–27,30,31,34–40,42,45]: - Limited awareness and knowledge of HL (difference between individual and OHL). - Lack of HL training. - Limited application of HL practices. Positive experiences [3,31,34,36,40,42]: - Patient-centred attitude and commitment to provide high quality care. - Awareness of HL issues and (self-reported) application of HL practices. - OHL-assessment reported to increase awareness and understanding of OHL barriers, especially assessment with patients.	OHL problems identified across organizations [17,25,30,31,35,38,42,43]: - OHL not a strategic priority, although its importance is acknowledged. - Organizational cultures vary in fostering organizational change and quality improvement. - OHL policies and structures lacking; e.g., to improve patient centredness, empowerment, and comprehensible communication. - Lack of systematic routine procedures to address HL problems, coordination and delivery of care, community resources, and to engage patients.
Delivery of OHL-interventions	Some positive patient outcomes after organization-wide OHL-interventions [25–27,30,41]: - Small to greater improvement of individual HL levels after educational interventions. - Behaviour changes after intervention with community volunteers. - Some positive impact of patient–provider interventions. - Increased patient engagement/input on improving written health information and services.	Positive intermediate outcomes on competency, communication, and practices after organization-wide OHL-interventions [25–27,30,32,33,41,42]: - Greater commitment and competency to address health literacy and communication after training. - Increased application of health literacy practices. - Improved provider-patient interaction. Intermediate outcomes on written communication [29,32,41,42]: - Wider assessments and revision of materials - Positive, but varying, improvement regarding comprehensibility and actionability of materials.	Positive intermediate organizational outcomes after organization-wide OHL-interventions [25–27,30,32,33,41,42]: - Embedding of OHL into organizational processes as strategic priorities, frameworks, and policies. - Organization-wide platform to revise materials. - Redesign of service procedures to improve health literacy screening, access, and patient engagement. - Design of more comprehensible websites. - Staff capacity building on HL, comprehensible communication, and self-management. Limited improvement reported [25,28,29,32,42,43]: - Struggle to define priorities and action plans - Navigation and protocols on communication. - Sustainable and routine application of HL practices.

Table 3. Factors and strategies influencing assessment and delivery of OHL-interventions.

Stage	Outcome Level		
	Patient Level	Professional Level	Organizational Level
OHL-assessment	Facilitators [3,24,25,30,42] - Involving patients in assessment Barriers [42] - Lack of patient-perspective - Effort to recruit patients	Facilitators [3,22,28,31,34,42,43]: - Introduction meetings to increase HL awareness and staff buy-in. - OHL-assessment perceived as relevant and feasible. - Tool features: adaptable, clear structure, feasible to use. - Staff commitment Barriers [28,34,37–39,42,43]: - Assessments perceived as lengthy and resource-intensive - Turnover and part-time working staff - Assessment requiring more time than anticipated - Limited knowledge of quality improvement	Facilitators [3,28,31,34,35,39,42,43]: - Comprehensive assessments - Assessments applied in stepwise and flexible manner. - Change champion and project-committees - Support from leaders and researchers. - Culture and strategies for quality improvement. Barriers [17,28,34,37–39,42,43]: - Limited resources. - Limited knowledge of quality improvement. - Variety in departments increases difficulty of HL assessment.
Delivery of OHL-interventions	Facilitator [25–27,30,41] - Patient engagement in evaluating information and health services. - Patients taking part in interventions to improve outcomes	Facilitators [25–27,30,32,33,41,42]: - Staff commitment - Staff involved in co-design of interventions, planning processes, and quality improvement cycles. - Staff meetings to discuss HL - Staff having knowledge of change strategies and quality improvement Barriers [28,29,42,43]: - Staff with limited knowledge of health literacy concept	Facilitators [25–27,30,32,33,41,42]: - Support from leaders and researchers. - Accountability. - Organization-wide approach: strategic and collaborative planning and development of program logic models combining top-down and bottom-up approaches. - Detailed, coordinated and concrete action plans - Co-design process to develop and pilot interventions - Quality improvement cycles to pilot test and refine interventions. - Practices affiliated with larger health systems Barriers [28,29,32,42,43]: - Limited leadership support - Limited resources - Lack of systematic approach to coordinate implementation.

Table 3. Cont.

Stage	Outcome Level		
	Patient Level	Professional Level	Organizational Level
			- Time required for implementation activities - Bureaucratic and technological barriers - Lack of coordination with other quality improvement initiatives - Restrictions related to navigation guidelines

Critical facilitators regarding the delivery of OHL-interventions were reported to be: leadership support, an organization-wide approach, a change champion and project committee, sufficient resources, professional commitment and competencies, and patient engagement, in order to achieve improvement at professional and organizational levels, see Table 3 [25–27,30–33,41,42]. An organization-wide approach, supported by senior management, was reported to stimulate the development of program logic models, strategic prioritization, and planning of OHL improvement [25,30,32]. These organizations often reported having simultaneously used top-down and bottom-up strategies to increase staff commitment to and knowledge of change strategies and quality improvement [25,30,32]. Co-design strategies and PDCA cycles were applied to develop, refine, and test interventions [25,30,32]. In contrast to the assessment phase, patients seemed to be less engaged in the application of interventions [25,42]. Only in the studies of Vellar et al. (2017) and Mastroianni et al. (2019) [30,41] were patients systematically involved in processes to improve navigation and patient-information materials. In the research project of Beauchamp et al. (2018) [25], small samples of patients were involved in the development and testing of interventions. Studies that found OHL-interventions to have only a limited impact reported that their implementation periods were brief, and affected by barriers such as lack of a change champion and coordinated planning processes [29,43], as well as limited time, resources and leadership support [22,28,29,43].

4. Discussion

The aim of this scoping review was to summarize the evidence regarding: (1) outcomes of OHL-interventions at patient, professional and organizational levels; (2) factors and strategies that influence the implementation and outcomes of OHL-interventions. We selected 24 articles, which included 17 original research projects (fully) based on qualitative and quantitative descriptive studies. With regard to the outcomes we: (a) identified OHL-related problems across patient-, professional- and organizational levels [3,25,32,34,36–38,42]; and (b) found that application of organization-wide OHL-interventions resulted in some improvement of patient outcomes [25–27,30–32,41], and greater change in intermediate outcomes at professional and organizational levels [25–27,30,32,33,41,42]. However, some studies reported only limited change [28,29,43], and no studies reported improvement on more distal outcomes. We found that several critical factors and strategies facilitated organization-wide outcomes of OHL [25–27,30–33,41,42]: leadership support, an organization-wide approach, an innovation culture, a change champion, commitment and adequate capacity of staff, and patient engagement.

Compared with the earlier reviews of Farmanova et al. [19] and Lloyd et al. (2018) [20], our findings confirmed the evidence regarding identified OHL-related problems, and we observed greater progress on the impact of organization-wide OHL interventions [25–27,30–33,41,42]. A first point regarding our evidence is that the number of OHL-pro-blems identified across a variety of countries underlines the need to use comprehensive frameworks to improve organizational health literacy in health care settings [14,35,46–50]. The progress we observed related particularly to recent studies, which showed how a single health literacy project led to development of a health literate organization by employing a systematic and organization-wide approach. These studies strengthened the evidence particularly on three points: (1) patient outcomes showed some evidence of increased health literacy, understanding of information, and participation in health care [25–27,30,41]; (2) outcomes among health professionals showed evidence of improved competencies and practices to address health literacy [25,30,32,42]; (3) intermediate organizational outcomes showed evidence of embedding of OHL into policies and structures, staff training, and interventions to improve screening, communication and patient engagement [25–27,30–33,41,42]. This review thus indicates a growing awareness of how to achieve sustainable improvement on various OHL-domains, and supports the findings in recent reviews by Zanobini et al. (2020) [18] and Meggetto et al. (2020) [51].

Our review points to several critical facilitators and strategies that can promote health literacy friendly organizations in the long term: leadership support, an organization-wide approach, an innovation culture, a change champion, commitment and capacity of staff, and patient engagement [25–27,30–33,41,42]. These facilitators correspond with findings reported in other studies on innovation in health care settings [52–56] and universal processes for organizational change [19,20]. In our review, some studies reported limited outcomes because they had a shorter duration (six months) [28,29,43], struggled with coordination, staff turnover, and a lack of a change champion as well as leadership support and resources [28,29,43]. Other studies in our review suggest that a systematic organization-wide approach is more promising [25–27,30–33,41,42]. These implementation strategies involved simultaneous use of top-down and bottom-up strategies to engage staff and patients; such strategies have been widely used in the field of health promotion [32,57]. This observation underlines the frameworks of Trezona (2017) [47] and Zanobini (2020) [18] in the sense that various OHL-domains are interconnected and need to be targeted simultaneously in order to initiate a cyclical and widening process of improving the quality of health care by making organizations responsive to health literacy [51]. These findings have thus strengthened the evidence base for implementation of OHL-interventions.

However, our review also shows the evidence for OHL-interventions still to be generally weak, particularly regarding their effects on more distal outcomes like improved health or cost-effectiveness [18,20]. The first, general, issue regards the total lack of studies with an experimental design: studies conducted only baseline measurements, or had small samples when investigating change over time, and did not compare outcomes with control settings. Second, the instruments for measuring OHL outcomes did not include information on reliability and validity, although some instruments [34,44] indicated having face validity, and were used in different settings and countries [20]. Recently, several instruments were designed to assess a wide spectrum of OHL-domains [34,44,46,47], and one of these was reported to have satisfactory reliability and validity [49,58]. Although these instruments did not evaluate the outcomes of interventions, they may have the potential to be used for benchmarking and for investigating change over time [49].

The particular weakness of the evidence for OHL-interventions is that their impact is still unclear regarding more distal outcomes like patient health outcomes, quality of care, and cost reduction. This may be explained by several factors. First, in our review, mea-surement of more distal outcomes among larger samples of patients was lacking. However, we noted that, in some studies, small groups of patients were engaged in the development and evaluation of interventions [25,30,41], which resulted in improvement of health literacy levels, and in understanding and self-management of patients. Second, it seems plausible that the impact of organization-wide OHL interventions results first in intermediate outcomes among professionals and organizations, outcomes which may be influenced by many factors [14]. Zanobini [18] for example reports that (single) interventions directly targeted at patients result in improved outcomes in patient satisfaction, knowledge, and skills. In sum, promising outcomes may result from studies that combine patient-targeted interventions with systematic approaches directed at professional and organizational levels, and include measurement of distant patient outcomes, quality of care, and cost-effectiveness.

4.1. Strengths and Limitations

Several strengths of this study can be noted. We conducted a comprehensive search strategy and selection procedure to include relevant studies in the review. The fact that the selected studies were conducted in various health care organizations and countries is promising for the generalizability of the results. However, several limitations should be mentioned. First, the approach of a scoping review did not include a quality assessment of the selected studies; this limited the potential to connect content and quality. Second, we focused on peer-reviewed articles which had abstracts in English; this may have led to missing relevant studies from the grey literature or studies published in other languages. We are, however, confident that we have selected the most relevant ones. A final limitation is that publication bias may have influenced this review: studies reporting negative results could be difficult to get published. However, we identified several studies which explicitly reported the problems encountered, and consider the influence of publication bias to be limited.

4.2. Implications

Organization-wide implementation of OHL-interventions can improve intermediate outcomes among professionals and organizations, and has the potential to mitigate health literacy problems among patients. We recommend: (1) assessing OHL problems using a comprehensive and valid instrument; (2) starting with implementation of easy-to-achieve interventions; (3) using a systematic approach to achieve greater organizational change, simultaneously applying bottom-up and top-down approaches; (4) taking into account the critical facilitators of implementation: a change champion vs a project committee, lea-dership support, sufficient resources, patient involvement, and competent and committed staff.

In order to strengthen evidence on OHL-interventions, we need studies with a more rigorous design to evaluate their effectiveness, and which use OHL-instruments that have adequate reliability and validity and are suitable for the European context [14,18,20]. Furthermore, more distal patient-related outcomes like quality of care, safety, and cost-effectiveness should be evaluated.

Health care organizations have primarily focused on treatment, but there is an increasing recognition of their role in health promotion and prevention in order to address health inequalities in the broader social context [14,15,25]. OHL-interventions are one approach to improve outcomes for individuals with limited health literacy. Other effective strategies may be school-based health literacy education, mass-media communication or empowering individual people as well as communities, and building health literacy competencies of (future) health professionals [59]. As such, OHL-interventions are probably most effective in combination with these other approaches, but this evidently requires further study.

A contextual factor that must be acknowledged in relation to this scoping review is that the period of the literature search preceded the start of the COVID-19 pandemic. The importance of health literacy came to the fore during the COVID-19 pandemic, as the resilience of communities and the relationship of citizens to health care providers depend on it, particularly in crisis situations. This underlines the relevance of this scoping review on OHL-interventions. The COVID-19 pandemic is likely to have influenced the field of OHL-intervention research as health care organizations have, to a greater or lesser extent, faced several periods of crisis due to exceptional service demands. The nature of this influence is unknown. Therefore, we recommend that future studies investigate the influence of the COVID-19 pandemic on the research related to organizational health literacy. Organization-wide OHL-interventions have previously required longer time periods, of several years, for changes to be implemented successfully and sustained. Since the onset of the pandemic in March 2020, health care organizations may have responded in one of two ways: putting the implementation of OHL-interventions on hold or embracing OHL quickly in response to the situation. The COVID-19 pandemic has shown that health settings can accelerate innovation, but whether this holds for OHL-interventions is to be determined.

5. Conclusions

Delivery of organization-wide OHL-interventions resulted in some improvement in patient-related outcomes and changes at the professional and organizational levels and may be a promising approach to mitigate health literacy problems. Critical success factors for organization-wide implementation are leadership support, simultaneous top-down and bottom-up approaches, a change champion and project committee, and staff commitment. Efforts to implement organization-wide OHL-interventions should take into account these critical success factors. Organization-wide interventions were reported to achieve more positive change on OHL-domains, but evidence regarding OHL-outcomes needs strengthening.

Supplementary Materials: The following are available online at https://www.mdpi.com/article/10.3390/ijerph182211906/s1, Table S1: Overview detailed search strategy.

Author Contributions: Conceptualization, M.S.K., S.A.R. and A.F.d.W.; methodology, M.S.K., S.A.R., J.S. and A.F.d.W.; software, M.S.K.; validation, A.F.d.W., M.S.K., J.S.; formal analysis, M.S.K. and A.F.d.W.; investigation, M.S.K.; resources, M.S.K.; data curation, M.S.K.; writing—original draft preparation, M.S.K.; writing—review and editing, S.A.R., J.S. and A.F.d.W.; visualization, M.S.K.; supervision, S.A.R.; project administration, M.S.K.; funding acquisition, A.F.d.W. All authors have read and agreed to the published version of the manuscript.

Funding: This study immediately builds upon the work of the IROHLA project, 2013–2016, which was coordinated by the University Medical Center Groningen and has received external funding from the European Union's Seventh Framework Programme (FP7/2007-2013) under grant agreement #305831.

Acknowledgments: The authors would like to thank Truus van Ittersum for her contribution to the search strategy.

Conflicts of Interest: The authors declare no conflict of interest.

References

1. Sørensen, K.; Pelikan, J.M.; Röthlin, F.; Ganahl, K.; Slonska, Z.; Doyle, G.; Fullam, J.; Kondilis, B.; Agrafiotis, D.; Uiters, E.; et al. Health Literacy in Europe: Comparative Results of the European Health Literacy Survey (HLS-EU). *Eur. J. Public Health* **2015**, *25*, 1053–1058. [CrossRef] [PubMed]
2. Kwan, B.; Frankish, J.; Rootman, I.; Zumbo, B.; Kelly, K.; Begoray, D.; Kazanjian, A.; Mullet, J.; Hayes, M. *The Development and Validation of Measures of "Health Literacy" in Different Populations*; University of Britisch Columbia, Institute of Health Promotion Research: Vancouver, BC, Canada; University of Victoria, Centre for Community Health Promotion Research: Victoria, BC, Canada, 2006.
3. Groene, R.O.; Rudd, R.E. Results of a Feasibility Study to Assess the Health Literacy Environment: Navigation, Written, and Oral Communication in 10 Hospitals in Catalonia, Spain. *J. Commun. Healthc.* **2011**, *4*, 227–237. [CrossRef]
4. Goto, A.; Lai, A.Y.; Rudd, R.E. Health Literacy Training for Public Health Nurses in Fukushima: A Multi-Site Program Evaluation. *Jpn. Med. Assoc. J. JMAJ* **2015**, *58*, 69–77.
5. Rudd, R.E.; Comings, J.P.; Hyde, J.N. Leave No One Behind: Improving Health and Risk Communication Through Attention to Literacy. *J. Health Commun.* **2003**, *730*, 37–41. [CrossRef]
6. Berkman, N.D.; Sheridan, S.L.; Donahue, K.E.; Halpern, D.J.; Crotty, K. Low Health Literacy and Health Outcomes: An Updated Systematic Review. *Ann. Intern. Med.* **2011**, *155*, 97–107. [CrossRef] [PubMed]
7. Williams, A.M.; Muir, K.W.; Rosdahl, J.A. Readability of Patient Education Materials in Ophthalmology: A Single-Institution Study and Systematic Review. *BMC Ophthalmol.* **2016**, *16*, 133. [CrossRef] [PubMed]
8. Pires, C.; Vigário, M.; Cavaco, A. Readability of Medicinal Package Leaflets: A Systematic Review. *Rev. Saude Publica* **2015**, *49*, 1–13. [CrossRef] [PubMed]
9. Van der Heide, I.; Heijmans, M.; Schuit, A.J.; Uiters, E.; Rademakers, J. Functional, Interactive and Critical Health Literacy: Varying Relationships with Control over Care and Number of GP Visits. *Patient Educ. Couns.* **2015**, *98*, 998–1004. [CrossRef]
10. Heijmans, M.; Waverijn, G.; Rademakers, J.; van der Vaart, R.; Rijken, M. Functional, Communicative and Critical Health Literacy of Chronic Disease Patients and Their Importance for Self-Management. *Patient Educ. Couns.* **2015**, *98*, 41–48. [CrossRef]
11. Rudd, R. The Evolving Concept of Health Literacy: New Directions for Health Literacy Studies. *J. Commun. Healthc.* **2015**, *8*, 7–9. [CrossRef]
12. Koh, H.K.; Brach, C.; Harris, L.M.; Parchman, M.L. A Proposed "health Literate Care Model" Would Constitute a Systems Approach to Improving Patients' Engagement in Care. *Health Aff.* **2013**, *32*, 357–367. [CrossRef] [PubMed]
13. Brach, C.; Keller, D.; Hernandez, L.M.; Baur, C.; Parker, R.; Dreyer, B.; Schyve, P.; Lemerise, A.J.; Schillinger, D. Ten Attributes of Health Literate Health Care Organizations. *NAM Perspect. Discuss. Pap.* **2012**. [CrossRef]
14. Brach, C. The Journey to Become a Health Literate Organization: A Snapshot of Health System Improvement. *Stud. Health Technol. Inform.* **2017**, *240*, 203–237. [PubMed]
15. Palumbo, R. Leveraging Organizational Health Literacy to Enhance Health Promotion and Risk Prevention: A Narrative and Interpretive Literature Review. *Yale J. Biol. Med.* **2021**, *94*, 115–128.
16. Annarumma, C.; Palumbo, R. Contextualizing Health Literacy to Health Care Organizations: Exploratory Insights. *J. Health Manag.* **2016**, *18*, 611–624. [CrossRef]
17. Palumbo, R.; Annarumma, C.; Musella, M. Exploring the Meaningfulness of Healthcare Organizations: A Multiple Case Study. *Int. J. Public Sect. Manag.* **2017**, *30*, 503–518. [CrossRef]

18. Zanobini, P.; Lorini, C.; Baldasseroni, A.; Dellisanti, C.; Bonaccorsi, G. A Scoping Review on How to Make Hospitals Health Literate Healthcare Organizations. *Int. J. Environ. Res. Public Health* **2020**, *17*, 1036. [CrossRef] [PubMed]
19. Farmanova, E.; Bonneville, L.; Bouchard, L. Organizational Health Literacy: Review of Theories, Frameworks, Guides, and Implementation Issues. *Inquiry* **2018**, *55*, 1–17. [CrossRef]
20. Lloyd, J.E.; Song, H.J.; Dennis, S.M.; Dunbar, N.; Harris, E.; Harris, M.F. A Paucity of Strategies for Developing Health Literate Organisations: A Systematic Review. *PLoS ONE* **2018**, *13*, 1–17. [CrossRef]
21. Arksey, H.; O'Malley, L. Scoping Studies: Towards a Methodological Framework. *Int. J. Soc. Res. Methodol.* **2005**, *8*, 19–32. [CrossRef]
22. Grabeel, K.L.; Beeler, C. Taking the Pulse of the University of Tennessee Medical Center's Health Literacy Knowledge. *Med. Ref. Serv. Q.* **2018**, *37*, 89–96. [CrossRef]
23. Grabeel, K.L.; Russomanno, J.; Oelschlegel, S.; Tester, E.; Heidel, R.E. Computerized versus Hand-Scored Health Literacy Tools: A Comparison of Simple Measure of Gobbledygook (SMOG) and Flesch-Kincaid in Printed Patient Education Materials. *J. Med. Libr. Assoc.* **2018**, *106*, 38–45. [CrossRef]
24. Tester, E.; Grabeel, K.L.; Oelschlegel, S.; Heidel, R.E.; Russomanno, J. Call to Action: Librarians Promoting Health Literacy Assessments in Oral Communication. *J. Hosp. Librariansh.* **2019**, *19*, 129–143. [CrossRef]
25. Beauchamp, A.; Batterham, R.W.; Dodson, S.; Astbury, B.; Elsworth, G.R.; McPhee, C.; Jacobson, J.; Buchbinder, R.; Osborne, R.H. Systematic Development and Implementation of Interventions to OPtimise Health Literacy and Access (Ophelia). *BMC Public Health* **2017**, *17*, 230. [CrossRef] [PubMed]
26. Goeman, D.; Conway, S.; Norman, R.; Morley, J.; Weerasuriya, R.; Osborne, R.H.; Beauchamp, A. Optimising Health Literacy and Access of Service Provision to Community Dwelling Older People with Diabetes Receiving Home Nursing Support. *J. Diabetes Res.* **2016**, *2016*, 1–12. [CrossRef] [PubMed]
27. Jessup, R.L.; Osborne, R.H.; Buchbinder, R.; Beauchamp, A. Using Co-Design to Develop Interventions to Address Health Literacy Needs in a Hospitalised Population. *BMC Health Serv. Res.* **2018**, *18*, 989. [CrossRef]
28. Mabachi, N.M.; Cifuentes, M.; Barnard, J.; Brega, A.G.; Albright, K.; Weiss, B.D.; Brach, C.; West, D. Demonstration of the Health Literacy Universal Precautions Toolkit. *J. Ambul. Care Manag.* **2016**, *39*, 199–208. [CrossRef]
29. Brega, A.G.; Freedman, M.A.G.; LeBlanc, W.G.; Barnard, J.; Mabachi, N.M.; Cifuentes, M.; Albright, K.; Weiss, B.D.; Brach, C.; West, D.R. Using the Health Literacy Universal Precautions Toolkit to Improve the Quality of Patient Materials. *J. Health Commun.* **2015**, *20* (Suppl. 2), 69–76. [CrossRef] [PubMed]
30. Vellar, L.; Mastroianni, F.; Lambert, K. Embedding Health Literacy into Health Systems: A Case Study of a Regional Health Service. *Aust. Health Rev.* **2017**, *41*, 621–625. [CrossRef]
31. Weaver, N.L.; Wray, R.J.; Zellin, S.; Gautam, K.; Jupka, K. Advancing Organizational Health Literacy in Health Care Organizations Serving High-Needs Populations: A Case Study. *J. Health Commun.* **2012**, *17* (Suppl. 3), 55–66. [CrossRef]
32. Wray, R.; Weaver, N.; Adsul, P.; Gautam, K.; Jupka, K.; Zellin, S.; Goggins, K.; Vijaykumar, S.; Hansen, N.; Rudd, R. Enhancing Organizational Health Literacy in a Rural Missouri Clinic: A Qualitative Case Study. *Int. J. Health Care Qual. Assur.* **2019**, *32*, 788–804. [CrossRef] [PubMed]
33. Cawthon, C.; Mion, L.C.; Willens, D.E.; Roumie, C.L.; Kripalani, S. Implementing Routine Health Literacy Assessment in Hospital and Primary Care Patients. *Jt. Comm. J. Qual. Patient Saf.* **2014**, *40*, 68–76. [CrossRef]
34. DeWalt, D.A.; Broucksou, K.A.; Hawk, V.; Brach, C.; Hink, A.; Rudd, R.; Callahan, L. Developing and Testing the Health Literacy Universal Precautions Toolkit. *Nurs. Outlook* **2011**, *59*, 85–94. [CrossRef] [PubMed]
35. Dietscher, C.; Pelikan, J. Gesundheitskompetente Krankenbehandlungsorganisationen. *Prävent. Gesundh.* **2016**, *11*, 53–62. [CrossRef]
36. Horowitz, A.M.; Maybury, C.; Kleinman, D.V.; Radice, S.D.; Wang, M.Q.; Child, W.; Rudd, R.E. Health Literacy Environmental Scans of Community-Based Dental Clinics in Maryland. *Am. J. Public Health* **2014**, *104*, 85–93. [CrossRef] [PubMed]
37. Lambert, M.; Luke, J.; Downey, B.; Crengle, S.; Kelaher, M.; Reid, S.; Smylie, J. Health Literacy: Health Professionals' Understandings and Their Perceptions of Barriers That Indigenous Patients Encounter. *BMC Health Serv. Res.* **2014**, *14*, 1–10. [CrossRef]
38. Martinez-Donate, A.P.; Halverson, J.; Simon, N.-J.; Strickland, J.S.; Trentham-Dietz, A.; Smith, P.D.; Linskens, R.; Wang, X. Identifying Health Literacy and Health System Navigation Needs among Rural Cancer Patients: Findings from the Rural Oncology Literacy Enhancement Study (ROLES). *J. Cancer Educ.* **2013**, *28*, 573–581. [CrossRef]
39. O'Neal, K.S.; Crosby, K.M.; Miller, M.J.; Murray, K.A.; Condren, M.E. Assessing Health Literacy Practices in a Community Pharmacy Environment: Experiences Using the AHRQ Pharmacy Health Literacy Assessment Tool. *Res. Soc. Adm. Pharm.* **2013**, *9*, 564–596. [CrossRef]
40. Smith, D.L.; Hedrick, W.; Earhart, H.; Galloway, H.; Arndt, A. Evaluating Two Health Care Facilities' Ability to Meet Health Literacy Needs: A Role for Occupational Therapy. *Occup. Ther. Health Care* **2010**, *24*, 348–359. [CrossRef]
41. Mastroianni, F.; Chen, Y.C.; Vellar, L.; Cvejic, E.; Smith, J.K.; McCaffery, K.J.; Muscat, D.M. Implementation of an Organisation-Wide Health Literacy Approach to Improve the Understandability and Actionability of Patient Information and Education Materials: A Pre-Post Effectiveness Study. *Patient Educ. Couns.* **2019**, *102*, 1656–1661. [CrossRef]

42. Kaper, M.; Sixsmith, J.; Meijering, L.; Vervoordeldonk, J.; Doyle, P.; Barry, M.M.; de Winter, A.F.; Reijneveld, S.A. Implementation and Long-Term Outcomes of Organisational Health Literacy Interventions in Ireland and the Netherlands: A Longitudinal Mixed-Methods Study. *Int. J. Environ. Res. Public Health* **2019**, *16*, 4812. [CrossRef]
43. Shoemaker, S.J.; Staub-DeLong, L.; Wasserman, M.; Spranca, M. Factors Affecting Adoption and Implementation of AHRQ Health Literacy Tools in Pharmacies. *Res. Soc. Adm. Pharm.* **2013**, *9*, 553–563. [CrossRef]
44. Rudd, R.E.; Anderson, J.E. *The Health Literacy Environment of Hospitals and Health Centers. Partners for Action: Making Your Healthcare Facility Literacy-Friendly*; Health and Adult Literacy and Learning Initiative, Harvard School of Public Health: Boston, MA, USA, 2006.
45. Shoemaker, S.J.; Wolf, M.S.; Brach, C. Development of the Patient Education Materials Assessment Tool (PEMAT): A New Measure of Understandability and Actionability for Print and Audiovisual Patient Information. *Patient Educ. Couns.* **2014**, *96*, 395–403. [CrossRef] [PubMed]
46. Trezona, A.; Dodson, S.; Fitzsimon, E.; LaMontagne, A.D.; Osborne, R.H. Field-Testing and Refinement of the Organisational Health Literacy Responsiveness Self-Assessment (Org-HLR) Tool and Process. *Int. J. Environ. Res. Public Health* **2020**, *17*, 1000. [CrossRef] [PubMed]
47. Trezona, A.; Dodson, S.; Osborne, R.H. Development of the Organisational Health Literacy Responsiveness (Org-HLR) Framework in Collaboration with Health and Social Services Professionals. *BMC Health Serv. Res.* **2017**, *17*, 513. [CrossRef]
48. Trezona, A.; Dodson, S.; Osborne, R.H. Development of the Organisational Health Literacy Responsiveness (Org-HLR) Self-Assessment Tool and Process. *BMC Health Serv. Res.* **2018**, *18*, 694. [CrossRef] [PubMed]
49. Kowalski, C.; Lee, S.Y.D.; Schmidt, A.; Wesselmann, S.; Wirtz, M.A.; Pfaff, H.; Ernstmann, N. The Health Literate Health Care Organization 10 Item Questionnaire (HLHO-10): Development and Validation. *BMC Health Serv. Res.* **2015**, *15*, 1–9. [CrossRef] [PubMed]
50. Pelikan, J.M.; Dietscher, C. Warum Sollten Und Wie Können Krankenhäuser Ihre Organisationale Gesundheitskompetenz Verbessern? [Why Should and How Can Hospitals Improve Their Organizational Health Literacy?]. *Bundesgesundheitsblatt Gesundheitsforsch. Gesundh.* **2015**, *58*, 989–995. [CrossRef]
51. Meggetto, E.; Kent, F.; Ward, B.; Keleher, H. Factors Influencing Implementation of Organizational Health Literacy: A Realist Review. *J. Health Organ. Manag.* **2020**, *34*, 385–407. [CrossRef]
52. Fleuren, M.; Wiefferink, K.; Paulussen, T. Determinants of Innovation within Health Care Organizations: Literature Review and Delphi Study. *Int. J. Qual. Health Care* **2004**, *16*, 107–123. [CrossRef]
53. Fleuren, M.A.H.; Paulussen, T.G.W.M.; Van Dommelen, P.; Van Buuren, S. Towards a Measurement Instrument for Determinants of Innovations. *Int. J. Qual. Health Care* **2014**, *26*, 501–510. [CrossRef]
54. Carroll, C.; Patterson, M.; Wood, S.; Booth, A.; Rick, J.; Balain, S. A Conceptual Framework for Implementation Fidelity. *Implement. Sci.* **2007**, *2*, 1–9. [CrossRef]
55. Hasson, H. Systematic Evaluation of Implementation Fidelity of Complex Interventions in Health and Social Care. *Implement. Sci.* **2010**, *5*, 1–9. [CrossRef]
56. Hasson, H.; Blomberg, S.; Dunér, A. Fidelity and Moderating Factors in Complex Interventions: A Case Study of a Continuum of Care Program for Frail Elderly People in Health and Social Care. *Implement. Sci.* **2012**, *7*, 1–11. [CrossRef] [PubMed]
57. Van Daele, T.; van Audenhove, C.; Hermans, D.; van den Bergh, O.; van den Broucke, S. Empowerment Implementation: Enhancing Fidelity and Adaptation in a Psycho-Educational Intervention. *Health Promot. Int.* **2014**, *29*, 212–222. [CrossRef] [PubMed]
58. Hayran, O.; Özer, O. Organizational Health Literacy as a Determinant of Patient Satisfaction. *Public Health* **2018**, *163*, 20–26. [CrossRef] [PubMed]
59. Geboers, B.; Reijneveld, S.A.; Koot, J.A.R.; de Winter, A.F. Moving towards a Comprehensive Approach for Health Literacy Interventions: The Development of a Health Literacy Intervention Model. *Int. J. Environ. Res. Public Health* **2018**, *15*, 1268. [CrossRef]

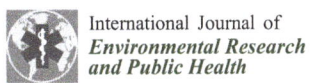

Review

Ethnic Inequalities in Healthcare Use and Care Quality among People with Multiple Long-Term Health Conditions Living in the United Kingdom: A Systematic Review and Narrative Synthesis

Brenda Hayanga [1,*], Mai Stafford [2] and Laia Bécares [1]

1. School of Education and Social Work, University of Sussex, Essex House, Falmer, Brighton BN1 9RH, UK; l.becares@sussex.ac.uk
2. The Health Foundation, 8 Salisbury Square, London EC4Y 8AP, UK; mai.stafford@health.org.uk
* Correspondence: b.hayanga@sussex.ac.uk

Citation: Hayanga, B.; Stafford, M.; Bécares, L. Ethnic Inequalities in Healthcare Use and Care Quality among People with Multiple Long-Term Health Conditions Living in the United Kingdom: A Systematic Review and Narrative Synthesis. *Int. J. Environ. Res. Public Health* **2021**, *18*, 12599. https://doi.org/10.3390/ijerph182312599

Academic Editor: Stuart Gilmour

Received: 27 August 2021
Accepted: 24 November 2021
Published: 29 November 2021

Publisher's Note: MDPI stays neutral with regard to jurisdictional claims in published maps and institutional affiliations.

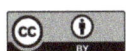

Copyright: © 2021 by the authors. Licensee MDPI, Basel, Switzerland. This article is an open access article distributed under the terms and conditions of the Creative Commons Attribution (CC BY) license (https://creativecommons.org/licenses/by/4.0/).

Abstract: Indicative evidence suggests that the prevalence of multiple long-term conditions (i.e., conditions that cannot be cured but can be managed with medication and other treatments) may be higher in people from minoritised ethnic groups when compared to people from the White majority population. Some studies also suggest that there are ethnic inequalities in healthcare use and care quality among people with multiple long-term conditions (MLTCs). The aims of this review are to (1) identify and describe the literature that reports on ethnicity and healthcare use and care quality among people with MLTCs in the UK and (2) examine how healthcare use and/or care quality for people with MLTCs compares across ethnic groups. We registered the protocol on PROSPERO (CRD42020220702). We searched the following databases up to December 2020: ASSIA, Cochrane Library, EMBASE, MEDLINE, PsycINFO, PubMed, ScienceDirect, Scopus, and Web of Science core collection. Reference lists of key articles were also hand-searched for relevant studies. The outcomes of interest were patterns of healthcare use and care quality among people with MLTCs for at least one minoritised ethnic group, compared to the White majority population in the UK. Two reviewers, L.B. and B.H., screened and extracted data from a random sample of studies (10%). B.H. independently screened and extracted data from the remaining studies. Of the 718 studies identified, 14 were eligible for inclusion. There was evidence indicating ethnic inequalities in disease management and emergency admissions among people with MLTCs in the five studies that counted more than two long-term conditions. Compared to their White counterparts, Black and Asian children and young people had higher rates of emergency admissions. Black and South Asian people were found to have suboptimal disease management compared to other ethnic groups. The findings suggest that for some minoritised ethnic group people with MLTCs there may be inadequate initiatives for managing health conditions and/or a need for enhanced strategies to reduce ethnic inequalities in healthcare. However, the few studies identified focused on a variety of conditions across different domains of healthcare use, and many of these studies used broad ethnic group categories. As such, further research focusing on MLTCs and using expanded ethnic categories in data collection is needed.

Keywords: ethnic inequalities; healthcare use; care quality; multiple long-term conditions; UK

1. Introduction

Long-term conditions (also known as chronic conditions) are health conditions that are currently uncurable and consequently are managed with medication and other therapies (e.g., cardiovascular disease, diabetes and depression) [1,2]. In the UK, it is estimated that between 23% and 27% of the population live with two or more long-term conditions, and this number is expected to rise in the coming decades [2–4]. These trends present a challenge not only for individuals but also for society and entire healthcare systems [5,6]. People with multiple long-term conditions (MLTCs) are more likely to have increased disability, poorer functioning, reduced well-being, lower quality of life and higher mortality [6,7]. The relationship between MLTCs and increased healthcare costs is well documented [8]. Further, the challenges in providing high quality care for people with MLTCs are recognized [9]. People with MLTCs have increased exposure to healthcare services and systems, which are often fragmented and/or tailored towards managing single health conditions, thereby hindering the holistic management of MLTCs [7]. This uncoordinated care may lead to extra obligations for patients and healthcare staff, threats to patient safety and an increase in patient-level frustration [10,11].

This study focuses on people from minoritised ethnic groups with MLTCs and how their patterns of healthcare use and care quality vary from their White counterparts. In line with other studies, we use the term minoritised ethnic group to refer to people who do not self-identify as belonging to the White majority ethnic group [12,13]. Commonly used acronyms such as BAME (Black, Asian and Minority Ethnic) can be exclusionary as they single out specific ethnic groups [14,15]. Other terms such as 'minority' can be associated with diminished status if we consider that, historically, the narrative of 'minorities' marked troubled histories of immigration control, policing, racial violence, inferiorisation and discrimination that were characteristic of daily life for early migrants to the UK from Africa, the Caribbean and Asia [16]. The term 'minoritised' places emphasis on how social positions are social constructions rather than practices and outcomes that are natural and inevitable [17].

There is some evidence to suggest that people from minoritised ethnic groups in the UK are at an increased risk of developing MLTCs when compared to the White majority population, and they are also more likely to develop MLTCs at an earlier age [18,19]. The findings from a recent review indicate a higher prevalence of MLTCs in some minoritised ethnic groups compared to their White counterparts [20]. These ethnic inequalities in MLTCs are likely to reflect broader economic and social inequalities, which in turn are driven by racism and racial discrimination [21,22]. These same mechanisms can lead to inequities in access and use of healthcare and care quality, which can lead to negative outcomes for people with MLTCs [23]. Studies of single conditions report that, in general, people from minoritised ethnic groups are less likely to access specialist services and less likely to report positive experiences of primary care when compared to their White counterparts [24–26]. It is possible that people with MLTCs from minoritised ethnic groups may face similar experiences when using healthcare services. Findings from a recent ethnographic study conducted by Revealing Reality for the Taskforce on Multiple Conditions give insight into how ethnic inequalities in healthcare use and care quality can arise [23]. The study explored the lives of people with MLTCs experiencing health inequity and disadvantage, living in some of the most deprived wards in the UK. This study illustrated how wider societal processes (e.g., deprivation and suboptimal healthcare provision) intersect with individual level processes (e.g., poor literacy skills, language difficulties, competing priorities) to negatively impact people's ability to access and utilise healthcare services, adhere to treatment regimens and ultimately manage their MLTCs [23].

Whilst the aforementioned study gives insight into the experiences of people with MLTCs, including those from minoritised ethnic groups, their focus was not on uncovering ethnic inequalities. It is important to examine ethnic variations in healthcare use and healthcare quality among people with MLTCs. Findings of such an exploration can illuminate ethnic inequalities and inform actions to redress the health disadvantage faced by particular populations [27], which, if ignored, can result in the widening of existent ethnic inequalities. Given the increasing ethnic diversity of the UK population [28], a detailed examination of the association between MLTCs, healthcare and ethnicity in the UK is warranted.

Past reviews of healthcare use and care quality, which have included studies reporting on differences across ethnic groups, have focused on a particular domain of healthcare (e.g., access to healthcare [29]) or health services for a particular group of conditions (e.g., somatic healthcare service related to screening, general practitioners, specialists, emergency rooms and hospital care [30]). In one review, the authors synthesised the best evidence for improving healthcare quality for people from minoritised ethnic groups [31]. However, the focus of these reviews was not on people with MLTCs [29–31]. To our knowledge, no review has synthesised evidence on ethnic inequalities in healthcare use and care quality among people with MLTCs living in the UK. Such an undertaking can highlight areas where inequalities are evident and inform discussions and efforts to address them. Therefore, the aims of this review are (1) to identify and describe the literature that reports on ethnicity and healthcare use and care quality among people with MLTCs living in the UK and (2) to examine how healthcare use and/or care quality for people with MLTCs compares across ethnic groups in studies counting more than two long-term conditions.

2. Methods

2.1. Search Strategy

In line with the Preferred Reporting Items for Systematic review and Meta-Analysis Protocols (PRISMA-P) [32], we registered the protocol for this review on PROSPERO (CRD42020220702). Between October and December 2020, we searched the following databases for studies that compared healthcare use and/or care quality across different ethnic groups of people with MLTCs living in the UK: ASSIA, Cochrane Library, EMBASE, MEDLINE, PsycINFO, PubMed, ScienceDirect, Scopus and Web of Science core collection. We also conducted a search on OpenGrey to ensure that relevant grey literature was not excluded. We supplemented the electronic search with a manual search of the key studies identified. We contacted relevant authors when full texts were not available.

We followed the conventions of each search engine and used search terms that denoted the key concepts in this review: Ethnicity (e.g., "Ethnic Groups" [Mesh] OR "BME" OR "BAME"), Multiple health conditions (e.g., "Multiple Chronic Conditions" OR Comorbid* OR Multimorbidity), Health inequality (e.g., "Health Equity" [Mesh] OR "Healthcare disparit*" [MeSH] OR Inequalit*), Healthcare use (e.g., "Delivery of Healthcare" [Mesh] OR "Tertiary Healthcare" [Mesh]), Care quality (e.g., "Quality of Healthcare" [Mesh] OR "Patient Acceptance of Healthcare" [Mesh] OR "Patient Satisfaction" [Mesh]) and the geographical location (e.g., "United Kingdom" [MeSH Terms] OR "UK") (See Appendix A for a full list of search terms).

2.2. Selection Criteria

We did not restrict the start of the search to any particular period in time and included only UK studies, published in English, reporting on healthcare use and/or care quality among people with MLTCs, across different ethnic groups of people living in the UK [33]. Our justification for focusing on studies in the UK was driven by the recognition that the UK has a unique healthcare system that is publicly funded, with a range of comprehensive services that are (mostly) free at the point of use [34]. Further, it has a diverse minoritised ethnic group population [35]. These factors would complicate comparisons with other countries with different healthcare, political, and economic systems and population structures.

In the extant literature, MLTCs are defined and operationalised in different ways. Some use the term MLTCs synonymously with the term multimorbidity (here defined as the presence of two or more long-term health conditions [3,36]). Others also incorporate the term comorbidity (i.e., the presence of any distinct additional co-existing ailment in an individual with an index condition under investigation [37,38]). Given these definitions, we included studies that counted only two conditions (e.g., diabetes and depression) as well as those that counted two or more long-term conditions. However, to address the second aim we excluded studies that counted only two conditions and focused on those that also counted more than two long-term conditions as they are more likely to give insight into those with complex medical needs and greater use of healthcare [39,40].

Healthcare use and care quality are broad concepts that encapsulate different domains. Healthcare use can be defined as the quantification or description of the use of services by persons for the purpose of preventing and curing health problems, promoting maintenance of health and well-being, or obtaining information about one's health status and prognosis [41]. Indicators of healthcare use include GP consultations, hospital visits including inpatient, outpatient and day visits, hospital admissions, accidents and emergency department visits, diagnoses, prescriptions, referrals, immunisations and screening [29,42,43]. In contrast, healthcare quality has been defined as the degree to which healthcare services increase the chances of desired health outcomes for people and are aligned with current professional knowledge [44]. Indicators of care quality include effectiveness, patient-centeredness, efficiency, equity of care and principles such as acceptability, trust, responsiveness, safety, waiting times, patient experience, satisfaction with accessibility, humaneness of care, number of readmissions and cultural appropriateness [45,46]. We included studies regardless of the domain of healthcare use and care quality under investigation.

We imported the studies retrieved from the electronic search to Endnote X8. We first removed the duplicates. Following this, B.H. and L.B. screened a random sample (10%) of the titles and abstracts. Differences were resolved through discussion. B.H. proceeded to independently screen the remaining studies. The same process was repeated when screening the full texts.

2.3. Data Extraction

B.H. and L.B. extracted data from a random sample (10%) of the studies identified. Disagreements were settled by discussion. B.H. independently extracted data from the remaining studies. We extracted relevant information from the included studies using a structured form, which included the following items: study identifier, study design, geographical location, data source, sample size, population characteristics (e.g., age and gender profile, ethnic group categories), type and number of MLTCs, confounding variables and healthcare use and care quality domains and results.

2.4. Outcomes

The outcomes of interest were patterns of healthcare use and care quality among people with MLTCs for at least one minoritised ethnic group, compared to the White majority population.

2.5. Data Analysis

Owing to the lack of a common definition of healthcare use and care quality, the different domains of healthcare use and care quality assessed, the variety of conditions explored and the different ethnic group categories assessed in the included studies, we conducted a narrative synthesis of the findings. We present the findings of the synthesis in themes, and supplement the reporting with tables and figures. The findings are presented in two sections. First, we provide an overview of the studies that report healthcare use and care quality across ethnic groups of people with MLTCs, including the participant characteristics, domains of healthcare and care quality assessed, and types of health conditions under investigation. Second, we present the evidence of ethnic inequalities in healthcare use among people with MLTCs from the studies that went beyond counting only two long-term conditions. We use the terminology used by authors to describe ethnic categories in their studies.

3. Results

3.1. Overview of Included Studies

We identified 621 titles from the electronic search (See Figure 1, which is based on PRISMA guidelines [47]). After removal of duplicates and studies identified as ineligible from the title or abstract, 42 papers were eligible for further evaluation. A further 28 studies were excluded because, despite reporting on the key concepts of interest (i.e., MLTCS, ethnicity, healthcare use), some reported MLTCs and healthcare use separately ($n = 21$), others reported inequalities in healthcare for one health condition ($n = 5$) and others did not compare healthcare use across the different ethnic groups ($n = 2$). Consequently, 14 studies were included in the review, with five of these studies contributing to the evidence on ethnic inequalities in healthcare use in people with MLTCs living in the UK. These were studies in which the authors counted more than two long-term conditions and not just two conditions. The former are more likely to illuminate patterns of ethnic inequality among those with complex medical needs and greater use of healthcare [39,40].

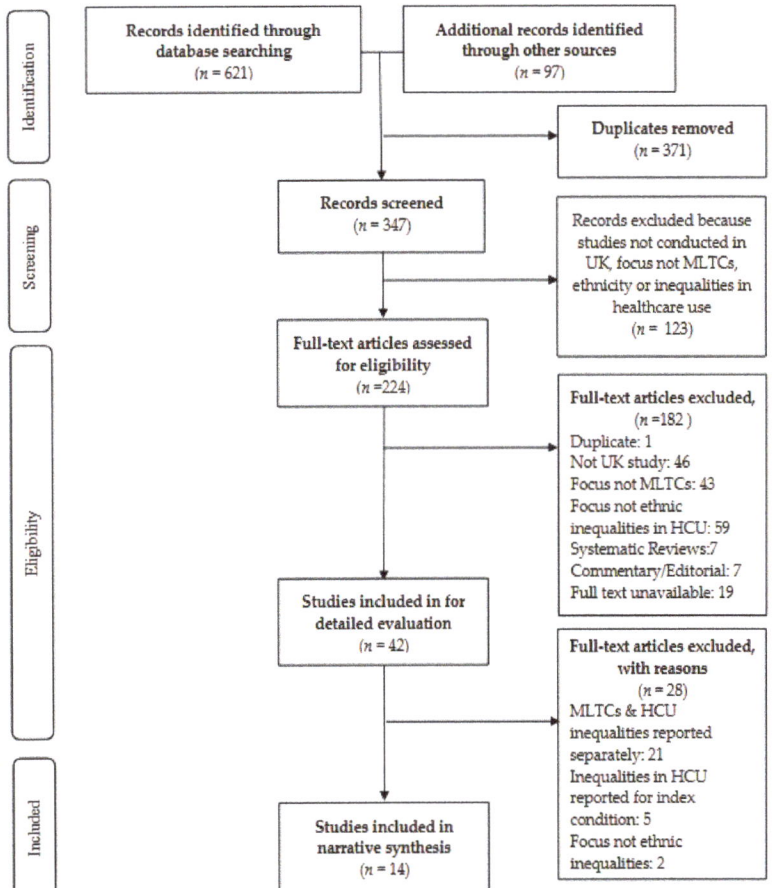

Figure 1. PRISMA flowchart [47].

The 14 studies included in this review were published between 2001 and 2021. There were three national studies [48–50] and 11 local studies conducted in Birmingham [51], Leicester [52] and London [53–60]. The number of participants in the included studies ranged from 45 to nearly 61.5 million. The majority of studies used patient records. In eight of the 14 studies, data from primary care records were analysed [48,54,56–61]. The remaining studies used hospital records ($n = 2$) [49,50] and records from specialist services such as Diabetes Outpatient Clinics ($n = 2$) [52,55]. One study used data from the Comorbidity Dual Diagnosis Study [53], and another used data from a community-based Mental Health and Substance Misuse services survey [51].

3.2. Participant Characteristics

3.2.1. Ethnic Group Identification

Nine of the 14 included studies explicitly reported how ethnicity was identified (64%). Of these, participants self-reported their ethnic identity in seven studies [53–57,60,61]. In one study, ethnicity was assigned by keyworkers [51], and in another study, computerised name recognition software was used to identify South Asian people [52].

3.2.2. Ethnic Group Categorisation

Of the 14 included studies, two compared ethnic variations in healthcare use among people with MLTCs between two ethnic group categories. Of these studies, White people were compared to Black [58] and South Asian people [52]. Three studies categorised their participants into three ethnic group categories [54–56], and two studies compared outcomes across four ethnic groups [53,57]. The remaining studies grouped their participants into five or more ethnic group categories ($n = 7$) [48–51,59–61].

3.2.3. Missing Ethnicity Data

Information concerning missing ethnicity data was available in nine of the 14 included studies (64%). In two of these studies, those with missing ethnicity data were labelled as missing/unknown and included in the analyses [48,49]. In the remaining seven studies, participants with missing ethnicity data were excluded from the analyses [51,54–57,59,60]. One study excluded participants who were of 'Other' ethnicity due to the heterogeneity by ethnicity within the group [60]. Only one study conducted sensitivity analyses to ascertain if the results would differ if those with missing ethnicity data were excluded [48].

3.2.4. Gender and Age

There were 11 studies that reported the gender profile of the participants. One study included only female participants [61], and the remaining ten studies included both male and female participants [48,51–56,58–60]. Of the 14 included studies, six reported the mean age and standard deviation (SD). The average age of participants in these studies ranged from 26.8 (SD = 5.9) years to 66 (SD = 8.5) years [48,52,53,55,60,61]. Four studies included participants aged 18 years and above [51,54,57,59]. In one study, participants were aged 25 years and above [56], and in another, they were aged 16 years and above. [58]. The focus of one study was on children and young people aged between 10 years and 24 years [49], while another study included participants aged 10 years and over [50].

3.3. Domains of Healthcare Use and Care Quality Assessed in Included Studies

Table 1 below lists the domains and sub-domains of healthcare use and care quality assessed in the included studies. The most frequently assessed domain was disease management/monitoring ($n = 6$). Of these studies, the authors examined ethnic differences in diabetes management and cardiovascular risk factors monitoring among people with MLTCs. These were measured by assessing HbA1c levels, cholesterol levels, smoking status, protein urea levels and Body Mass Index, [52,54,55,57,58,60]. One study assessed ethnic differences in health screening, including mammography and cervical smears, among people with psychosis and comorbidities [58]. There were three studies that reported on ethnic differences in prescriptions among people with MLTCs [55,57,61]. Another three studies reported on the use of hospital services, including admission and length of hospital stay [49,50,53]. Few studies looked at disease progression ($n = 2$), mortality/risk of mortality ($n = 2$) and quality of treatment ($n = 2$). One study assessed the use of Mental Health and Substance Misuse services among people with severe mental health problems who use substances problematically [51].

Table 1. Domains and sub-domains of healthcare use and care quality assessed in included studies.

Domains of Healthcare Use/Care Quality	Number of Studies	Sub-Domains of Healthcare Use and Care Quality
Disease management/monitoring	6	<ul><li>Monitoring glycaemic control/HbA1c levels [52,54,55,57,60]</li><li>Monitoring of cholesterol levels [54,55,57,58]</li><li>Monitoring of blood pressure levels [54,57,58]</li><li>Monitoring of smoking habit [55,58]</li><li>Body Mass Index [58]</li><li>Monitoring of protein urea levels [55]</li><li>Cervical smears [58]</li><li>Mammography [58]</li></ul>
Prescriptions	3	<ul><li>Statins [57]</li><li>Anti-depressants and anxiolytics [61]</li><li>ACE inhibitors, β-blockers, calcium channel blockers, α-blockers, diuretics [55]</li></ul>
Use of hospital services	3	<ul><li>Emergency admission [49]</li><li>Hospital admission [53]</li><li>Alcohol-related admissions [50]</li><li>Length of stay in hospital [53]</li></ul>
Mortality/Risk of Mortality	2	<ul><li>In-hospital mortality [48]</li><li>Risk of death [56]</li></ul>
Disease progression	2	<ul><li>Rate of renal decline [55,56]</li></ul>
Treatment quality	2	<ul><li>Incorrect treatment [59]</li><li>Complex treatment [55]</li></ul>
Tertiary service utilisation	1	<ul><li>Use of Mental Health and Substance Misuse services [51]</li></ul>

3.4. Studies Reporting on Ethnic Differences in Patterns of Healthcare Use and Care Quality among People with Multiple Long-Term Conditions Living in the UK

Of the 14 included studies, 12 studies (86%) specified an index condition when reporting on ethnic differences in healthcare use and care quality among people with MLTCs (Table 2). The most frequently cited index conditions were diabetes (n = 6) [48,52,54–56,60] and mental health conditions (n = 4) [51,53,58,61]. One study focused on people with hypertension [59], and another assessed alcohol-related conditions as a comorbidity [50].

Two studies (14%) did not specify an index condition when examining ethnic inequalities in patterns of healthcare use and care quality among people with MLTCs. Of these studies, one assessed risk factor management among people with cardiovascular multimorbidity [57], while the other assessed emergency admissions and long-term conditions in children and young people [49].

3.5. Evidence of Ethnic Inequalities in Healthcare Use among People with Multiple Long-Term Conditions

In this review, five studies also counted more than two long-term conditions and are likely to give us insight into people with complex healthcare needs and greater use of healthcare [39,40]. Four studies focused on disease management, and one study focused on use of hospital services, in particular, emergency admissions. It would be inappropriate to combine their results because the studies represent different domains of healthcare use. Consequently, we discuss these two domains separately in the following section.

Table 2. Characteristics of included studies.

Study ID	Study Design	Geographical Location	Data Source	Sample Size	Participant Characteristics	Ethnic Group Categories	Number of Conditions	Index Condition	Sub-Domain of Healthcare	Covariates
Afuwape, 2006 [53]	Retrospective cohort	Local	Comorbidity Dual Diagnosis Study	213	%Female: 16; Mean Age: 37 years	White, Black Caribbean, Black African, Black British	2	Psychotic illness	Hospital admission, length of stay in hospital, service satisfaction	-
Barron, 2020 [48]	Cross-sectional	National	General practice records	61,414,470	%Female: 50.1; Mean Age (SD): 40.9 (23.2)	Asian, Black, Mixed, Other, White, Unknown	2	Diabetes,	In-hospital mortality	-
Barry, 2015 [50]	Cross-sectional	National	Hospital Episode Statistics	264,870	%Female: NR; Age: 10+ years	White British, White Irish, Black Caribbean, Black African, SA—Pakistani and Bangladeshi, SA—Indian	2	Alcohol-related health conditions	Hospital admissions	-
Das-Munshi, 2021 [60]	Longitudinal study	Local	Primary care records	56,770	%Female: 46; Mean Age (SD): 63 (14)	White British, Irish, Black African, Black Caribbean, Bangladeshi, Indian, Pakistani, Chinese	2	Diabetes	Glycaemic management	age, gender, deprivation
Earle, 2001 [55]	Retrospective case note review	Local	Diabetes Outpatient Clinic	45	%Female: 36; Mean Age (SD): 66 (8.5)	Indo-Asian, African-Caribbean, Caucasian	2	Diabetes	Systolic and diastolic blood pressure, glycaemic control, and usage of ACE inhibitors, β-blockers, calcium channel blockers, α-blockers, diuretics, rate of renal decline, antihypertensive regimen	-

Table 2. *Cont.*

Study ID	Study Design	Geographical Location	Data Source	Sample Size	Participant Characteristics	Ethnic Group Categories	Number of Conditions	Index Condition	Sub-Domain of Healthcare	Covariates
Graham, 2001 [51]	Cross-sectional	Local	Community-based Mental Health and Substance Misuse services	498	%Female: 22.2; Age: 18+ years	White UK, African-Caribbean, Asian, European, Irish, Mixed race, Black other, Other	2	Severe mental illness	Use of Mental Health and Substance Misuse services	-
Mathur, 2018 [56]	Observational community-based cohort study with nested case-control	Local	General practice records	99,648	%Female: 56; Age: 25+ years	White, South Asian, Black	2	Diabetes	Rate of decline, and risk of death	age, sex and baseline measures of HbA1c, eGFR, CVD, ACE/ARB and diabetes duration
Prady, 2016 [61]	Cross-sectional	Local	Primary care records	2234	%Female: 100; Mean Age (SD): 26.8 (5.9)	White British, Pakistani, Mixed, Indian, White non-British, Black, Bangladeshi, Other	2	Common mental disorders	Drug prescription for common mental disorders	-
Schofield, 2012 [59]	Cross-sectional	Local	Lambeth DataNet	28,320	%Female: 50.9; Age: 18+ years	White, Mixed, Asian or Asian British, Black or Black British, Chinese or Other	2	Hypertension	NICE recommended treatment	-
Alshamsan, 2011 [54]	Cross-sectional	Local	Electronic medical records	6690	%Female: 49.1; Age: 18 years	White, Black, South Asian	10	Diabetes	Diabetes management (HbA1c, total cholesterol, and blood pressure levels)	age, sex, diabetes duration, BMI, socioeconomic status, and practice level clustering

79

Table 2. Cont.

Study ID	Study Design	Geographical Location	Data Source	Sample Size	Participant Characteristics	Ethnic Group Categories	Number of Conditions	Index Condition	Sub-Domain of Healthcare	Covariates
Mathur, 2011 [57]	Cross-sectional	Local	Primary care records	6274	%Female: NR; Age: 18+ years	White, South Asian, Black, Other	5	-	Cardiovascular multimorbidity risk management, cholesterol, blood pressure, blood glucose levels HbA1c levels, statin prescriptions	age and sex, clustered by general practice
Mehta, 2011 [52]	Cross-sectional study	Local	Outpatient diabetes clinic	5664	%Female: 45.6; Mean Age (SD): 33 (13)	South Asian, White European	12	Diabetes	Diabetes management (glycaemic control)	-
Pinto, 2010 [58]	Cross-sectional study	Local	Lambeth DataNet	1090	%Female: 39.9; Age: 16+ years	White, Black	5	Psychosis	Health screening and chronic disease monitoring measures (record of cervical smears, mammograms, cholesterol testing, blood pressure readings and smoking status); BMI recorded	age and IMD-2004 score
Wijlaars, 2018 [49]	Cross-sectional study	National	Hospital Episode Statistics	763,199	%Female: NR; Age range: 10–24 years	White, Black, Asian, Mixed, Unknown	9	-	Emergency admission	age, sex, IMD, transition

ACE: Angiotensin-converting-enzyme inhibitors; ARB: Angiotensin II Receptor Blockers; BMI: Body Mass Index; CVD: Cardiovascular disease; eGFR: estimated glomerular filtration rate; HbA1c: Haemoglobin A1c; IMD: Index of Multiple Deprivation; NICE: National Institute for Health and Care Excellence; NR: Not reported; SD: Standard Deviation.

3.5.1. Ethnic Inequalities in Disease Management among People with Multiple Long-Term Conditions

The four studies that suggest that there are ethnic inequalities across different domains of disease management among people with MLTCs are local studies that analysed data from primary care records using a cross-sectional study design, where the authors assessed the outcomes at a single point in time [52,54,57,58]. The sample sizes ranged from 1090 participants to 6690 participants, and comparisons were made between White participants and Black [54,57,58], South Asian [52,54,57], Asian [49] and those who self-identified as belonging to Mixed [49,57] and 'Other' ethnic groups [57]. Three of these studies specified an index condition: diabetes [52,54] and psychosis [58]. Mehta and colleagues (2011) assessed the relationship between glycaemic control, chronic disease comorbidity and ethnicity in people with diabetes. They found that among patients with Type 2 diabetes mellitus, the excess odds of having suboptimal glycaemic control (HbA1c $\geq$ 7%) was 1.86 (95% CI: 1.49 to 2.32) for South Asians, with a comorbidity relative to White Europeans. Taking into consideration cardiac disease comorbidity and non-cardiac disease comorbidity, South Asians (compared to White Europeans) with Type 2 diabetes had an excess risk of having suboptimal glycaemic control, with odds ratios of 1.91 (95% CI: 1.49 to 2.44) and 2.27 (95% CI: 1.50 to 3.43), respectively.

Alshamsan and colleagues (2011) set out to examine ethnic inequalities in diabetes management among people with and without comorbid health conditions after a period of sustained investment in quality improvement in the UK [54]. After adjusting for age, sex, diabetes duration, BMI, socioeconomic status and practice level clustering, they found that the presence of two or more cardiovascular comorbidities was associated with similar blood pressure control among White people and South Asian patients when compared with White people without comorbidity [54]. The mean difference in systolic blood pressure was +1.5 mmHg (95% Confidence Interval (CI): −0.3–3.3) and +1.4 mmHg (95% CI: −0.8–3.6), respectively [54]. In contrast, the presence of two or more cardiovascular comorbidities was associated with worse blood pressure control among Black patients, with a mean difference in systolic blood pressure of +6.2 mmHg (95% CI: 3.5–8.5) [54].

Similarly, Mathur and colleagues (2011) investigated the likelihood of reaching clinical targets for blood pressure, total serum cholesterol and glycated haemoglobin by ethnic group for patients with MLTCs [57]. Their results show that after adjusting for age, sex and clustering by general practice, among those with three to five cardiovascular morbidities, Black patients were less likely to meet their blood pressure target, with adjusted odds ratios (AORs) of 0.63 (95% CI: 0.53 to 0.75) [57]. However, there were no differences apparent between White and South Asian patients [57]. Among those with three to five morbidities, both South Asian and Black patients were less likely to reach an HbA1c target of $\leq$7.5% compared to White patients, with adjusted odds ratios of 0.69 (95% CI: 0.60 to 0.79) and 0.79 (95% CI: 0.67 to 0.93), respectively [57]. For total serum cholesterol in patients with three to five morbidities, South Asian patients were consistently more likely to reach the target of $\leq$4 mmol/L than patients of White ethnicity, with adjusted odds ratios of 1.65 (95% CI: 1.49 to 1.83), but Black patients were less likely to meet the cholesterol target (AOR: 0.83 (95% CI: 0.71 to 0.97)) [57]. Patterns in statin prescribing mirrored those for control of total cholesterol; compared to White patients, South Asian patients were more likely to be prescribed statin, but Black patients were less likely to be prescribed statin [57].

The findings from Pinto and colleagues (2010) also point to ethnic inequalities in disease management in people with MLTCs. They investigated ethnic differences in the primary care management of patients with psychosis and analysed health screening and monitoring rates according to the presence of comorbidity [58]. After adjusting for age and area-level deprivation, no significant differences were evident between White and Black patients in relation to cholesterol tests, blood pressure reading, BMI, smoking status and mammogram screening rates [58]. However, they found lower cervical smear rates in Black women with previously abnormal cervical smears, with an odds ratio of 0.22 (95% CI: 0.07–0.69) [58].

3.5.2. Ethnic Inequalities in Emergency Admission among People with Multiple Long-Term Conditions

The findings of one study are suggestive of ethnic inequalities in hospital admissions, in particular, emergency admissions, in people with MLTCs [49]. The study conducted by Wijlaars and colleagues (2018) was a national cross-sectional study that used hospital records. The 763,199 children and young people who took part in this study were categorised into the following ethnic groups: White, Black, Asian, Mixed and Unknown [49]. The authors set out to explore whether changes in emergency admission rates during transition from paediatric to adult hospital services differed in children and young people (aged between 10 and 24 years) with and without underlying long-term conditions [49]. They considered emergency admission to be a clinically important indicator of poor health, which might be affected by the quality of healthcare received from the community during transition [49]. They excluded pregnancy-related admissions and injury-related admissions, with the exception of intentional self-harm, which could signify an underlying mental health condition [49]. After adjusting for age, sex, deprivation and transition, Black and Asian ethnicity were associated with an increase in emergency admission rates for children and young people with LTCs (Incidence Rate Ratio (IRR): 2.49, 99% CI: 2.39 to 2.60)) and Asian ethnicity (IRR: 1.13, 99% CI: 1.08 to 1.19) [49]. This study also found that across the whole sample, the rates of emergency admission increased at the age when young people transition from paediatric care to adult healthcare [49].

4. Discussion

4.1. Summary of Findings

Of the studies that counted more than two long-term conditions, there were no studies that reported on care quality and few explored ethnic inequalities in healthcare use among people with MLTCs. The findings from these few studies indicate that there are ethnic inequalities in emergency admission and some aspects of disease management among people with MLTCs. Both Asian and Black children and young people with MLTCs were more likely to have higher rates of emergency admissions when compared to their White counterparts [49]. The findings also suggest that some minoritised ethnic groups with MLTCs are at particular risk of suboptimal disease management. In particular, Black people with MLTCs were found to be less likely to be prescribed statins and to reach set targets for blood pressure, HbA1c levels and total serum cholesterol levels when compared to other ethnic groups [54,57]. In addition, Black women with MLTCs and previously abnormal smears had lower cervical smear rates compared to White women [58]. In contrast, South Asian patients with MLTCs were more likely to have better control of their blood pressure and total serum cholesterol, but less likely to meet targets for HbA1c levels when compared to patients with MLTCs from other ethnic groups [52,54,57]. However, given the few studies identified, the different domains of healthcare use under investigation and the different health conditions explored, our conclusions are tentative.

4.2. Comparison with Other Reviews

To our knowledge, this is the first review of studies reporting on ethnic inequalities in these domains of healthcare use among people with MLTCs in the UK. Therefore, it is difficult to make comparisons with other reviews that focus on different populations or particular dimensions of healthcare use. However, some of the findings of this review complement those of other reviews of ethnic inequalities in healthcare use that have not focused on MLTCs. For example, the evidence from a review conducted by Dixon-Woods and colleagues (2005) found that utilisation of primary care was generally high among most minoritised ethnic group populations, though there were important exceptions [29]. Just as in this review, they found that uptake of some preventative services (e.g., breast and cervical screening) was relatively lower for minoritised ethnic group people [29]. Their findings also suggest that there are important variations within and between minoritised ethnic groups in their utilisation of healthcare [29]. This variation was also evident in our review, as South Asian patients with MLTCs had better blood pressure and cholesterol control compared to Black patients with MLTCs [57].

4.3. Mechanisms

The association between MLTCs, socioeconomic status and healthcare use has been reported; people with MLTCs living in poverty have been found to be less likely to use health services than those with financial resources [62]. Given the close link between ethnicity and socioeconomic disadvantage [29], it is important to consider socio-economic disadvantage when interpreting ethnic inequalities in healthcare. Of the five studies that also counted more than two long-term health conditions, two adjusted for area-level deprivation and one adjusted for socioeconomic status (and other factors, e.g., age, sex and cardiovascular risk) [49,54,58]. Ethnic inequalities in disease management were still evident after adjustment of socio-economic deprivation (and other factors on the explanatory pathway), with Black people reported to have poorer disease management [54,58], and Black and Asian children more likely to have increased rates of emergency admission [49]. While Mathur and colleagues did not adjust for individual level deprivation, their analysis focused on populations living in the eight most socially deprived localities in Britain [57].

That ethnic inequalities for some groups still persisted after adjustment of deprivation (and other factors) in some of these studies suggests that the observed inequalities are likely to be driven by other factors. Given the complex, intersecting processes that shape the development of MLTCs and determine the use of healthcare and care quality [18,27], the mechanisms underlying the observed ethnic inequalities are likely to be the result of the interplay of several processes. Individual-level factors, such as poor management among some people [54] and cultural barriers to effective self-management [52], have been proposed as reasons underlying observed ethnic differences. However, we argue that understanding ethnic inequalities in healthcare use requires an appreciation of the ways in which individual-level processes (e.g., ethnicity and class) intersect with macrolevel processes (e.g., racism and discrimination) to produce inequalities [63]. International studies have illustrated how racism and negative discriminatory practices can result in mistrust of healthcare professionals and create barriers to compliance with treatment, timely diagnoses and treatment and healthcare use [64–66]. These processes can impact efforts to manage MLTCs among minoritised ethnic group populations, thereby resulting in ethnic inequalities. Further evidence is provided by Ben and colleagues (2017), who conducted a systematic review and meta-analysis of quantitative studies reporting on the associations between self-reported racism and different dimensions of healthcare service utilisation [67]. They found that people experiencing racism were approximately two to three times more likely to report reduced trust in healthcare systems and professionals, lower satisfaction with health services and perceived care quality, and compromised communication and relationships with healthcare providers [67]. As such, the influences of racism and discrimination cannot be ignored, as they directly and indirectly create conditions that disadvantage many from minoritised ethnic groups, which in turn can result in ethnic inequalities in healthcare use.

4.4. Strengths and Limitations

A limitation of this review is that a single reviewer initially screened the titles and abstracts and excluded irrelevant studies, which might have introduced a level of reviewer bias. It is therefore possible that we may have missed relevant studies [68]. However, a manual search of the reference list of key studies was conducted to increase the likelihood of identifying as many relevant studies as possible. In addition, a subset of studies (10%) were double-screened and extracted prior to the independent screening and extraction to reduce reviewer bias. While the interest in MLTCs and associations with healthcare utilisation, costs and healthcare systems has grown over the last decade [33], the guidelines to optimise care for people with MLTCs are fairly recent. For example, in 2016, the National Institute for Health and Care Excellence published guidance for healthcare professionals, people with MLTCs and their families/carers [69]. Thus, there has not been much time to assess care quality among people with MLTCs, and thus studies in this area are sparse. Those that have done so have not explored ethnic inequalities in care quality [70,71]. As such, they were not included in this review. Relatedly, there were no qualitative studies that met the inclusion criteria; therefore, the findings of this review are based on the evidence from quantitative studies. It is important to remember that evidence from qualitative studies is equally important as it gives us an in-depth understanding of the experiences of people with MLTCs while illuminating the processes that can lead to inequalities in healthcare use and care quality as reported above [23]. The findings from these studies can help healthcare systems adapt to the needs of people with MLTCs, thereby improving their health [72].

Despite these limitations, this review has several strengths. First, the review was informed by the PRISMA guidelines to facilitate the transparent reporting of the review process [47,73]. Second, we conducted the electronic search across a range of databases to locate (un)published studies and hand-searched the reference lists of relevant studies and systematic reviews to reduce the likelihood of missing key studies. Third, when synthesising the results of studies that contributed to the evidence of ethnic inequalities in healthcare use and care quality among people with MLTCs, we only included studies that also counted more than two long-term conditions to give us insight into ethnic inequalities in healthcare use among people with complex healthcare needs [40].

This review also highlighted the limitations of the studies conducted in this area. For example, the review has illuminated the limited range of long-term conditions considered. The majority of studies included in this review focused on index conditions, particularly diabetes [52,54,56], mental health conditions [51,53,58,61] and cardiovascular disease [59]. As such, we have a partial understanding of ethnic inequalities in healthcare use among people with MLTCs. In addition, many of these studies categorised their participants into broad ethnic categories. In the five studies that contributed to the evidence of ethnic inequalities in healthcare use among people with MLTCs, minoritised ethnic group people were often clustered into Black [49,54,57,58], South Asian [52,54,57], Asian [49], Mixed [49,57] and Other [57] ethnic categories. It is important to note that in certain circumstances, combining individual ethnic groups into larger categories can facilitate the identification of broad patterns, given that some may have shared experiences of racism, discrimination, marginalisation and social exclusion [53]. However, these broad ethnic categories may mask the extent of intra-ethnic inequalities. For example, as reported above, Black people with MLTCs may be at particular risk of poor disease management [54,57,58]. However, the Black ethnic group population is diverse, and healthcare use and care quality might vary among the different subgroups. Findings from Afuwape and colleagues (2006) exemplify this notion [53]. They examined the characteristics of a community cohort with psychosis and comorbid substance misuse by ethnic group and found that Black Caribbean people had the longest mean contact with mental health services compared to Black African, Black Other and White patients [53]. This study highlights the value of disaggregating broad ethnic group categories. This nuanced approach is more likely to lead to the identification of those who are most vulnerable to developing MLTCs and in greatest need of intervention, and moves away from essentialising minoritised populations.

It is likely that reported ethnic inequalities are underestimated. The studies that contributed to evidence of ethnic inequalities in disease management and emergency admission all analysed data from patient records from primary and secondary care. Ethnicity recording across the National Health Service has improved markedly over the past decade [74]. However, there is evidence that ethnicity coding for patients who self-identify as White British is recorded correctly, but there are higher levels of incorrect coding of the ethnicity of patients from minoritised ethnic groups [75]. Others have also found that in most cases, hospital records over-represent 'Other' ethnic group categories while under-representing 'Mixed' ethnic groups and some specific ethnic groups [76]. Incomplete or inaccurate recording of ethnicity data makes it difficult to reliably assess health needs, access and outcomes across different ethnic groups [76]. Many of the studies included in this review excluded people in the 'Other' ethnic group. It is therefore possible that these studies underestimate the true extent of ethnic inequalities in emergency admission and disease management among people with MLTCs.

4.5. Implications

The observed inequalities in disease management across ethnic groups suggest that universal coverage and investment in quality initiatives may not be adequate and that enhanced strategies or targeted interventions are needed to improve equity of disease management across populations [52,54]. It is possible that the observed ethnic inequalities in emergency admission among children and young people with MLTCs from minoritised ethnic groups might not only be due to a higher level of ill health but also the poor management of health conditions in primary care. This finding also suggests that ethnic inequalities in healthcare use and care quality start early in the life course. However, further research is required to unpack these findings.

As mentioned previously, the minoritised ethnic group population in the UK is diverse and consists of those born outside the UK and those born in the UK [28]. With different migration histories, the length of residence in the UK among those born outside the UK will vary and may impact healthcare utilisation. Interestingly, studies exploring the association between healthcare use and the number of years spent in the UK have found mixed evidence [77–79]. One study found no differences in healthcare use between non-UK-born migrants and the UK-born population [79]. Another reported that international migrants were less likely to have used secondary care than established residents and within-England migrants [77]. These findings mirror those of Saunders and colleagues (2021), who found that newly arrived migrants have lower healthcare utilisation levels than the UK-born population, a pattern partially explained by younger age and lower levels of ill health [78]. However, these studies do not explicitly focus on populations with MLTCs. Given that none of the studies included in the review considered length of residence in the UK, further research is required to ascertain whether there is an association between length of residence, healthcare use among people with MLTCs and observed ethnic inequalities reported in this review.

The limitations of the studies identified in this review reflect the methodological challenges of investigating ethnic inequalities in healthcare use and care quality among people with MLTCs [29]. Evidently, more work is required to develop a comprehensive understanding of the extent of ethnic inequalities in healthcare use and care quality among people with MLTCs living in the UK. Future studies would need to consider how best to address the challenge of varying definitions for healthcare use and care quality. They would need to include people with a range of MLTCs and include more ethnic group categories, including marginalised White populations (e.g., Gypsy, Roma and Traveller communities), who have been reported to have poor health outcomes when compared to people from other communities [80,81]. They would also need to assess ethnic variations in other domains of healthcare and account for both individual-level and area-level deprivation and how they intersect with other factors. Such studies would add to the sparse evidence base in this area and allow for national and international comparisons.

In this review, studies that counted more than two long-term conditions that reported on care quality were lacking. If we consider that the assessment of care quality among people with MLTCs is in its infancy, this finding is not surprising. However, future studies should also aim to explore ethnic inequalities in care quality. Studies that adopt a longitudinal approach to analysing ethnic inequalities in healthcare use and care quality are required. These studies would give insight into the longitudinal association of MLTCs, healthcare use and care quality delivered with health outcomes across different ethnic groups [7,27]. Future studies would also benefit from conceptualising and analysing ethnic inequalities in healthcare use and care quality in people with MLTCs through an intersectional lens that considers the complex, multifaceted processes [63] that lead to the development of MLTCs and influence healthcare use and care quality. Such work could illuminate the extent to which key explanatory pathways, including racism and discrimination, contribute to the development of ethnic inequalities. The findings of such analyses could inform discussions on how ethnic inequalities in healthcare use and care quality among people with MLTCs can be effectively addressed.

5. Conclusions

This review identified few studies reporting on ethnic inequalities in healthcare use among people with MLTCs living in the UK. It illustrates a sparse evidence base, characterised by studies focusing on different health conditions and different domains of healthcare, which precludes us from drawing any firm conclusions. Indeed, the few studies identified are suggestive of ethnic inequalities in emergency admissions and particular domains of disease management among people with MLTCs. However, the methodological limitations of the studies identified in this review hamper our understanding of the full extent of ethnic inequalities in healthcare use and care quality among people with MLTCs. Based on these limitations, we call for action and have provided directions for future studies that we hope will provide evidence that can inform targeted prevention and management strategies to reduce inequalities in healthcare use and care quality among people with MLTCs.

Author Contributions: L.B. and M.S. formulated the overarching research goals and aims of the systematic review. L.B., M.S. and B.H. planned the methodological approach and developed the protocol. B.H. formulated the search terms in discussion with L.B. and M.S. B.H. conducted the search, imported the results and removed the duplicate studies. B.H. and L.B. screened and extracted data from a random sample of studies (10%). B.H. screened and extracted data from the remaining studies. B.H. conducted the narrative synthesis with substantial methodological and intellectual input from L.B. and M.S. B.H. prepared the manuscript and wrote the initial draft. L.B. and M.S. critically reviewed and commented on the initial and subsequent drafts. When reviewing the manuscripts, both L.B. and M.S. verified the data from the studies that contributed to the evidence of ethnic inequalities in healthcare use and care quality among people with multiple long-term conditions. All authors had full access to the included studies. B.H. submitted the manuscript for publication. All authors have read and agreed to the published version of the manuscript.

Funding: This work is funded by The Health Foundation [AIMS 1874695].

Institutional Review Board Statement: Not applicable, this study did not involve humans.

Informed Consent Statement: Not applicable, this study did not involve humans.

Data Availability Statement: This study did not report any supporting data.

Conflicts of Interest: M.S. is employed by The Health Foundation. The authors declare no conflict of interest.

Appendix A

Table A1. Search terms used when searching Applied Social Sciences Index and Abstracts.

10	MLTCs + Ethnicity + inequality + quality care + country	(((MAINSUBJECT.EXACT.EXPLODE ("Mixed ethnicity") OR MAINSUBJECT.EXACT. EXPLODE ("Ethnicity") OR ab,ti,if ("Ethnic Group?" OR "african continental ancestry group" OR Arab OR Africa? OR Afro? OR Asian OR "Asian Continental Ancestry Group" OR "Asylum seeker" OR Bangladesh? OR Black OR "BME" OR "BAME" OR Caribbean OR China OR Chinese OR Cultur? OR Divers? OR Ethnic? OR Gypsy OR India? OR Irish OR Migrant OR Minorit? OR Mixed OR "Mixed ethnic?" OR "Multiple ethnic?" OR Multi rac? OR 'Other White' OR Pakistan? OR Roma OR "White Other" OR Refugee? OR race OR racial? OR "South Asian" OR "European Continental Ancestry Group")) AND (MAINSUBJECT.EXACT ("England and Wales") OR MAINSUBJECT.EXACT ("Channel Islands") OR MAINSUBJECT.EXACT ("UK") OR MAINSUBJECT.EXACT ("Scotland") OR MAINSUBJECT.EXACT ("England") OR MAINSUBJECT.EXACT ("Northern Ireland") OR MAINSUBJECT.EXACT ("Wales") OR ti, ab, if ("United Kingdom" OR "UK" OR England OR Wales OR Scotland OR "Northern Ireland" OR Britain OR "Great Britain")) AND (ti, ab, if ("Multiple Chronic Conditions" OR Co morbid? OR Multi morbidity OR Multi patholog? OR "multiple condition?" OR "Multiple health condition?" OR "Multiple health problems" OR "Multiple medical conditions" OR "Multiple medical problems" OR "Pluri$patholog?" OR Polymorbid? OR "multiple illness?" OR "Multiple Chronic Health Conditions" OR "Multiple Chronic Medical Conditions" OR "multiple chronic illness?") OR MAINSUBJECT.EXACT.EXPLODE ("Comorbidity"))) NOT (MAINSUBJECT.EXACT. EXPLODE ("USA") OR MAINSUBJECT.EXACT.EXPLODE ("North America") OR MAINSUBJECT.EXACT.EXPLODE ("Canada") OR MAINSUBJECT.EXACT.EXPLODE ("Australia") OR MAINSUBJECT.EXACT.EXPLODE ("New Zealand") OR MAINSUBJECT.EXACT. EXPLODE ("South America") OR MAINSUBJECT.EXACT.EXPLODE ("Central America") OR ti, ab, if ("Americas" OR "USA" OR America OR "North America" OR Canada OR Australia OR "New Zealand"))) AND (ti, ab, if ("Health Equity" OR "Healthcare disparit?" OR Inequalit? OR disparit? OR "Healthcare Disparit?" OR "Health care Disparit?" OR "Health-care Disparit?" OR "Health Care Inequalit?" OR "Healthcare Inequalit?" OR "Health-care Inequalit?" OR "inequalit? in healthcare" OR "inequalit? in health care" OR "inequality in health-care" OR "disparit? in healthcare" OR "disparit? in health care" OR "disparit? in health-care" OR "inequit?" OR "health inequit?") OR MAINSUBJECT.EXACT ("Health inequalities")) AND (ti, ab, if ("Quality of Health Care" OR "Patient Acceptance of Health Care" OR "Patient Satisfaction" OR "Health Care Quality, Access, and Evaluation" OR "Care Quality" OR "Quality of care" OR "Quality of health care" OR "quality of health-care" OR "Quality of healthcare" OR "healthcare quality" OR "health-care quality" OR "health care quality" OR "quality health service" OR "health service quality" OR satisfaction OR dissatisfaction OR satisfied OR dissatisfied OR "effectiveness" OR safety OR responsiveness OR acceptab? OR appropriate? OR timeliness) OR MAINSUBJECT.EXACT. EXPLODE ("Quality of care"))

Table A1. Cont.

9	MLTCs + Ethnicity + Healthcare use + inequality + country	((((MAINSUBJECT.EXACT.EXPLODE ("Mixed ethnicity") OR MAINSUBJECT.EXACT. EXPLODE ("Ethnicity") OR ab,ti,if ("Ethnic Group?" OR "african continental ancestry group" OR Arab OR Africa? OR Afro? OR Asian OR "Asian Continental Ancestry Group" OR "Asylum seeker" OR Bangladesh? OR Black OR "BME" OR "BAME" OR Caribbean OR China OR Chinese OR Cultur? OR Divers? OR Ethnic? OR Gypsy OR India? OR Irish OR Migrant OR Minorit? OR Mixed OR "Mixed ethnic?" OR "Multiple ethnic?" OR Multi rac? OR 'Other White' OR Pakistan? OR Roma OR "White Other" OR Refugee? OR race OR racial? OR "South Asian" OR "European Continental Ancestry Group")) AND (MAINSUBJECT.EXACT ("England and Wales") OR MAINSUBJECT.EXACT ("Channel Islands") OR MAINSUBJECT.EXACT ("UK") OR MAINSUBJECT.EXACT ("Scotland") OR MAINSUBJECT.EXACT ("England") OR MAINSUBJECT.EXACT ("Northern Ireland") OR MAINSUBJECT.EXACT ("Wales") OR ti, ab, if ("United Kingdom" OR "UK" OR England OR Wales OR Scotland OR "Northern Ireland" OR Britain OR "Great Britain")) AND (ti, ab, if ("Multiple Chronic Conditions" OR Co morbid? OR Multi morbidity OR Multi patholog? OR "multiple condition?" OR "Multiple health condition?" OR "Multiple health problems" OR "Multiple medical conditions" OR "Multiple medical problems" OR "Pluri$patholog?" OR Polymorbid? OR "multiple illness?" OR "Multiple Chronic Health Conditions" OR "Multiple Chronic Medical Conditions" OR "multiple chronic illness?") OR MAINSUBJECT.EXACT.EXPLODE ("Comorbidity"))) NOT (MAINSUBJECT.EXACT. EXPLODE ("USA") OR MAINSUBJECT.EXACT.EXPLODE ("North America") OR MAINSUBJECT.EXACT.EXPLODE ("Canada") OR MAINSUBJECT.EXACT.EXPLODE ("Australia") OR MAINSUBJECT.EXACT.EXPLODE ("New Zealand") OR MAINSUBJECT.EXACT. EXPLODE ("South America") OR MAINSUBJECT.EXACT.EXPLODE ("Central America") OR ti, ab, if ("Americas" OR "USA" OR America OR "North America" OR Canada OR Australia OR "New Zealand"))) AND (ti, ab, if ("Health Equity" OR "Healthcare disparit?" OR Inequalit? OR disparit? OR "Healthcare Disparit?" OR "Health care Disparit?" OR "Health-care Disparit?" OR "Health Care Inequalit?" "Healthcare Inequalit?" OR "Health-care Inequalit?" OR "inequalit? in healthcare" OR "inequalit? in health care" OR "inequality in health-care" OR "disparit? in healthcare" OR "disparit? in health care" OR "inequit?" OR "health inequit?") OR MAINSUBJECT.EXACT ("Health inequalities")) AND (ti, ab, if ("Delivery of Health Care" OR "Tertiary Healthcare" OR "Primary Health Care" OR "Health Care Quality, Access, and Evaluation" [Mesh] OR "Community Health Services" OR Healthcare OR health-care OR "health care" OR "health service" OR "health centre" OR "Health centre" OR "medical care" OR "National Health Service" OR "NHS" OR A E OR "Accident and emergency" OR "Acute healthcare" OR "Acute health care" OR "Acute health-care" OR "Acute hospital care" OR "urgent care" OR "emergency care" OR "primary care" OR "general practitioner" OR "GP" OR "General pract? visit" OR "GP visit?" OR "GP consult?" OR "General pract? consult?" OR "medical consult?" "GP services" OR "General practitioner services" OR "physician visit" OR "Family Physician" OR Dental OR Dentist OR dentistry OR "Eye care" OR Optician OR "Oral health" OR Pharmacy OR pharmacies OR "pharmacy service" OR "Secondary care" OR Hospital OR "Hospital visit" OR "hospital admission" OR "Day patient" OR in-patient OR "inpatient" OR outpatient OR out-patient OR referral OR therap? OR "Preventative healthcare" OR "preventative health care" OR "preventative health-care" OR "preventative service" OR "preventative medicine" OR "health outreach" OR screen? OR vaccinat? OR "Palliative care" OR "Case manag?" OR "Community care" OR "Community nurse" OR "Community services?" OR "Tertiary care" OR "tertiary health care" OR "tertiary healthcare" OR "tertiary health-care" OR specialist OR "specialist health service" OR "Mental health service" OR "sexual health service") OR MAINSUBJECT.EXACT.EXPLODE ("Health care"))
8	quality care	ti, ab, if ("Quality of Health Care" OR "Patient Acceptance of Health Care" OR "Patient Satisfaction" OR "Health Care Quality, Access, and Evaluation" OR "Care Quality" OR "Quality of care" OR "Quality of health care" OR "quality of health-care" OR "Quality of healthcare" "healthcare quality" OR "health-care quality" OR "health care quality" OR "quality health service" OR "health service quality" OR satisfaction OR dissatisfaction OR satisfied Or dissatisfied OR "effectiveness" OR safety OR responsiveness OR acceptab? OR appropriate? OR timeliness) OR MAINSUBJECT.EXACT.EXPLODE ("Quality of care")

Table A1. Cont.

7	healthcare utilisation	ti, ab, if ("Delivery of Health Care" OR "Tertiary Healthcare" OR "Primary Health Care" OR "Health Care Quality, Access, and Evaluation" [Mesh] OR "Community Health Services" OR Healthcare OR health-care OR "health care" OR "health service" OR "health centre" OR "Health centre" OR "medical care" OR "National Health Service" OR "NHS" OR A&E OR "Accident and emergency" OR "Acute healthcare" OR "Acute health care" OR "Acute health-care" OR "Acute hospital care" OR "urgent care" OR "emergency care" OR "primary care" OR "general practitioner" OR "GP" OR "General pract? visit" OR "GP visit?" OR "GP consult?" OR "General pract? consult?" OR "medical consult?" "GP services" OR "General practitioner services" OR "physician visit" OR "Family Physician" OR Dental OR Dentist OR dentistry OR "Eye care" OR Optician OR "Oral health" OR Pharmacy OR pharmacies OR "pharmacy service" OR "Secondary care" OR Hospital OR "Hospital visit" OR "hospital admission" OR "Day patient" OR in-patient OR "inpatient" OR outpatient OR out-patient OR referral OR therap? OR "Preventative healthcare" OR "preventative health care" OR "preventative health-care" OR "preventative service" OR "preventative medicine" OR "health outreach" OR screen? OR vaccinat? OR "Palliative care" OR "Case manag?" OR "Community care" OR "Community nurse" OR "Community services?" OR "Tertiary care" OR "tertiary health care" OR "tertiary healthcare" OR "tertiary health-care" OR specialist OR "specialist health service" OR "Mental health service" OR "sexual health service") OR MAINSUBJECT.EXACT.EXPLODE ("Health care")
6	Health inequality	ti, ab, if ("Health Equity" OR "Healthcare dispari?"OR Inequalit? OR disparit? OR "Healthcare Disparit?" OR "Health care Disparit?" OR "Health-care Disparit?" OR "Health Care Inequalit?" "Healthcare Inequalit?" OR "Health-care Inequalit?" OR "inequalit? in healthcare" OR "inequalit? in health care" OR "inequality in health-care" OR "disparit? in healthcare" OR "disparit? in health care" OR "disparit? in health-care" OR "inequit?" OR "health inequit?") OR MAINSUBJECT.EXACT ("Health inequalities")
5	MLTCs + Ethnicity + Country	(#1 AND #2 AND #3) NOT #4 ((MAINSUBJECT.EXACT.EXPLODE ("Mixed ethnicity") OR MAINSUBJECT.EXACT.EXPLODE ("Ethnicity") OR ab,ti,if ("Ethnic Group?" OR "african continental ancestry group" OR Arab OR Africa? OR Afro? OR Asian OR "Asian Continental Ancestry Group" OR "Asylum seeker" OR Bangladesh? OR Black OR "BME" OR "BAME" OR Caribbean OR China OR Chinese OR Cultur? OR Divers? OR Ethnic? OR Gypsy OR India? OR Irish OR Migrant OR Minorit? OR Mixed OR "Mixed ethnic?" OR "Multiple ethnic?" OR Multi$rac? OR 'Other White' OR Pakistan? OR Roma OR "White Other" OR Refugee? OR race OR racial? OR "South Asian" OR "European Continental Ancestry Group")) AND (MAINSUBJECT. EXACT ("England and Wales") OR MAINSUBJECT.EXACT ("Channel Islands") OR MAINSUBJECT.EXACT ("UK") OR MAINSUBJECT.EXACT ("Scotland") OR MAINSUBJECT. EXACT ("England") OR MAINSUBJECT.EXACT ("Northern Ireland") OR MAINSUBJECT. EXACT ("Wales") OR ti, ab, if ("United Kingdom" OR "UK" OR England OR Wales OR Scotland OR "Northern Ireland" OR Britain OR "Great Britain")) AND (ti, ab, if ("Multiple Chronic Conditions" OR Co$morbid? OR Multi$morbidity OR Multi$patholog? OR "multiple condition?" OR "Multiple health condition?" OR "Multiple health problems" OR "Multiple medical conditions" OR "Multiple medical problems" OR "Pluri$patholog?" OR Polymorbid? OR "multiple illness?" OR "Multiple Chronic Health Conditions" or "Multiple Chronic Medical Conditions" OR "multiple chronic illness?") OR MAINSUBJECT.EXACT.EXPLODE ("Comorbidity"))) NOT (MAINSUBJECT.EXACT.EXPLODE ("USA") OR MAINSUBJECT.EXACT.EXPLODE ("North America") OR MAINSUBJECT.EXACT.EXPLODE ("Canada") OR MAINSUBJECT.EXACT. EXPLODE ("Australia") OR MAINSUBJECT.EXACT.EXPLODE ("New Zealand") OR MAINSUBJECT.EXACT.EXPLODE ("South America") OR MAINSUBJECT.EXACT. EXPLODE ("Central America") OR ti, ab, if ("Americas" OR "USA" OR America OR "North America" OR Canada OR Australia OR "New Zealand"))
4	excluded countries	MAINSUBJECT.EXACT.EXPLODE ("USA") OR MAINSUBJECT.EXACT.EXPLODE ("North America") OR MAINSUBJECT.EXACT.EXPLODE ("Canada") OR MAINSUBJECT.EXACT. EXPLODE ("Australia") OR MAINSUBJECT.EXACT.EXPLODE ("New Zealand") OR MAINSUBJECT.EXACT.EXPLODE ("South America") OR MAINSUBJECT.EXACT. EXPLODE ("Central America") OR ti, ab, if ("Americas" OR "USA" OR America OR "North America" OR Canada OR Australia OR "New Zealand")

Table A1. *Cont.*

3	Country	(MAINSUBJECT.EXACT ("England and Wales") OR MAINSUBJECT.EXACT ("Channel Islands") OR MAINSUBJECT.EXACT ("UK") OR MAINSUBJECT.EXACT ("Scotland") OR MAINSUBJECT.EXACT ("England") OR MAINSUBJECT.EXACT ("Northern Ireland") OR MAINSUBJECT.EXACT ("Wales")) OR ti, ab, if ("United Kingdom" OR "UK" OR England OR Wales OR Scotland OR "Northern Ireland" OR Britain OR "Great Britain")
2	Ethnicity	(MAINSUBJECT.EXACT.EXPLODE ("Mixed ethnicity") OR MAINSUBJECT.EXACT. EXPLODE ("Ethnicity")) OR ab,ti,if ("Ethnic Group?" OR "african continental ancestry group" OR Arab OR Africa? OR Afro? OR Asian OR "Asian Continental Ancestry Group" OR "Asylum seeker" OR Bangladesh? OR Black OR "BME" OR "BAME" OR Caribbean OR China OR Chinese OR Cultur? OR Divers? OR Ethnic? OR Gypsy OR India? OR Irish OR Migrant OR Minorit? OR Mixed OR "Mixed ethnic?" OR "Multiple ethnic?" OR Multi$rac? OR 'Other White' OR Pakistan? OR Roma OR "White Other" OR Refugee? OR race OR racial? OR "South Asian" OR "European Continental Ancestry Group")
1	Multiple long-term conditions (MLTCs)	ti, ab, if ("Multiple Chronic Conditions" OR Co$morbid? OR Multi$morbidity OR Multi$patholog? OR "multiple condition?" OR "Multiple health condition?" OR "Multiple health problems" OR "Multiple medical conditions" OR "Multiple medical problems" OR "Pluri$patholog?" OR Polymorbid? OR "multiple illness?" OR "Multiple Chronic Health Conditions" or "Multiple Chronic Medical Conditions" OR "multiple chronic illness?") OR MAINSUBJECT.EXACT.EXPLODE ("Comorbidity")

References

1. Moriarty, J. *Long Term Conditions*; Briefing Paper; Race Equality Foundation: London, UK, 2021.
2. Stafford, M.; Steventon, A.; Thorlby, R.; Fisher, R.; Turton, C.; Deeny, S. Briefing: Understanding the Health Care Needs of People with Multiple Health Conditions [Online]. 2018. Available online: https://www.health.org.uk/sites/default/files/upload/publications/2018/Understanding%20the%20health%20care%20needs%20of%20people%20with%20multiple%20health%20conditions.pdf (accessed on 2 June 2021).
3. National Institute for Health and Care Excellence. Multimorbidity [Online]. 2018. Available online: https://cks.nice.org.uk/topics/multimorbidity/ (accessed on 2 June 2021).
4. Kingston, A.; Robinson, L.; Booth, H.; Knapp, M.; Jagger, C. Projections of multi-morbidity in the older population in England to 2035: Estimates from the Population Ageing and Care Simulation (PACSim) model. *Age Ageing* **2018**, *47*, 374–380. [CrossRef]
5. Whitty, C.J.M.; MacEwen, C.; Goddard, A.; Alderson, D.; Marshall, M.; Calderwood, C.; Atherton, F.; McBride, M.; Atherton, J.; Stokes-Lampard, H.; et al. Rising to the challenge of multimorbidity. *BMJ* **2020**, *368*, l6964. [CrossRef] [PubMed]
6. Barnett, K.; Mercer, S.W.; Norbury, M.; Watt, G.; Wyke, S.; Guthrie, B. Epidemiology of multi-morbidity and implications for health care, research and medical education: A cross-sectional study. *Lancet Online* **2012**, *380*, 37–43. [CrossRef]
7. The Academy of Medical Sciences. Multimorbidity: A Priority for Global Health Research. 2018. Available online: https://acmedsci.ac.uk/file-download/82222577 (accessed on 27 July 2021).
8. Soley-Bori, M.; Ashworth, M.; Bisquera, A.; Dodhia, H.; Lynch, R.; Wang, Y.; Fox-Rushby, J. Impact of multimorbidity on healthcare costs and utilisation: A systematic review of the UK literature. *Br. J. Gen. Pract.* **2021**, *71*, e39–e46. [CrossRef] [PubMed]
9. Sinnott, C.; Mc Hugh, S.; Browne, J.; Bradley, C. GPs' perspectives on the management of patients with multimorbidity: Systematic review and synthesis of qualitative research. *BMJ Open* **2013**, *3*, e003610. [CrossRef] [PubMed]
10. Gill, A.; Kuluski, K.; Jaakkimainen, L.; Naganathan, G.; Upshur, R.; Wodchis, W.P. "Where do we go from here?" Health system frustrations expressed by patients with multimorbidity, their caregivers and family physicians. *Healthc. Policy* **2014**, *9*, 73–89. [CrossRef]
11. Hays, R.; Daker-White, G.; Esmail, A.; Barlow, W.; Minor, B.; Brown, B.; Blakeman, T.; Sanders, C.; Bower, P. Threats to patient safety in primary care reported by older people with multimorbidity: Baseline findings from a longitudinal qualitative study and implications for intervention. *BMC Health Serv. Res.* **2017**, *17*, 754. [CrossRef]
12. Saltus, R.; Pithara, C. "Care from the heart": Older minoritised women's perceptions of dignity in care. *IJMHSC* **2015**, *11*, 57–70. [CrossRef]
13. Solomon, D.; Tariq, S.; Alldis, J.; Burns, F.; Gilson, R.; Sabin, C.; Sherr, L.; Pettit, F.; Dhairyawan, R. Ethnic inequalities in mental health and socioeconomic status among older women living with HIV: Results from the PRIME Study. *STI* **2021**, in press. [CrossRef]
14. Saeed, A.; Rae, E.; Neil, R.; Connell-Hall, V.; Munro, F. To BAME or not to BAME: The Problem with Racial Terminology in the Civil Service. 2019. Available online: https://www.civilserviceworld.com/news/article/to-bame-or-not-to-bame-the-problem-with-racial-terminology-in-the-civil-service (accessed on 1 November 2021).
15. Bunglawala, Z. Civil Service Blog: Please, don't Call Me BAME or BME! 2019. Available online: https://civilservice.blog.gov.uk/2019/07/08/please-dont-call-me-bame-or-bme/ (accessed on 1 November 2021).
16. Brah, A. *Cartographies of Diaspora: Contesting Identities*; Routledge: London, UK, 1996.

17. Dawson, E. *Equity, Exclusion and Everyday Science Learning: The Experiences of Minoritised Groups*; Routledge: Abingdon, UK, 2019.
18. Verest, W.; Galenkamp, H.; Spek, B.; Snijder, M.B.; Stronks, K.; van Valkengoed, I.G.M. Do ethnic inequalities in multimorbidity reflect ethnic differences in socioeconomic status? The HELIUS study. *Eur. J. Public Health* **2019**, *29*, 687–693. [CrossRef] [PubMed]
19. Guy's and St Thomas' Charity. From One to Many. *Exploring People's Progression to Multiple Long-Term Conditions in an Urban Environment*. 2018. Available online: https://www.gsttcharity.org.uk/sites/default/files/GSTTC_MLTC_Report_2018.pdf (accessed on 16 May 2021).
20. Hayanga, B.; Bécares, L.; Stafford, M. *A Systematic Review and Narrative Synthesis of Ethnic Inequalities in Multiple Long-Term Health Conditions in the United Kingdom*; School of Education and Social Work, University of Sussex: Brighton, UK, [Manuscript submitted for publication].
21. Impact on Urban Health. Easing Pressures, How Work, Money and Homes Can Make Our Cities Healthier and Fairer. 2021. Available online: https://urbanhealth.org.uk/insights/reports/easing-pressures-how-work-money-and-homes-can-make-our-cities-healthier-and-fairer (accessed on 5 August 2021).
22. Nazroo, J.Y. The structuring of ethnic inequalities in health: Economic position, racial discrimination, and racism. *Am. J. Public Health* **2003**, *93*, 277–284. [CrossRef] [PubMed]
23. The Richmond Group of Charities, Impact on Urban Health. You only Had to Ask. What People with Multiple Conditions Say about Health Equity. A Report from the Taskforce on Multiple Conditions. July 2021. Available online: https://richmondgroupofcharities.org.uk/sites/default/files/youonlyhadtoask_fullreport_july2021_final.pdf (accessed on 29 July 2021).
24. Livingston, G.; Leavey, G.; Kitchen, G.; Manela, M.; Sembhi, S.; Katona, C. Accessibility of health and social services to immigrant elders: The Islington Study. *Br. J. Psychiatry* **2002**, *180*, 369–374. [CrossRef] [PubMed]
25. Raleigh, V.; Holmes, J. The Health of People from Ethnic Minority Groups in England [Online]. 2021. Available online: https://www.kingsfund.org.uk/publications/health-people-ethnic-minority-groups-england#Diabetes (accessed on 25 May 2021).
26. Race Disparity Unit. Patient Experience of Primary Care: GP Services. 2019. Available online: https://www.ethnicity-facts-figures.service.gov.uk/health/patient-experience/patient-experience-of-primary-care-gp-services/latest#by-ethnicity (accessed on 29 July 2021).
27. Essink-Bot, M.-L.; Lamkaddem, M.; Jellema, P.; Nielsen, S.S.; Stronks, K. Interpreting ethnic inequalities in healthcare consumption: A conceptual framework for research. *Eur. J. Public Health* **2012**, *23*, 922–926. [CrossRef] [PubMed]
28. Rees, P.; Wohland, P.; Norman, P.; Boden, P. Ethnic population projections for the UK, 2001–2051. *J. Pop Res.* **2012**, *29*, 45–89. [CrossRef]
29. Dixon-Woods, M.; Kirk, D.; Agarwal, S.; Annandale, E.; Arthur, T.; Harvey, J.; Hsu, R.; Katbamna, S.; Olsen, R.; Smith, L.; et al. Vulnerable Groups and Access to Health Care: A Critical Interpretive Review. 2005. Available online: https://www.menshealthforum.org.uk/sites/default/files/pdf/sdovulnerablegroups2005.pdf (accessed on 23 July 2021).
30. Norredam, M.; Nielsen, S.S.; Krasnik, A. Migrants' utilization of somatic healthcare services in Europe—A systematic review. *Eur. J. Public Health* **2009**, *20*, 555–563. [CrossRef]
31. Beach, M.C.; Gary, T.L.; Price, E.G.; Robinson, K.; Gozu, A.; Palacio, A.; Smarth, C.; Jenckes, M.; Feuerstein, C.; Bass, E.B.; et al. Improving health care quality for racial/ethnic minorities: A systematic review of the best evidence regarding provider and organization interventions. *BMC Public Health* **2006**, *6*, 104. [CrossRef] [PubMed]
32. Moher, D.; Shamseer, L.; Clarke, M.; Ghersi, D.; Liberati, A.; Petticrew, M.; Shekelle, P.; Stewart, L.A.; PRIMSA-P Group. Preferred reporting items for systematic review and meta-analysis protocols (PRISMA-P) 2015 statement. *Syst. Rev.* **2015**, *4*, 1. [CrossRef]
33. Fortin, M.; Stewart, M.; Poitras, M.E.; Almirall, J.; Maddocks, H. A systematic review of prevalence studies on multimorbidity: Toward a more uniform methodology. *Ann. Fam. Med.* **2012**, *10*, 142–151. [CrossRef] [PubMed]
34. Robertson, R. How Does the NHS Compare Internationally? *Big Election Questions*. 2017. Available online: https://www.kingsfund.org.uk/publications/articles/big-election-questions-nhs-international-comparisons (accessed on 28 May 2021).
35. Coleman, D. Projections of the Ethnic Minority Populations of the United Kingdom 2006–2056. *Pop Dev. Rev.* **2010**, *36*, 441–486. [CrossRef] [PubMed]
36. National Institute for Health Research. Multiple Long-Term Conditions (Multimorbidity): Making Sense of the Evidence [Online]. 2021. Available online: https://evidence.nihr.ac.uk/collection/making-sense-of-the-evidence-multiple-long-term-conditions-multimorbidity/ (accessed on 2 June 2021).
37. Feinstein, A.R. The pre-therapeutic classification of co-morbidity in chronic disease. *J. Chronic Dis.* **1970**, *23*, 455–468. [CrossRef]
38. Department of Health. Comorbidities. A Framework of Principles for System-Wide Action. Available online: https://assets.publishing.service.gov.uk/government/uploads/system/uploads/attachment_data/file/307143/Comorbidities_framework.pdf (accessed on 25 October 2021).
39. Cassell, A.; Edwards, D.; Harshfield, A.; Rhodes, K.; Brimicombe, J.; Payne, R.; Griffin, S. The epidemiology of multimorbidity in primary care: A retrospective cohort study. *Br. J. Gen. Pract.* **2018**, *68*, e245–e251. [CrossRef] [PubMed]
40. Harrison, C.; Britt, H.; Miller, G.; Henderson, J. Examining different measures of multimorbidity, using a large prospective cross-sectional study in Australian general practice. *BMJ Open* **2014**, *4*, e004694. [CrossRef] [PubMed]
41. Carrasquillo, O. Health Care Utilization. In *Encyclopedia of Behavioral Medicine*; Gellman, M.D., Turner, J.R., Eds.; Springer: New York, NY, USA, 2013; pp. 909–910.

42. Arueira Chaves, L.; de Souza Serio dos Santos, D.M.; Rodrigues Campos, M.; Luiza, V.L. Use of health outcome and health service utilization indicators as an outcome of access to medicines in Brazil: Perspectives from a literature review. *Public Health Rev.* **2019**, *40*, 5. [CrossRef] [PubMed]
43. Camenzind, P.A. Explaining regional variations in health care utilization between Swiss cantons using panel econometric models. *BMC Health Serv. Res.* **2012**, *12*, 62. [CrossRef]
44. Agency for Healthcare Research and Quality. Understanding Quality Measurement. 2021. Available online: https://www.ahrq.gov/patient-safety/quality-resources/tools/chtoolbx/understand/index.html#:~{}:text=The%20Institute%20of%20Medicine%20defines%20health%20care%20quality,as%20having%20the%20following%20properties%20or%20domains%3A%20Effectiveness (accessed on 27 October 2021).
45. Institute of Medicine. *Crossing the Quality Chasm: A New Health System for the 21st Century*; National Academy Press: Washington, DC, USA, 2001.
46. Hanefeld, J.; Powell-Jackson, T.; Balabanova, D. Understanding and measuring care quality: Dealing with complexity. *Bull. World Health Organ.* **2017**, *95*, 368–374. [CrossRef]
47. Moher, D.; Liberati, A.; Tetzlaff, J.; Altman, D.G.; The PRISMA Group. Preferred reporting items for systematic reviews and meta analyses: The PRISMA statement. *PLoS Med.* **2009**, *6*, e1000097. [CrossRef]
48. Barron, E.; Bakhai, C.; Kar, P.; Weaver, A.; Bradley, D.; Ismail, H.; Knighton, P.; Holman, N.; Khunti, K.; Sattar, N.; et al. Associations of type 1 and type 2 diabetes with COVID-19-related mortality in England: A whole-population study. *Lancet Diabetes Endocrinol.* **2020**, *8*, 813–822. [CrossRef]
49. Wijlaars, L.P.M.M.; Hardelid, P.; Guttmann, A.; Gilbert, R. Emergency admissions and long-term conditions during transition from paediatric to adult care: A cross-sectional study using Hospital Episode Statistics data. *BMJ Open* **2018**, *8*, e021015. [CrossRef]
50. Barry, E.; Laverty, A.A.; Majeed, A.; Millett, C. Ethnic group variations in alcohol-related hospital admissions in England: Does place matter? *Ethn. Health* **2015**, *20*, 557–563. [CrossRef]
51. Graham, H.L.; Maslin, J.; Copello, A.; Birchwood, M.; Mueser, K.; McGovern, D.; Georgiou, G. Drug and alcohol problems amongst individuals with severe mental health problems in an inner city area of the UK. *Soc. Psychiatry Psychiatr. Epidemiol.* **2001**, *36*, 448–455. [CrossRef] [PubMed]
52. Mehta, R.L.; Davies, M.J.; Ali, S.; Taub, N.A.; Stone, M.A.; Baker, R.; McNally, P.G.; Lawrence, I.G.; Khunti, K. Association of cardiac and non-cardiac chronic disease comorbidity on glycaemic control in a multi-ethnic population with type 1 and type 2 diabetes. *Postgrad. Med. J.* **2011**, *87*, 763–768. [CrossRef]
53. Afuwape, S.A.; Johnson, S.; Craig, T.J.K.; Miles, H.; Leese, M.; Mohan, R.; Thornicroft, G. Ethnic differences among a community cohort of individuals with dual diagnosis in South London. *J. Ment. Health* **2006**, *15*, 551–567. [CrossRef]
54. Alshamsan, R.; Majeed, A.; Vamos, E.P.; Khunti, K.; Curcin, V.; Rawaf, S.; Millett, C. Ethnic differences in diabetes management in patients with and without comorbid medical conditions: A cross-sectional study. *Diabetes Care* **2011**, *34*, 655–657. [CrossRef] [PubMed]
55. Earle, K.; Porter, K.; Ostberg, J.; Yudkin, J. Variation in the progression of diabetic nephropathy according to racial origin. *Nephrol. Dial. Transplant.* **2001**, *16*, 286–290. [CrossRef] [PubMed]
56. Mathur, R.; Dreyer, G.; Yaqoob, M.M.; Hull, S.A. Ethnic differences in the progression of chronic kidney disease and risk of death in a UK diabetic population: An observational cohort study. *BMJ Open* **2018**, *8*, e020145. [CrossRef]
57. Mathur, R.; Hull, S.A.; Badrick, E.; Robson, J. Cardiovascular multimorbidity: The effect of ethnicity on prevalence and risk factor management. *Br. J. Gen. Pract.* **2011**, *61*, e262–e270. [CrossRef]
58. Pinto, R.; Ashworth, M.; Seed, P.; Rowlands, G.; Schofield, P.; Jones, R. Differences in the primary care management of patients with psychosis from two ethnic groups: A population-based cross-sectional study. *Fam. Pract.* **2010**, *27*, 439–446. [CrossRef]
59. Schofield, P.; Baawuah, F.; Seed, P.T.; Ashworth, M. Managing hypertension in general practice: A cross-sectional study of treatment and ethnicity. *Br. J. Gen. Pract.* **2012**, *62*, e703–e709. [CrossRef]
60. Das-Munshi, J.; Schofield, P.; Ashworth, M.; Gaughran, F.; Hull, S.; Ismail, K.; Robson, J.; Stewart, R.; Mathur, R. Inequalities in glycaemic management in people living with type 2 diabetes mellitus and severe mental illnesses: Cohort study from the UK over ten year. *BMJ Open Diabetes Res. Care* **2021**, *9*, e002118. [CrossRef]
61. Prady, S.L.; Pickett, K.E.; Gilbody, S.; Petherick, E.S.; Mason, D.; Sheldon, T.A.; Wright, J. Variation and ethnic inequalities in treatment of common mental disorders before, during and after pregnancy: Combined analysis of routine and research data in the Born in Bradford cohort. *BMC Psychiatry* **2016**, *16*, 99. [CrossRef]
62. Kwon, I.; Shin, O.; Park, S.; Kwon, G. Multi-Morbid Health Profiles and Specialty Healthcare Service Use: A Moderating Role of Poverty. *IJERPH* **2019**, *16*, 1956. [CrossRef]
63. Collins, P.; Bilge, S. *Intersectionality*; Polity Press: Cambridge, UK, 2016.
64. Rivenbark, J.G.; Ichou, M. Discrimination in healthcare as a barrier to care: Experiences of socially disadvantaged populations in France from a nationally representative survey. *BMC Public Health* **2020**, *20*, 31. [CrossRef]
65. Adegbembo, A.O.; Tomar, S.L.; Logan, H.L. Perception of racism explains the difference between Blacks' and Whites' level of healthcare trust. *Ethn. Dis.* **2006**, *16*, 792–798.
66. Sabbah, W.; Gireesh, A.; Chari, M.; Delgado-Angulo, E.K.; Bernabé, E. Racial Discrimination and Uptake of Dental Services among American Adults. *Int. J. Environ. Res. Public Health* **2019**, *16*, 1558. [CrossRef] [PubMed]

67. Ben, J.; Cormack, D.; Harris, R.; Paradies, Y.C. Racism and health service utilisation: A systematic review and meta-analysis. *PLoS ONE* **2017**, *12*, e0189900. [CrossRef] [PubMed]
68. Stoll, C.R.T.; Izadi, S.; Fowler, S.; Green, P.; Suls, J.; Colditz, G.A. The value of a second reviewer for study selection in systematic reviews. *Res. Synth. Methods* **2019**, *10*, 539–545. [CrossRef]
69. National Institute for Health and Care Excellence. Multimorbidity: Clinical Assessment and Management. *NICE Guideline [NG56]*. 2016. Available online: https://www.nice.org.uk/guidance/ng56 (accessed on 16 August 2021).
70. Salisbury, C.; Man, M.S.; Bower, P.; Guthrie, B.; Chaplin, K.; Gaunt, D.M.; Brookes, S.; Fitzpatrick, B.; Gardner, C.; Hollinghurst, S.; et al. Management of multimorbidity using a patient-centred care model: A pragmatic cluster-randomised trial of the 3D approach. *Lancet* **2018**, *392*, 41–50. [CrossRef]
71. Mann, C.; Shaw, A.; Wye, L.; Salisbury, C.; Guthrie, B. A computer template to enhance patient-centredness in multimorbidity reviews: A qualitative evaluation in primary care. *Br. J. Gen. Pract.* **2018**, *68*, e495. [CrossRef] [PubMed]
72. Van der Aa, M.J.; van den Broeke, J.R.; Stronks, K.; Plochg, T. Patients with multimorbidity and their experiences with the healthcare process: A scoping review. *J. Comorb.* **2017**, *7*, 11–21. [CrossRef] [PubMed]
73. Page, M.J.; McKenzie, J.E.; Bossuyt, P.M.; Boutron, I.; Hoffmann, T.C.; Mulrow, C.D.; Shamseer, L.; Tetzlaff, J.M.; Akl, E.A.; Brennan, S.E.; et al. The PRISMA 2020 statement: An updated guideline for reporting systematic reviews. *BMJ* **2021**, *372*, n71. [CrossRef] [PubMed]
74. Mathur, R.; Bhaskaran, K.; Chaturvedi, N.; Leon, D.A.; vanStaa, T.; Grundy, E.; Smeeth, L. Completeness and usability of ethnicity data in UK-based primary care and hospital databases. *J. Public Health* **2014**, *36*, 684–692. [CrossRef]
75. Saunders, C.L.; Abel, G.A.; El Turabi, A.; Ahmed, F.; Lyratzopoulos, G. Accuracy of routinely recorded ethnic group information compared with self-reported ethnicity: Evidence from the English Cancer Patient Experience survey. *BMJ Open* **2013**, *3*, e002882. [CrossRef]
76. Scobie, S.; Spencer, J.; Raleig, V. Ethnicity coding in English health service datasets. 2021. Available online: https://www.nuffieldtrust.org.uk/files/2021-06/1622731816_nuffield-trust-ethnicity-coding-web.pdf (accessed on 28 November 2021).
77. Steventon, A.; Bardsley, M. Use of secondary care in England by international immigrants. *J. Health Serv. Res. Policy* **2011**, *16*, 90–94. [CrossRef] [PubMed]
78. Saunders, C.L.; Steventon, A.; Janta, B.; Stafford, M.; Sinnott, C.; Allen, L.; Deeny, S.R. Healthcare utilization among migrants to the UK: Cross-sectional analysis of two national surveys. *J. Health Serv. Res. Policy* **2021**, *26*, 54–61. [CrossRef] [PubMed]
79. Jayaweera, H.; Quigley, M.A. Health status, health behaviour and healthcare use among migrants in the UK: Evidence from mothers in the Millennium Cohort Study. *Soc. Sci. Med.* **2010**, *71*, 1002–1010. [CrossRef] [PubMed]
80. Parry, G.; Van Cleemput, P.; Peters, J.; Walters, S.; Thomas, K.; Cooper, C. Health status of Gypsies and Travellers in England. *J. Epidemiol. Community Health* **2007**, *61*, 198–204. [CrossRef]
81. Bécares, L. Which ethnic groups have the poorest health? In *Ethnic Identity and Inequalities in Britain*; Jivraj, S., Simpson, L., Eds.; Policy Press: Bristol, UK, 2015.

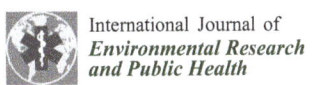

Protocol

Which Non-Pharmaceutical Primary Care Interventions Reduce Inequalities in Common Mental Health Disorders? A Protocol for a Systematic Review of Quantitative and Qualitative Studies

Louise Tanner [1,*], Sarah Sowden [1], Madeleine Still [1], Katie Thomson [1,2], Clare Bambra [1,2] and Josephine Wildman [1,2]

[1] Population Health Sciences Institute, Newcastle University, Newcastle NE1 8PB, UK; sarah.sowden@newcastle.ac.uk (S.S.); madeleine.still@newcastle.ac.uk (M.S.); katie.thomson@newcastle.ac.uk (K.T.); clare.bambra@newcastle.ac.uk (C.B.); josephine.wildman@newcastle.ac.uk (J.W.)

[2] National Institute for Health Research (NIHR) Applied Research Collaboration (ARC) for the North-East and North Cumbria (NENC), Newcastle Upon Tyne NE3 3XT, UK

* Correspondence: louise.tanner@newcastle.ac.uk

Abstract: Common mental health disorders (CMDs) represent a major public health concern and are particularly prevalent in people experiencing disadvantage or marginalisation. Primary care is the first point of contact for people with CMDs. Pharmaceutical interventions, such as antidepressants, are commonly used in the treatment of CMDs; however, there is concern that these treatments are over-prescribed and ineffective for treating mental distress related to social conditions. Non-pharmaceutical primary care interventions, such as psychological therapies and "social prescribing", provide alternatives for CMDs. Little is known, however, about which such interventions reduce social inequalities in CMD-related outcomes, and which may, unintentionally, increase them. The aim of this protocol (PROSPERO registration number CRD42021281166) is to describe how we will undertake a systematic review to assess the effects of non-pharmaceutical primary care interventions on CMD-related outcomes and social inequalities. A systematic review of quantitative, qualitative and mixed-methods primary studies will be undertaken and reported according to the PRISMA-Equity guidance. The following databases will be searched: Assia, CINAHL, Embase, Medline, PsycInfo and Scopus. Retrieved records will be screened according to pre-defined eligibility criteria and synthesised using a narrative approach, with meta-analysis if feasible. The findings of this review will guide efforts to commission more equitable mental health services.

Keywords: mental disorders; healthcare disparities; primary health care; systematic review; health inequalities; PROGRESS-Plus

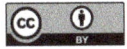

1. Introduction

Common mental health disorders (CMDs), such as depressive disorders and anxiety disorders, are a major global healthcare problem, causing a large amount of suffering and imposing huge economic costs; for example, mental health problems are estimated to cost the global economy around GBP 105 billion a year [1]. In many countries, including the United States, Canada, Australia and European countries such as France and the UK, primary care is usually the first point of contact for people with mental health problems. Most patients with a mental health problem are seen only in primary care [2–4], and in the UK, mental ill health comprises a third of GP appointments [5]. Pharmaceutical interventions, such as antidepressants, are commonly used, and are frequently effective in the treatment of CMDs. However, there is concern amongst healthcare professionals that pharmaceutical treatments are over-prescribed or inappropriately used, resulting in the medicalising of everyday stresses and distress caused by socioeconomic deprivation [6–8].

Antidepressant prescriptions show an increasing trend [9] that has outpaced the rise in the prevalence of CMDs [10]. There is also evidence that some indicators of disadvantage and marginalisation, such as unemployment, are associated with increased antidepressant use independent of a diagnosis of depression [11].

Non-pharmaceutical interventions provide alternative treatment options for mental distress. In England, for example, the Improving Access to Psychological Treatment (IAPT) service was developed by the National Health Service with the aim of integrating psychological therapies into primary care [12,13]. More recently, "social prescribing" is being formally embedded into primary care to provide an alternative for patients with mental health disorders (and other chronic health conditions) [14]. Social prescribing aims to improve patients' health and wellbeing by offering them support and linkage to community-based services that provide support with social needs and health behaviours [15,16].

With the aim of applying an equity lens to healthcare interventions, the Cochrane and Campbell Equity Methods group developed the PROGRESS-Plus framework to identify a range of sociodemographic characteristics that stratify health outcomes [17]. A number of PROGRESS-Plus domains have been found to be associated with the prevalence of mental health problems. There are sex differences in rates of mental ill health, with women having higher rates of anxiety and depression [18] and higher rates of substance-abuse-related mental health problems in men [19]. Mental health outcomes have also been found to be associated with one's place of residence, including in terms of access to green space [20] and living in areas of socioeconomic disadvantage [21]. Differential rates of mental health problems have also been found to be associated with race and ethnicity [22–24], occupation [25–27], religious identity [28–30], social capital [31], educational attainment [27,30], age [30], disability status [32] and sexual orientation [33]. Mental ill health is a particular problem in areas of socioeconomic deprivation, where mental health problems can be both a cause and effect of poverty and of social problems such as unemployment, homelessness, debt and violence [30].

In addition to experiencing higher rates of CMDs, people living with disadvantage and marginalisation are less able to access and benefit from treatments for conditions such as anxiety and depression [16,34]. In the UK, as in other high-income countries [35], addressing both mental ill health and health inequalities are key policy objectives, as evidenced in the NHS Long-term Plan [36] and the narrative surrounding the NHS response to the COVID-19 pandemic [37]. For these reasons, there is a pressing need for evidence about which interventions will reduce inequalities in treatment outcomes and which may, unintentionally, increase them. This systematic review will examine evidence on primary care interventions that are likely to decrease, or potentially increase, health inequalities in treatment access and outcomes for patients experiencing CMDs. Findings will guide the commissioning of more equitable mental health services.

In line with PRISMA-E guidelines [38–40], as the first stage of this equity-focused review, a framework for conceptualising primary care interventions and mental health inequalities was developed (Figure 1). The framework outlines the three types of non-pharmaceutical interventions considered in this review:

1. Social prescribing (for example, arts activities, healthy eating, housing and financial advice);
2. New models of care (for example, integration of primary and secondary healthcare, or the integration of health and social care);
3. New methods of clinical practice (for example, clinical psychologists integrated with general practice teams or extended consultation times).

The framework considers the potential domains of inequality addressed by an intervention, the approach taken, and factors that may impact the effectiveness of any given intervention in reducing inequalities in mental health outcomes. It was developed based on an existing framework used in a previous equity-focused review [41] and will be revised iteratively [42] as evidence from the systematic review emerges.

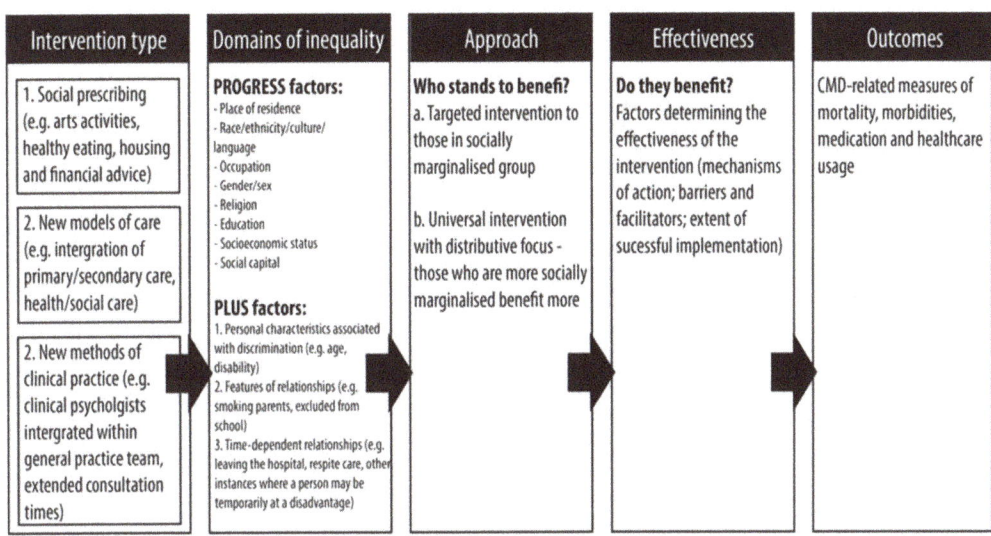

Figure 1. Framework for addressing inequalities in CMD-related health outcomes in relation to the PROGRESS-Plus domains [17,43,44], adapted from Sowden et al. [41].

2. Materials and Methods

The review will be carried out following established criteria for the good conduct and reporting of equity-focused systematic reviews using PRISMA-E guidelines [38–40] and reporting here conforms to the standards of the Preferred Reporting Items for Systematic Reviews and Meta-analysis Protocols (PRISMA-P) (see Supplementary File S1) [45]. The protocol for this systematic review was registered on the PROSPERO database on 23rd September 2021 (registration number: CRD42021281166) [46].

2.1. Research Questions

The main research question to be addressed in this review is:

Which non-pharmaceutical primary care interventions reduce inequalities in CMD-related adverse health outcomes?

Review sub-questions are:

1. Which non-pharmaceutical primary care interventions reduce the occurrence of CMD-related adverse health outcomes amongst populations in the most disadvantaged groups in relation to the PROGRESS-Plus framework?
2. Which non-pharmaceutical primary care interventions reduce inequalities in CMD-related adverse health outcomes between people from the least and most disadvantaged groups?
3. What are the mechanisms by which non-pharmaceutical primary care interventions impact CMD-related adverse health outcomes and inequalities?
4. What are the barriers and facilitators to the implementation of non-pharmaceutical primary care interventions in disadvantaged groups?

2.2. Objectives

The objectives of this systematic review are to:

- Locate studies reporting data for the effects of non-pharmaceutical primary care interventions on CMD-related health outcomes and inequalities, using systematic searches of bibliographic databases and sources of grey literature and systematic screening methods;
- Quantify the effects of non-pharmaceutical primary care interventions on CMD-related health outcomes and inequalities;

- Identify which aspects of the identified interventions influence CMD-related health outcomes and inequalities and the mechanisms (including barriers and facilitators) by which these factors exert their effects;
- Assess the methodological quality of the synthesised evidence;
- Identify policy implications and areas for further research in relation to the review findings.

2.3. Inclusion Criteria

The following criteria (summarised in Table 1) will be applied to each full text in order to assess their eligibility for inclusion in the review.

Table 1. Summary of inclusion and exclusion criteria.

Inclusion	Exclusion
Population: People with a common mental disorder (CMD) [a], who are being treated in primary care.	**Population:** Studies exclusively involving participants with alternative mental or physical health conditions.
Intervention: Non-pharmaceutical interventions delivered by or referred to from primary care teams. These will include: - Activities and support services provided by the voluntary sector; - New models of care or methods of clinical practice in relation to patient care; - Psychological interventions.	**Intervention:** Studies exclusively investigating the effects of pharmaceutical interventions.
Comparators: **Population** - Comparisons before and after the intervention amongst individuals from health disadvantaged population sub-groups; - Comparisons between health-disadvantaged and non-disadvantaged population sub-groups. **Intervention** - Comparisons between non-pharmaceutical primary care intervention versus no or alternative intervention.	

Outcomes:
Quantitative measures of:
- Healthcare use related to CMDs;
- Medication use related to CMDs;
- CMD screening and assessment tools
- Self-reported qualitative data on:
  - Mechanisms by which interventions impact on mental health;
  - Barriers and facilitators to implementing interventions.	

Study design: Quantitative, qualitative and mixed methods primary studies.	**Study design:** Editorials and letters.
Context: Studies published in English language in an OECD high-income country.	

[a] CMDs of interest in this review are: anxiety, depression, somatoform disorders, post-traumatic stress disorder or post-natal depression.

2.3.1. Population

The population of interest consists of people who are being treated in primary care in any high-income country defined by The Organisation for Economic Co-operation and Development (OECD) [47] whose characteristics in relation to one or more of the PROGRESS-Plus factors [48] are reported. Included studies must indicate that all or some participants have a CMD, which must be one of the following disorders, defined by Lund (2020): anxiety, depression, somatoform disorder, post-traumatic stress disorder or postnatal depression [49]. Participants are not required to have received a CMD diagnosis; presence of a CMD may be indicated using data from mental health screening tools (e.g., the Self-Reporting Questionnaire (SRQ-20)). The mental health status of participants may be reported narratively (e.g., in the title, participant characteristics or inclusion criteria) or in the baseline characteristics table. We will exclude studies exclusively involving participants with the following more severe and less common conditions, defined by Lund (2020): psychosis, dementias, child and adolescent mental disorders, conversion disorders, body dysmorphic disorders, personality disorders, eating disorders, suicide, self-harm, substance use disorders, intellectual disability, epilepsy and developmental disorders [49].

We will include studies reporting interventions that have been delivered exclusively to a disadvantaged population subgroup covered by the PROGRESS-Plus criteria (e.g., where participants are all from an ethnic minority group). We will also include studies involving participants with other specific characteristics (e.g., persons with specific exposures such as victims of abuse) if one or more of their PROGRESS-Plus characteristics are also reported. Furthermore, studies that report interventions that have been delivered universally to people from disadvantaged and non-disadvantaged backgrounds (e.g., older versus younger persons; individuals from low- versus high-income households) will be included if the authors report a sub-group analysis of the differential effectiveness of the intervention between population sub-groups (e.g., persons with and without disabilities).

2.3.2. Intervention

Interventions delivered by or referred to from primary care teams (including GPs and allied health professionals based in GP practices and community pharmacies) will be included.

For the purpose of this review, a broad definition of non-pharmaceutical primary care interventions will be used, including referral of individuals to activities and support services provided by the voluntary sector as well as new models of care or methods of clinical practice in relation to patient care. We will include psychological interventions, such as Cognitive Behavioural Therapy.

Studies exclusively investigating the effects of pharmaceutical interventions will be excluded. However, where a pharmaceutical intervention is one component of a multifaceted, integrative, holistic approach to treatment and care, the overall intervention will be included.

The intervention must have been either delivered exclusively to a disadvantaged population sub-group covered by the PROGRESS-PLUS criteria (e.g., older persons; individuals with disabilities) or reported a sub-group analysis of the differential effectiveness of the intervention between population sub-groups (e.g., older versus younger adults; persons with and without disabilities).

2.3.3. Comparators

Population

We will include studies reporting data on CMD-related health outcomes in relation to at least one type of inequality from the PROGRESS-PLUS criteria [48], i.e., place of residence (e.g., rural/urban location); race/ethnicity/culture/language; occupation; gender/sex; religion; education; socioeconomic status including social capital [48].

Eligible studies may present data enabling between-group comparisons (e.g., between persons who received the intervention from low- versus high-income households) or within-group comparisons (e.g., before and after the intervention, amongst individuals who are all from low-income households).

Intervention

Data from included studies comparing the effectiveness of intervention versus no or alternative intervention (including alternative similar interventions and variations in the format, duration and intensity of the intervention as well as usual treatment vs. novel one) will also be extracted where available and included in the synthesis.

2.3.4. Outcomes

Relevant outcomes from quantitative studies will include measures of morbidity which are directly related to CMDs (e.g., the number of health care consultations and measures of medication usage for CMDs) in addition to assessments from validated mental health screening tools, including but not limited to the State–Trait Anxiety Inventory (STAI) [50], the Perceived Stress Scale (PSS) [51], the Positive and Negative Affect Schedule (PANAS) [52], the Warwick–Edinburgh Mental Well-being Scale (WEMWBS) [53], the Self-Reporting Questionnaire (SRQ-20) [54] or the General Health Questionnaire (GHQ) [55]. We will also include adapted versions of these mental health screening tools that have been validated in other languages (e.g., the Spanish and Dutch versions of the PANAS) [56,57], as well as validated tools that have been developed for use in high-income countries outside of the UK, if the study is reported in English.

The overall impact of the interventions of interest will be assessed by comparing the occurrence of CMD-related adverse health outcomes before and after the intervention amongst health-disadvantaged population subgroups. Health inequalities will be assessed by comparing CMD-related adverse health outcomes between the most and least health-disadvantaged groups.

From qualitative studies, we will extract information providing insights on the mechanisms by which non-pharmaceutical primary care interventions could impact CMD outcomes and inequalities, in addition to barriers and facilitators to the successful implementation of these programmes.

2.3.5. Study Design

Quantitative primary studies, including randomised controlled trials (RCTs), other intervention studies (e.g., quasi-experimental), longitudinal studies (e.g., cohort and panel studies), repeated cross-sectional studies and ecological studies [58], will be included in the review in addition to qualitative [59] and mixed-methods primary studies.

2.3.6. Context

In order to be included in the review, studies must be written in English language and have been published in an OECD high-income county (studies that do not meet these criteria will be excluded during screening) [47].

2.4. Search Strategy

The following databases will be searched from their start until 1 June 2021 (host platforms in brackets): Applied Social Sciences Index and Abstracts (ASSIA; ProQuest)(Ann Arbor MI, USA); Cumulative Index to Nursing and Allied Health Literature (CINAHL) (EBSCO, USA); Embase (Ovid, London, UK); PsycInfo (EbscoHost, Ipswich MA, USA); Scopus (Elsevier, Amsterdam, The Netherlands). The draft search strategy for Medline is shown in Supplementary File S2.

The useful resource list of the Social Prescribing Network [60], the Social Interventions Research and Evaluations Network (SIREN) [61] and relevant charity websites will also be purposefully searched for relevant articles. Citing references will also be identified using Google Scholar's "cited by" feature. We will also screen the reference lists of reviews located during the searches which are deemed relevant to the research question, as well as any primary studies which are included in the review, to identify further potentially relevant studies. No limits on date or language will be placed on the searches.

Search strings for the relevant databases were built from existing search filters for PROGRESS-Plus [43] and mental health components [62]. Primary health care elements of the search were taken from that used in a Cochrane review of primary care treatment for alcohol and drugs [63]. The search strings for each database will be peer-reviewed by an experienced information specialist, using the PRESS checklist [64] prior to implementation.

2.5. Screening and Selection

Records located in the searches will be downloaded into an Endnote [65] library and de-duplicated. Rayyan software (Qatar Computing Research Institute, HBKU, Doha, Qatar) will be used to screen studies retrieved from the literature searches [66]. A two-stage process will be used to identify studies for inclusion in the review. First, titles and abstracts will be screened to identify studies relevant to the review topic. The full texts of potentially relevant studies will be sourced and assessed for eligibility in relation to pre-defined inclusion and exclusion criteria. One reviewer (MS) will screen each record, and a second member of the review team (LT) will check a random 10% sample at both stages of the screening process. Screening conflicts will be resolved via discussion and adjudication by a third reviewer (JMW, KT or SS) where necessary.

2.6. Data Extraction

Separate data-extraction forms will be created for quantitative, qualitative and mixed-methods studies. These will be based on existing tools and pre-piloted on a sample of studies deemed eligible for inclusion in the review, with modifications to ensure that all relevant information is captured. Extracted information from quantitative studies will include citation details (first author name and publication date), study characteristics (study aims, design, country and setting), population characteristics (PROGRESS-Plus and other reported characteristics), intervention details (type of intervention, mode and duration of delivery), comparators (pertaining to the population and intervention), outcomes and results (mean and SD values for each comparison group continuous data; number of events and sample size for each comparison group for categorical outcomes). We will extract additional data reported in the included studies which quantify the association between the exposures and outcomes of interest (e.g., results from correlational, regression and modelling studies). The qualitative-data-extraction form will include bibliographic information, methods (e.g., number of participants, data collection method), relevant findings, illustrations from the paper (e.g., participant quotes) and a suggested category or code for that finding. Data from each study will be extracted by one person and checked by a second person.

2.7. Quality Appraisal

Appropriate tools will be selected based on the study designs identified for inclusion in the review. The CASP tools [67] will be used to assess the quality of quantitative studies; a modified version of the relevant CASP tool will be used to quality appraise qualitative studies [68]. If eligible mixed-methods studies are identified, these will be critically appraised using the Mixed Methods Appraisal Tool (MMAT) [69]. Repeated cross-sectional studies will be assessed using the Appraisal tool for Cross-Sectional Studies (AXIS) [70]. All studies will be synthesised regardless of quality. A nominal scoring system will be devised to enable comparability of the overall quality between studies collecting the same type of data (i.e., quantitative, qualitative and mixed-methods). Based on the scoring system developed by the Cochrane Collaboration, studies will be rated as low quality, some concerns or high quality based on domain scores [71].

3. Results

Synthesis

The review will be reported according to the PRISMA-Equity guidance [40]. We will include a paragraph summarising the overall characteristics of included studies, including the number and percentage of studies with different characteristics (e.g., types of study, country of publication and participant characteristics). It is anticipated that heterogeneity will prevent the implementation of meta-analysis. However, if the quantitative data allow, pairwise meta-analysis will be performed using RevMan 5 [72]. For continuous outcomes, we will compare mean values, whereas the number of events and sample size will be extracted for binary outcomes to determine outcome rates. For studies presenting within-group comparisons (where an intervention has been delivered exclusively to a disadvantaged subgroup), we will compare mean values for continuous outcomes (e.g., mean anxiety scores) before versus after the intervention. For studies presenting between-group comparisons, we will compare changes from baseline values (where the data are available) for continuous variables and post-intervention data for binary variables (e.g., GP consultation rates) between population sub-groups. For the between-group comparisons, where there are data for >2 categories for a particular domain of inequality (e.g., low-, middle- and high-income households), we will compare the most and least disadvantaged population subgroups (e.g., highest- versus lowest-income households). Statistical heterogeneity will be assessed using the Chi^2 and Higgins I^2 statistics. Heterogeneity will be deemed to be present if the *p* value for the Chi^2 test is <0.10 or the Higgins I^2 statistic is >50%. A random-effects model will be implemented. If it is not feasible to undertake meta-analysis of the quantitative data, a vote-counting approach, such as a Harvest plot, will be used to graphically present the quantitative data. [73]

Thomas and Harden's (2008) three-stage approach to qualitative synthesis [74] will be used to thematically synthesise qualitative data. This will involve (1) coding the data line by line according to content and meaning; (2) grouping codes according to similarities and differences to produce descriptive themes; (3) generating analytical themes according to the reviewer's interpretation of the data in relation to the review question.

The results will be presented in relation to each domain of inequality for which relevant data were identified. The domain of inequality we are primarily interested in in this systematic review is socioeconomic status. Data in relation to this characteristic will be included in the synthesis preferentially over other PROGRESS-plus factors, if including evidence in relation to other social factors would be unmanageable within the time constraints of this project.

The Economic and Social Research Council's framework [75] will be used to write the narrative synthesis, combining the quantitative (effectiveness) results with the qualitative (mechanisms of action; barriers and facilitators) themes. This includes the following components:

- Developing a theory of how non-pharmaceutical primary care interventions reduce CMD-related adverse health outcomes and inequalities, why and for whom;
- Developing a preliminary synthesis of the data;
- Exploring relationships within and between studies;
- Assessing the robustness of the synthesis.

A Best Available Evidence approach [76] will be used to synthesise evidence from the quantitative studies. This will involve reporting evidence from studies with the most robust designs assessing the clinical effectiveness of interventions, prior to evidence from less-robust study designs. The following hierarchy will be used: (1) RCTs, other intervention studies (e.g., quasi-experimental); (2) individual-level longitudinal studies; (3) repeated cross-sectional studies; (4) ecological studies.

4. Discussion

CMDs are prevalent globally. In England, for example, 1 in 6 people report experiencing a common mental health problem (such as anxiety and depression) in any given week (data from 2014) [77]. Non-pharmaceutical primary care interventions provide alternative therapeutic options for mental distress to drug treatments. In order to support the use of such treatments for people with CMDs, their effectiveness must be assessed, as well as their impacts on health inequalities.

This systematic review will provide evidence regarding the effectiveness of non-pharmaceutical primary care interventions at reducing inequalities in CMD-related outcomes in relation to the PROGRESS-PLUS domains [48]. The mechanisms by which these interventions impact the outcomes of interest and barriers and facilitators to implementation will be explored. This will enable policy makers to identify non-pharmaceutical primary care interventions that are most effective at reducing inequalities in mental health outcomes and to determine which aspects of these interventions increase or decrease their effectiveness in different populations.

Limitations of the methods include potential language bias from excluding studies not published in the English language. Additionally, we will deviate from gold-standard methods by only having one reviewer screen, extract data and quality-appraise all of the articles and a second reviewer perform a 10% check.

Dissemination of findings will take place through a written report for stakeholders. The report findings will also be shared in two half-day workshops: one with practitioner stakeholders, including from the Clinical Commissioning Groups, Primary Care Networks and the Integrated Care Systems, and the other with members of the public. Dissemination workshops will also seek input from practitioners and public stakeholders into a bid for further funding. Two articles will be published in peer-reviewed journals.

5. Conclusions

Globally, CMDs create significant health and economic burdens. In many countries, patients with CMDs are predominantly treated in primary care. While many CMDs are treated with pharmaceutical interventions, non-pharmaceutical interventions, such as psychological therapies, are available as alternative treatments for people with anxiety and depressive disorders. Within primary care, new models of care and new methods of clinical practice, such as social prescribing, are also being developed to provide non-pharmaceutical options for patients with CMDs. However, the effects of these interventions on social inequalities in CMD-related health outcomes is unknown. This review will assess the impacts of non-pharmaceutical primary care interventions on social inequalities in CMD-related health outcomes, based on evidence from quantitative, qualitative and mixed-methods studies. The results will provide evidence to support the delivery of more equitable mental health services.

Supplementary Materials: The following are available online at https://www.mdpi.com/article/10.3390/ijerph182412978/s1, file S1: PRISMA-P 2015 checklist, file S2: draft search strategy for Medline.

Author Contributions: Conceptualization: J.W., C.B., K.T. and S.S.; Methodology: J.W., K.T., L.T., M.S., C.B. and S.S.; Writing (Original Draft Preparation): J.W., K.T., L.T., M.S. and S.S.; Writing (Review and Editing): J.W., K.T., L.T., M.S., C.B. and S.S. All authors have read and agreed to the published version of the manuscript.

Funding: This research is funded by NIHR Research Capability Funding (RCF) from NHS North of England Care System Support (NECS). S.S. is supported by Health Education England (HEE) and the National Institute for Health Research (NIHR) through an Integrated Clinical Academic Lecturer Fellowship (Ref CA-CL-2018-04-ST2-010) and RCF funding, NHS North of England Care System Support (NECS). This project is supported by the National Institute of Health Research (NIHR) Applied Research Collaboration (ARC) for the North East and North Cumbria (NENC). K.T. and J.W. are members of the NIHR ARC NENC. The views expressed are those of the authors and not necessarily those of the funders.

Conflicts of Interest: The authors declare no conflict of interest.

References

1. The Independent Mental Health Taskforce. The Five Year Forward View for Mental Health. 2016. Available online: https://www.england.nhs.uk/wp-content/uploads/2016/02/Mental-Health-Taskforce-FYFV-final.pdf (accessed on 22 November 2021).
2. Kendrick, T.; Burns, T.; Garland, C.; Greenwood, N.; Smith, P. Are specialist mental health services being targeted on the most needy patients? The effects of setting up special services in general practice. *Br. J. Gen. Pract.* **2000**, *50*, 121–126.
3. Reilly, S.T.; Planner, C.; Hann, M.; Reeves, D.; Nazareth, I.; Lester, H. The role of primary care in service provision for people with severe mental illness in the United Kingdom. *PLoS ONE* **2012**, *7*, e36468. [CrossRef] [PubMed]
4. Sundquist, J.; Ohlsson, H.; Sundquist, K.; Kendler, K.S. Common adult psychiatric disorders in Swedish primary care where most mental health patients are treated. *BMC Psychiatry* **2017**, *17*, 235. [CrossRef] [PubMed]
5. Puschner, B.; Kösters, M.; Bouché, L. *The epidemiology, burden and treatment of mental disorders in primary care. Mental Disorders in Primary Care: A Guide to Their Evaluation and Management*; Oxford University Press: Oxford, UK, 2017; pp. 1–20.
6. Shaw, I.; Woodward, L. The medicalisation of unhappiness? The management of mental distress in primary care. In *Constructions of Health and Illness*; Routledge: London, UK, 2017; pp. 124–136.
7. American Academy of Family Physicians. Mental Health Care Services by Family Physicians (Position Paper). 2021. Available online: https://www.aafp.org/about/policies/all/mental-health-services.html (accessed on 22 November 2021).
8. Hálfdánarson, Ó.; Zoega, H.; Aagaard, L.; Bernardo, M.; Brandt, L.; Fusté, A.C.; Furu, K.; Garuolienė, K.; Hoffmann, F.; Huybrechts, K.F.; et al. International trends in antipsychotic use: A study in 16 countries, 2005–2014. *Eur. Neuropsychopharmacol.* **2017**, *27*, 1064–1076. [CrossRef] [PubMed]
9. Bogowicz, P.; Curtis, H.J.; Walker, A.J.; Cowen, P.; Geddes, J.; Goldacre, B. Trends and variation in antidepressant prescribing in English primary care: A retrospective longitudinal study. *BJGP Open* **2021**, *5*. [CrossRef]
10. Spence, R.; Ariti, C.; Bardsley, M. Focus On: Antidepressant Prescribing. 2014. Available online: https://www.nuffieldtrust.org.uk/research/focus-on-antidepressant-prescribing (accessed on 22 November 2021).
11. Boyle, S.; Murphy, J.; Rosato, M.; Boduszek, D.; Shevlin, M. Predictors of antidepressant use in the English population: Analysis of the adult psychiatric morbidity survey. *Ir. J. Psychol. Med.* **2020**, *37*, 15–23. [CrossRef]
12. NHS England. Adult Improving Access to Psychological Therapies Programme. 2021. Available online: https://www.england.nhs.uk/mental-health/adults/iapt/ (accessed on 22 November 2021).
13. Petersen, I. Integrating task-sharing psychological treatments within primary health care services. In *Systems Considerations*; SAGE Publications Sage UK: London, UK, 2021.
14. Drinkwater, C.; Wildman, J.; Moffatt, S. Social prescribing. *BMJ* **2019**, *364*. [CrossRef]
15. Croxson, C.H.; Ashdown, H.F.; Hobbs, F.R. GPs' perceptions of workload in England: A qualitative interview study. *Br. J. Gen. Pract.* **2017**, *67*, e138–e147. [CrossRef]
16. The Devastating Cost of Treatment Delays. Available online: https://www.bma.org.uk/news-and-opinion/the-devastating-cost-of-treatment-delays (accessed on 29 November 2021).
17. O'Neill, J.; Tabish, H.; Welch, V.; Petticrew, M.; Pottie, K.; Clarke, M.; Evans, T.; Pardo, J.P.; Waters, E.; White, H.; et al. Applying an equity lens to interventions: Using PROGRESS ensures consideration of socially stratifying factors to illuminate inequities in health. *J. Clin. Epidemiol* **2014**, *67*, 56–64. [CrossRef]
18. Somers, J.M.; Goldner, E.M.; Waraich, P.; Hsu, L. Prevalence and incidence studies of anxiety disorders: A systematic review of the literature. *Can. J. Psychiatry* **2006**, *51*, 100–113. [CrossRef] [PubMed]
19. Cabezas-Rodríguez, A.; Utzet, M.; Bacigalupe, A. Which are the intermediate determinants of gender inequalities in mental health?: A scoping review. *Int. J. Soc. Psychiatry* **2021**, *2021*. [CrossRef] [PubMed]
20. Mitchell, R.J.; Richardson, E.A.; Shortt, N.K.; Pearce, J.R. Neighborhood environments and socioeconomic inequalities in mental well-being. *Am. J. Prev. Med.* **2015**, *49*, 80–84. [CrossRef] [PubMed]
21. Pearce, J.; Cherrie, M.; Shortt, N.; Deary, I.; Thompson, C.W. Life course of place: A longitudinal study of mental health and place. *Trans. Inst. Br. Geogr.* **2018**, *43*, 555–572. [CrossRef]
22. Sentell, T.; Shumway, M.; Snowden, L. Access to mental health treatment by English language proficiency and race/ethnicity. *J. Gen. Intern. Med.* **2007**, *22*, 289–293. [CrossRef]
23. Mclean, C.; Campbell, C.; Cornish, F. African-Caribbean interactions with mental health services in the UK: Experiences and expectations of exclusion as (re) productive of health inequalities. *Soc. Sci. Med.* **2003**, *56*, 657–669. [CrossRef]
24. Grey, T.; Sewell, H.; Shapiro, G.; Ashraf, F. Mental health inequalities facing UK minority ethnic populations: Causal factors and solutions. *J. Psychol. Issues Organ. C* **2013**, *3*, 146–157. [CrossRef]
25. Milner, A.; King, T.; LaMontagne, A.D.; Bentley, R.; Kavanagh, A. Men's work, women's work, and mental health: A longitudinal investigation of the relationship between the gender composition of occupations and mental health. *Soc. Sci. Med.* **2018**, *204*, 16–22. [CrossRef] [PubMed]
26. Canivet, C.; Aronsson, G.; Bernhard-Oettel, C.; Leineweber, C.; Moghaddassi, M.; Stengård, J.; Westerlund, H.; Östergren, P.-O. The negative effects on mental health of being in a non-desired occupation in an increasingly precarious labour market. *SSM - Popul. Heal.* **2017**, *3*, 516–524. [CrossRef] [PubMed]
27. Barr, B.; Kinderman, P.; Whitehead, M. Trends in mental health inequalities in England during a period of recession, austerity and welfare reform 2004 to 2013. *Soc. Sci. Med.* **2015**, *147*, 324–331. [CrossRef]

28. Dilmaghani, M. Religious identity and health inequalities in Canada. *J. Immigr. Minor. Health* **2017**, *20*, 1060–1074. [CrossRef]
29. Haque, A. Religion and mental health: The case of American Muslims. *J. Relig. Health* **2004**, *43*, 45–58. [CrossRef]
30. World Health Organization. Social Determinants of Mental Health. 2014. Available online: https://apps.who.int/iris/bitstream/handle/10665/112828/9789241506809_eng.pdf (accessed on 22 November 2021).
31. Pinxten, W.; Lievens, J. The importance of economic, social and cultural capital in understanding health inequalities: Using a Bourdieu-based approach in research on physical and mental health perceptions. *Sociol. Heal. Illn.* **2014**, *36*, 1095–1110. [CrossRef] [PubMed]
32. Emerson, E.; Hatton, C. Contribution of socioeconomic position to health inequalities of British children and adolescents with intellectual disabilities. *Am. J. Ment. Retard.* **2007**, *112*, 140–150. [CrossRef]
33. Semlyen, J.; King, M.; Varney, J.; Hagger-Johnson, G. Sexual orientation and symptoms of common mental disorder or low wellbeing: Combined meta-analysis of 12 UK population health surveys. *BMC Psychiatry* **2016**, *16*, 1–9. [CrossRef]
34. The Health Foundation. Inequalities in Health Care for People with Depression and/or Anxiety. 2021. Available online: https://www.health.org.uk/publications/long-reads/inequalities-in-health-care-for-people-with-depression-and-anxiety (accessed on 22 November 2021).
35. World Health Organization. Policy Frameworks. 2021. Available online: https://www.euro.who.int/en/health-topics/noncommunicable-diseases/mental-health/policy-frameworks (accessed on 22 November 2021).
36. NHS. NHS Long Term Plan. 2019. Available online: https://www.longtermplan.nhs.uk/ (accessed on 22 November 2021).
37. Stevens, S.; Pritchard, A. Third Phase of NHS Response to COVID-19. 2020. Available online: https://www.england.nhs.uk/coronavirus/wp-content/uploads/sites/52/2020/07/20200731-Phase-3-letter-final-1.pdf (accessed on 22 November 2021).
38. Tugwell, P.; Petticrew, M.; Kristjansson, E.; Welch, V.; Ueffing, E.; Waters, E.; Bonnefoy, J.; Morgan, A.; Doohan, E.; Kelly, M.P. Assessing equity in systematic reviews: Realising the recommendations of the Commission on Social Determinants of Health. *BMJ* **2010**, *341*. [CrossRef]
39. Welch, V.; Petticrew, M.; Petkovic, J.; Moher, D.; Waters, E.; White, H.; Tugwell, P.; Atun, R.; Awasthi, S.; Barbour, V.; et al. Extending the PRISMA statement to equity-focused systematic reviews (PRISMA-E 2012): Explanation and elaboration. *J. Clin. Epidemiol* **2016**, *70*, 68–89. [CrossRef] [PubMed]
40. Welch, V.; Petticrew, M.; Tugwell, P.; Moher, D.; O'Neill, J.; Waters, E.; White, H. PRISMA-Equity 2012 extension: Reporting guidelines for systematic reviews with a focus on health equity. *PLoS Med.* **2012**, *9*, e1001333. [CrossRef] [PubMed]
41. Sowden, S.; Nezafat-Maldonado, B.; Wildman, J.; Cookson, R.; Thomson, R.; Lambert, M.; Beyer, F.; Bambra, C. Protocol: Interventions to reduce inequalities in avoidable hospital admissions: Explanatory framework and systematic review protocol. *BMJ Open* **2020**, *10*, e035429. [CrossRef] [PubMed]
42. Kneale, D.; Thomas, J.; Harris, K. Developing and optimising the use of logic models in systematic reviews: Exploring practice and good practice in the use of programme theory in reviews. *PLoS ONE* **2015**, *10*, e0142187.
43. Prady, S.L.; Uphoff, E.P.; Power, M.; Golder, S. Development and validation of a search filter to identify equity-focused studies: Reducing the number needed to screen. *BMC Med. Res. Methodol.* **2018**, *18*, 1–9. [CrossRef]
44. Oliver, S.; Kavanagh, J.; Caird, J.; Lorenc, T.; Oliver, K.; Harden, A. Health Promotion, Inequalities and Young People's Health. A Systematic Review of Research. 2008. Available online: http://eppi.ioe.ac.uk/cms/LinkClick.aspx?fileticket=lsYdLJP8gBI%3d&tabid=2412&mid=4471&language=en-US (accessed on 8 December 2021).
45. Moher, D.; Shamseer, L.; Clarke, M.; Ghersi, D.; Liberati, A.; Petticrew, M.; Shekelle, P.; Stewart, L.A. Preferred reporting items for systematic review and meta-analysis protocols (PRISMA-P) 2015 statement. *Syst. Rev.* **2015**, *4*, 1–9. [CrossRef]
46. Which Non-Pharmaceutical Primary Care Interventions Reduce Inequalities in Common Mental Health Disorders? A Protocol for a Systematic Review of Quantitative and Qualitative Studies (PROSPERO 2021 CRD42021281166). 2021. Available online: https://www.crd.york.ac.uk/prospero/display_record.php?RecordID=281166 (accessed on 29 November 2021).
47. The World Bank Group. High Income. 2021. Available online: https://data.worldbank.org/country/XD (accessed on 22 November 2021).
48. Cochrane Methods Equity. PROGRESS-Plus. 2021. Available online: https://methods.cochrane.org/equity/projects/evidence-equity/progress-plus (accessed on 22 November 2021).
49. Lund, C.; Breen, A.; Flisher, A.J.; Kakuma, R.; Corrigall, J.; Joska, J.; Swartz, L.; Patel, V. Poverty and common mental disorders in low and middle income countries: A systematic review. *Soc. Sci. Med.* **2010**, *71*, 517–528. [CrossRef]
50. Spielberger, C.D.; Gorsuch, R.; Lushene, R.; Vagg, P.; Jacobs, G. *State-Trait Anxiety Inventory*; Mind Garden: Palo Alto, CA, USA, 1983.
51. Cohen, S.; Kamarck, T.; Mermelstein, R. Perceived stress scale. Measuring stress. In *A Guide for Health and Social Scientists*; Oxford University Press: Oxford, UK, 1994; Volume 10, pp. 1–2.
52. Thompson, E.R. Development and validation of an internationally reliable short-form of the positive and negative affect schedule (PANAS). *J. Cross-Cultural Psychol.* **2007**, *38*, 227–242. [CrossRef]
53. Tennant, R.; Hiller, L.; Fishwick, R.; Platt, S.; Joseph, S.; Weich, S.; Parkinson, J.; Secker, J.; Stewart-Brown, S. The Warwick-Edinburgh mental well-being scale (WEMWBS): Development and UK validation. *Health Qual. Life Outcomes* **2007**, *5*, 1–13. [CrossRef]

54. Scholte, W.F.; Verduin, F.; Van Lammeren, A.; Rutayisire, T.; Kamperman, A.M. Psychometric properties and longitudinal validation of the self-reporting questionnaire (SRQ-20) in a Rwandan community setting: A validation study. *BMC Med. Res. Methodol.* **2011**, *11*, 1–10. [CrossRef] [PubMed]
55. Sriram, T.; Chandrashekar, C.; Isaac, M.; Shanmugham, V. *The general health questionnaire (GHQ). Soc. Psychiatry and Psychiatric Epidemiology*; Springer International: Cham, Switzerland, 1989; Volume 24, pp. 317–320.
56. Díaz-García, A.; González-Robles, A.; Mor, S.; Mira, A.; Quero, S.; García-Palacios, A.; Baños, R.M.; Botella, C. Positive and Negative Affect Schedule (PANAS): Psychometric properties of the online Spanish version in a clinical sample with emotional disorders. *BMC Psychiatry* **2020**, *20*, 1–13. [CrossRef]
57. Engelen, U.; De Peuter, S.; Victoir, A.; Van Diest, U.; Van Den Bergh, O. Further validation of the Positive and Negative Affect Schedule (PANAS) and comparison of two Dutch versions. *Gedrag en Gezondheid* **2006**, *34*, 89.
58. Munnangi, S.; Boktor, S.W. *Epidemiology of Study Design*; StatPearls Publishing LLC.: Treasure Island, FL, USA, 2021.
59. Tenny, S.; Brannan, G.D.; Brannan, J.M. Qualitative Study. 2021. Available online: https://www.ncbi.nlm.nih.gov/books/NBK470395/ (accessed on 29 November 2021).
60. The Social Prescribing Network. Resources. 2018. Available online: https://www.socialprescribingnetwork.com/resources (accessed on 22 November 2021).
61. SIREN (Social Interventions Research and Evaluation Network). Make Health Whole. *Integrating Care. Improving Lives.* 2017–2021. Available online: https://makehealthwhole.org/resource/siren-social-interventions-research-evaluation-network/ (accessed on 22 November 2021).
62. Wilczynski, N.L.; Haynes, R.B.; Hedges, T. Optimal search strategies for identifying mental health content in MEDLINE: An analytic survey. *Ann. Gen. Psychiatry* **2006**, *5*, 1–7. [CrossRef]
63. Kaner, E.F.; Beyer, F.R.; Muirhead, C.; Campbell, F.; Pienaar, E.D.; Bertholet, N. Effectiveness of brief alcohol interventions in primary care populations. *Cochrane Database Syst Rev.* **2018**. [CrossRef]
64. McGowan, J.; Sampson, M.; Salzwedel, D.M.; Cogo, E.; Foerster, V.; Lefebvre, C. PRESS peer review of electronic search strategies: 2015 guideline statement. *J. Clin. Epidemiol.* **2016**, *1*, 40–46. [CrossRef]
65. The EndNote Team. *EndNote*, EndNote X9 ed.; Clarivate: Philadelphia, PA, USA, 2013.
66. Ouzzani, M.; Hammady, H.; Fedorowicz, Z.; Elmagarmid, A. Rayyan—A web and mobile app for systematic reviews. *Syst. Rev.* **2016**, *5*, 1–10. [CrossRef]
67. CASP. CASP Checklists. 2021. Available online: https://casp-uk.net/casp-tools-checklists/ (accessed on 22 November 2021).
68. Long, H.A.; French, D.P.; Brooks, J.M. Optimising the value of the critical appraisal skills programme (CASP) tool for quality appraisal in qualitative evidence synthesis. *Res. Methods Med. Health Sci.* **2020**, *1*, 31–42. [CrossRef]
69. Hong, Q.N.; Fàbregues, S.; Bartlett, G.; Boardman, F.; Cargo, M.; Dagenais, P.; Gagnon, M.-P.; Griffiths, F.; Nicolau, B.; O'Cathain, A.; et al. The Mixed Methods Appraisal Tool (MMAT) version 2018 for information professionals and researchers. *Educ. Inf.* **2018**, *34*, 285–291. [CrossRef]
70. Downes, M.J.; Brennan, M.; Williams, H.C.; Dean, R. Development of a critical appraisal tool to assess the quality of cross-sectional studies (AXIS). *BMJ Open* **2016**, *6*, e011458. [CrossRef] [PubMed]
71. The Cochrane Collaboration. RoB 2: A Revised Cochrane Risk-of-Bias Tool for Randomized Trials. 2021. Available online: https://methods.cochrane.org/bias/resources/rob-2-revised-cochrane-risk-bias-tool-randomized-trials (accessed on 22 November 2021).
72. The Cochrane Collaboration. *Review Manager (RevMan) [Computer Program]*, 5.4 ed.; Cochrane: London, UK, 2020.
73. Ogilvie, D.; Fayter, D.; Petticrew, M.; Sowden, A.; Thomas, S.; Whitehead, M. The harvest plot: A method for synthesising evidence about the differential effects of interventions. *BMC Med. Res. Methodol.* **2008**, *8*, 1–7. [CrossRef] [PubMed]
74. Thomas, J.; Harden, A. Methods for the thematic synthesis of qualitative research in systematic reviews. *BMC Med. Res. Methodol.* **2008**, *8*, 1–10. [CrossRef]
75. Popay, J.; Roberts, H.; Sowden, A.; Petticrew, M.; Arai, L.; Rodgers, M. Guidance on the conduct of narrative synthesis in systematic reviews. *Prod. ESRC Methods Programm. Vers.* **2006**, *1*, b92.
76. Petticrew, M.; Roberts, H. *Systematic Reviews in the Social Sciences: A Practical Guide*; Blackwell Publishing: Hoboken, NJ, USA, 2006.
77. McManus, S.; Bebbington, P.E.; Jenkins, R.; Brugha, T. *Mental Health and Wellbeing in England: The Adult Psychiatric Morbidity Survey 2014*; NHS Digital: Leeds, UK, 2016.

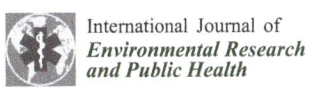

Article

'It All Kind of Links Really': Young People's Perspectives on the Relationship between Socioeconomic Circumstances and Health

Hannah Fairbrother [1,*], Nicholas Woodrow [2], Mary Crowder [2], Eleanor Holding [2], Naomi Griffin [3], Vanessa Er [4], Caroline Dodd-Reynolds [3], Matt Egan [4], Karen Lock [4], Steph Scott [5], Carolyn Summerbell [3], Rachael McKeown [6], Emma Rigby [6], Phillippa Kyle [3] and Elizabeth Goyder [2]

1. Health Sciences School, University of Sheffield, Sheffield S10 2LA, UK
2. ScHARR, University of Sheffield, Sheffield S1 4DA, UK; n.woodrow@sheffield.ac.uk (N.W.); m.crowder@sheffield.ac.uk (M.C.); e.holding@sheffield.ac.uk (E.H.); e.goyder@sheffield.ac.uk (E.G.)
3. Department of Sport and Exercise Science, Fuse | Durham University, Durham DH1 3HN, UK; naomi.c.griffin@durham.ac.uk (N.G.); caroline.dodd-reynolds@durham.ac.uk (C.D.-R.); carolyn.summerbell@durham.ac.uk (C.S.); phillippa.kyle@durham.ac.uk (P.K.)
4. Department of Health Services Research and Policy, London School of Hygiene and Tropical Medicine, London WC1E 7HT, UK; vanessa.er@lshtm.ac.uk (V.E.); matt.egan@lshtm.ac.uk (M.E.); karen.lock@lshtm.ac.uk (K.L.)
5. Population Health Sciences Institute, Faculty of Medical Sciences, Newcastle University, Newcastle upon Tyne NE1 4LP, UK; steph.scott@newcastle.ac.uk
6. Association for Young People's Health, London SE1 4YR, UK; rachael@youngpeopleshealth.org.uk (R.M.); emma@youngpeopleshealth.org.uk (E.R.)
* Correspondence: h.fairbrother@sheffield.ac.uk

Abstract: Meaningful inclusion of young people's perceptions and experiences of inequalities is argued to be critical in the development of pro-equity policies. Our study explored young people's perceptions of what influences their opportunities to be healthy within their local area and their understandings of health inequalities. Three interlinked qualitative focus group discussions, each lasting 90 to 100 min, with the same six groups of young people (*n* = 42) aged 13–21, were conducted between February and June 2021. Participants were recruited from six youth groups in areas of high deprivation across three geographical locations in England (South Yorkshire, the North East and London). Our study demonstrates that young people understand that health inequalities are generated by social determinants of health, which in turn influence behaviours. They highlight a complex interweaving of pathways between social determinants and health outcomes. However, they do not tend to think in terms of the social determinants and their distribution as resulting from the power and influence of those who create and benefit from health and social inequalities. An informed understanding of the causes of health inequalities, influenced by their own unique generational experiences, is important to help young people contribute to the development of pro-equity policies of the future.

Keywords: health inequalities; social inequalities; social determinants of health; young people; qualitative

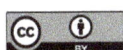

1. Introduction

There is a well-established relationship between socioeconomic position and health [1,2]. Health follows a socioeconomic gradient, where each step up the socioeconomic ladder is associated with better outcomes [3,4]. This patterning is longstanding and evident throughout the life course across a range of different outcomes at both micro and macro geographical levels [5–7]. In the UK, set against a backdrop of rising levels of poverty and the fallout of government austerity policies following the 2008 recession [8], the past decade has seen socioeconomically patterned health inequalities widen for both adults and children and young people [9,10]. More recently, the COVID-19 pandemic has exacerbated existing inequalities, with those lower down the socioeconomic ladder being disproportionately affected both in economic and health terms [11].

Central to many contemporary explanations for socioeconomically patterned health inequalities is the concept of Social Determinants of Health (SDH). The World Health Organisation's Commission on the Social Determinants of Health described the SDH as 'the conditions in which people are born, grow, live, work and age' and argued that 'the marked health inequities between countries are caused by the unequal distribution of power, income, goods, and services, globally and nationally' [7] (p. 1). However, while there is broad consensus as to the importance of the SDH, there is much less consistency in the way in which the concept is mobilised [12–14]. What we see is a range of discourses that draw upon the SDH but differ significantly in the way they explain *how* societal factors result in differences in health [15]. These differences in interpretation, Raphael (2011) argues, are not just about 'intellectual world views' but fundamentally affect how we seek to approach and redress health inequalities [12] (p. 223). Raphael (2011) proposes a spectrum of seven discourses to encapsulate the different ways of understanding (and responding to) the SDH (see Table 1) [12].

Table 1. Summary of Raphael's (2011) seven discourses of the social determinants of health (SDH).

Discourse Level	Key Point
One: SDH as identifying and supporting those in need of health and social services.	Identifying and targeting those at greatest need through service provision.
Two: SDH as identifying those with modifiable medical and behavioural risk factors.	Identifying behavioural risk factors (e.g., diet, physical activity, alcohol and tobacco use) and promoting positive 'lifestyle choices'.
Three: SDH as indicating the material living conditions that affect health.	Living conditions/circumstances affect health and choices either directly or indirectly through interrelated material, psychological and behavioural effects.
Four: SDH as indicating material living circumstances that differ as a function of group membership (class, gender and race).	Different (potential) axes of inequality can interact/intersect and compound each other to change people's experience of the SDH.
Five: SDH and their distribution result from public policy decisions made by governments and other societal institutions.	Public policy can create and maintain (or reduce and disrupt) the SDH.
Six: SDH and their distribution result from economic and political structures and justifying ideologies.	Political and economic structures shape policy decisions.
Seven: SDH and their distribution result from the power and influence of those who create and benefit from health and social inequalities.	Individuals and groups shape policy that protects and benefits them at the expense of others (e.g., tax structures that favour the wealthy).

According to Raphael (2011) and other key researchers in the field (such as Scott-Samuel and Smith (2015), a real reduction in apparently intractable health inequalities will only be possible by tackling inequitable political structures and the power and influence of the people that shape them (Discourse Level Six and Seven) [12,16]. To create a step-change, Raphael argues, we need to 'educate [...] the public that deteriorating quality SDH and inequitable SDH distributions result from the undue influence upon public policymaking of those creating and profiting from social and health inequalities' [12] (p. 230). The argument that we need to change public understandings is widespread [17] and reinforced by a recent collaboration between the Health Foundation and the Frameworks Institute, which sought to 'develop a deeper appreciation of the ways in which people understand and think about health in order to develop more effective approaches to communicating the evidence' [18]. Improving public awareness of health inequalities and the social determinants of health is argued to be vital for galvanizing support for change to the political status quo and the development of pro-equity policies [18].

Studies exploring public perceptions of the link between socioeconomic circumstance and health, however, are limited [17,19]. There is broad agreement regarding the importance of the SDH among the research community, with many narratives echoing the higher-level discourse of Raphael's (2011) typology through repeated critiques of a focus on lifestyle behaviours and neglect of the causal pathways of health inequalities and economic and environmental factors [12,20,21]; though see Dijkstra and Horstman's (2021) critique of social epidemiological research which constructs low socioeconomic status populations as 'inherently unhealthy and problematic' [22] (p. 6). However, public understanding of the factors shaping health has been argued to be limited [12,17,23]. This is supported by recent research by the Frameworks Institute which found that 'public discourse and policy action is limited in acknowledging the role that societal factors such as housing, education, welfare and work play in shaping people's long-term health' [18] (p. 1). Drawing on the Frameworks Institute's findings on young people's views, Marmot et al. (2020) characterised public understandings as individualistic, fatalistic and prone to divisive 'them and us' thinking [1] (p. 145). In contrast, in their review of the admittedly limited evidence base (a meta-ethnography of 17 qualitative studies), Smith and Anderson (2018) argue that people experiencing socioeconomic disadvantage do display an awareness of how socioeconomic hardship can lead to ill health [17]. The picture is thus mixed with contradictory findings regarding the perceived chasm between research consensus and public understanding. In the context of increasing socioeconomic and health inequalities over recent decades and particularly recently due to the COVID-19 pandemic (which has exacerbated existing, socially patterned inequalities through its interaction with inequalities in chronic disease and the social determinants of health including poor quality housing and lower access to healthcare in disadvantaged communities) [1,11,24], it is an opportune time to revisit public perceptions of how socioeconomic circumstances shape health. Further, Smith and Anderson (2018) highlight a dearth of studies exploring the views and experiences of young people [17] (see also Woodgate and Leach's (2010) study and Backett-Milburn et al.'s 2003 study [25,26]). This is an important gap in the evidence base [17,22,27,28]. Youth activism in other spheres such as climate change teaches us that young people have the potential to galvanize support for and contribute to significant policy change [29].

Study Aim

The aim of our research project was to explore young people's perceptions of what influences their opportunities to be healthy within their local area and their understandings of health inequalities. This paper presents key findings on young people's perspectives on the relationship between socioeconomic circumstances and health.

2. Materials and Methods

2.1. Overview

We undertook a series of three interlinked qualitative focus group discussions with six groups of young people (n = 42) aged 13–21, resulting in 18 focus group discussions in total. Participants were recruited from six youth groups across three geographical locations in England (South Yorkshire (SY), the North East (NE) and London (L)). All three locations fell within the most deprived quintile based on the 2019 English indices of multiple deprivation (IMD). Data generation took place between February and June 2021, during the COVID-19 pandemic. Due to the UK's lockdown and social distancing restrictions [30], the majority of focus groups were conducted online (n = 15). However, focus group discussions (n = 3) with one youth group in the North East were conducted face-to-face, once social distancing restrictions permitted, since the youth group did not have facilities to support online data generation in their building (e.g., computers, Wi-Fi) and not all the young people had the technologies to participate from home. Focus group discussions lasted between 90 and 100 min. Further details on the methodological and ethical challenges of this study are described elsewhere [31]. Ethical approval for the study was granted by the School of Health and Related Research (ScHARR) Ethics Committee at the University of Sheffield.

Throughout our project, we actively engaged with Mason's (2018) 'difficult questions' for qualitative research to help ensure the quality, rigour and methodological integrity of our study [32]. In relation to reliability, we seek to provide a detailed and transparent account of our sampling, recruitment, data generation and analysis. Our concerns for the validity of our method and interpretation focus on ensuring the fit between our method and 'tracing the route' (albeit a messy and non-linear one) of our interpretations.

2.2. Sampling and Recruitment

The focus groups involved young people from pre-existing youth organisations, and our sampling was shaped by each group's demographics. Given our focus on socioeconomic circumstances, we initially sought to work with youth groups in socioeconomically contrasting areas. Recognising that socioeconomic position permeates and intersects with other axes of inequality, we also sought to ensure that we worked with young people of different genders and ethnicities in both urban and rural areas (including coastal areas), and we approached youth groups that we thought would enable this. However, due to challenges of recruitment during a pandemic (with youth groups pausing and/or moving online) we had to take a pragmatic approach and work with youth groups with whom we already had established working relationships, all of which were in areas of high deprivation. The youth group workers we approached saw issues around health inequalities as pertinent in their areas and thus important to engage with. Further, while we initially aimed to work with young people aged 13–17, we took a flexible, inclusive approach as some of our youth groups also included young people over 18. We did not want to exclude young people outside of this range if they were keen to participate, particularly since the focus groups replaced their usual weekly meetings. Our inclusive approach also recognises that young people's transitions to adulthood in the UK have become increasingly elongated and less linear [33]. It is important to understand the concepts of 'youth' and 'adulthood' as not being simply a feature of age but also encompassing a variety of different experiences and understandings within this life phase [34]. The young people we worked with were all members of youth organisations, which, for us, was a primary criterion for participating in this study.

In this way, we adopted a purposive sampling strategy, designed to encapsulate a relevant range of perspectives [32]. Drawing on Braun and Clarke (2021), our sample was guided by the breadth and focus of the research question(s); the demands placed on participants; the depth of data likely to be generated; pragmatic constraints; and the analytic goals and purpose of the overall project [35]. Our approach coheres with Braun and Clarke's (2021) description of qualitative research as a 'situated, reflexive and theoretically embedded practice of knowledge generation' [35] (p. 210). This focus on the active construction of meaning opens up the potential to keep working towards new understandings. Our final sample consisted of 42 young people aged 13–21 and included young people of different genders and ethnicities in both urban and rural areas (including coastal areas) (see Table 2).

Youth workers invited group members to participate and shared an information video and project overview, and researchers attended sessions with the youth groups to talk through the study and build rapport. Any young person interested in taking part was given a more detailed information sheet. For potential participants under the age of 16, opt-in consent from parents/guardians was gained. Written consent was then gathered for all participating young people (either on paper or electronic). Participants were asked to provide basic demographic information, including their postcode, which we used to capture an overall average deprivation rank measure (average position out of the 32,844 small areas in England, with closer to 1 being more deprived) (see Table 2). Despite all the field sites falling in the most deprived quintile, the average participant position across the groups ranged from quintile 1 to 3.

Table 2. Sample demographics.

Sample	Number of Participants	Age	Gender	Ethnicity	Deprivation Position
Overall	42	Age range: 13–21 Average age: 16.7	18 Female 19 Male 2 Non-binary 2 Trans Male 1 Gender-Fluid	30 White British 6 Asian/Asian British 3 Black/Black British 2 Mixed/Multiple ethnic group 1 Chinese	Average participant position = 8096 (Quintile 2)
South Yorkshire 1 (SY1) (urban)	6	Age range: 15–17 Average age: 15.5	3 Female 2 Male 1 Gender-Fluid	6 White British	Average participant position = 8009 (Quintile 2)
South Yorkshire 2 (SY2) (urban)	8	Age range: 13–17 Average age: 15.1	3 Female 5 Male	8 White British	Average participant position = 9414 (Quintile 2)
North East 1 (NE1) (rural, coastal)	7	Age range: 15–17 Average age: 15.8	2 Female 1 Male 2 Non-binary 2 Trans Male	7 White British	Average participant position = 15004 (Quintile 3)
North East 2 (NE2) (rural, coastal)	8	Age range: 13–20 Average age: 15.75	8 Male	8 White British	Average participant position = 1351 (Quintile 1)
London 1 (L1) (urban)	10	Age range: 16–21 Average age: 18.7	8 Female 2 Male	1 White British 5 Asian/Asian British 3 Black/Black British 1 Mixed/Multiple ethnic group	Average participant position = 7065 (Quintile 2)
London 2 (L2) (urban)	3	Age range: all aged 20 Average age: 20	2 Female 1 Male	1 Asian/Asian British 1 Mixed/Multiple ethnic group 1 Chinese	Average participant position = 7734 (Quintile 2)

2.3. Data Generation

The stigmas around topics of health and inequality (where practices and situations are individualised and equated with deficit, passivity and irrational choice) make discussion of such topics challenging [36,37]. We employed focus group discussions to generate data and we gave careful consideration to the topic guides (activities and language used), as well as how support could be provided during and after the sessions [31]. While focus groups may prevent people sharing information due to concerns around privacy and stigma [38], they can help to reduce potential power differentials between researchers and participants and provide a space where people can discuss challenging topics with the support of others [39]. We ensured that we framed our questions so that participants could talk generally about young people in their area rather than feeling pressured into discussing their own personal experiences (e.g., 'What kind of things where you live support young people to be 'healthy'?'). Youth workers helped to facilitate the discussions alongside the research team. As well as having at least one youth worker involved in each session, we had four members of the research team in each online session and two members of the research team in each face-to-face session. There was at least one week between each of the three sessions for each group, which helped to avoid fatigue and to provide the opportunity for participants to reflect on and discuss the sessions with youth workers and peers.

Topic guides were piloted and revised as part of our Public Involvement and Engagement work with partner youth organisations (see Supplementary File S1: Topic Guides). Both online and face-to-face focus groups followed the same format (introductions, warm-up activity, main activity (in smaller breakout groups) and close and cool-down activity). The first focus group used a participatory concept mapping activity (for example see Jessiman et al. 2021 [40]) to explore perceptions of what influences young people's opportunities to be healthy in their local area (see Supplementary File S2 for an example of a map developed from participants' discussions). The second looked at understandings of inequalities in health. Participants were asked to discuss what they understood by the term 'health inequality' and asked to select and share their ideas about contemporary news articles relevant to health inequalities (e.g., free school meals, the uneven impact of COVID-19). The third focus group involved a discussion of the young people's key priorities for change in improving health in their area.

2.4. Data Analysis

In keeping with our open question framing (designed to avoid participants feeling pressured into disclosing personal stories), we employed thematic analysis, drawing on Braun and Clarke's (2006) framework [41]. In particular, our approach was guided by an emphasis on analysis as 'creative and active' [42] (p. 343) and an inherently 'interpretive, reflexive process' [42] (p. 332). The qualitative data management software system NVivo-12 was used to support data management. A coding frame (see Supplementary File S3: Coding Framework) was developed through HF, MC, VE, NG, EH and NW independently reading and adding descriptors to a selection of transcripts. Key codes and overarching themes were then discussed and agreed upon. The development of the coding framework was largely inductive, but an initial scaffolding was provided by key concepts in the literature and the research questions [17,43–46]. Following independent double coding of a selection of the transcripts ($n = 6$, two from each geographical area), we refined the framework before finally coding all transcripts. The development of a coding framework enabled multiple researchers in different locations to contribute to coding. The framework was used as a flexible starting point for analysis for this paper, which was carried out by the two lead authors (H.F. and N.W.). While we did not originally code our transcripts in relation to Raphael's (2011) SDH discourse framework [12], we mobilise this framework in the discussion of our findings as a helpful tool for illuminating *how* young people understand the relationship between socioeconomic circumstances and health.

We use verbatim extracts from the focus groups to illustrate the key findings. While we collected demographic data, this was anonymised at the point of collection to protect participant confidentiality. This means only the field site location and focus group session for each quote are provided (e.g., SY1.1 = South Yorkshire Group 1, session 1). Thus we are unable to identify individual quotes from participants but have endeavoured to present a range of young people's voices across and within all participant groups.

3. Results

3.1. Perceptions of Factors Linking Socioeconomic Position and Health

Participants in our study identified a number of different factors that they perceived to impact upon young people's opportunities to enjoy good health in their local area. Through the course of their discussions, they described how abilities to eat healthily, access health-promoting spaces and activities and housing conditions all influenced health and were all shaped by socioeconomic position. The exacerbating impact of COVID-19 upon these abilities was also discussed. These themes were salient across all youth groups.

3.1.1. Eating Healthily in Contexts of Deprivation

Young people described a range of barriers to eating healthily in contexts of deprivation: the cost of and access to 'healthy' food, the apparent ubiquity of 'unhealthy' food, time pressure and competing priorities for limited financial resources. There was a general consensus among participants that 'healthy food' (particularly fresh fruit and vegetables) was more expensive than 'unhealthy food' (particularly processed foods) and that this was a key source of inequality:

> 'you can get chocolate bars for £1, you can get KFC for £1, £2 for a whole meal [...] and then you go for the healthy meals and it's like £3, £4 for no reason. And then they ask, oh why is everyone not eating healthy food instead? How can we eat healthy food if the area doesn't even have any healthy food, it's, our environment is just full of unhealthy food.' (L1.1)

Many young people described poor access to healthy food within their local areas and contrasted this with the ubiquity of 'fast-food' take-away outlets. Young people from London in particular linked fast-food density to the socioeconomic context of the area:

'when I go to richer parts of London, for example, like, when I go to the City where my university is, the [Name of university], I don't see that many fast food shops around me but I see, like, when I'm in my own local area, [Name of location], there's so many fast food shops.' (L2.2)

They also described how this situation had worsened due to the COVID-19 lockdown measures, with spaces seen as 'unhealthy' (takeaways) noted to be quicker to open up than health-supporting spaces (youth clubs, gyms). Generally, limited financial resources alongside limited access created a context of *unaffordability*, which constrained consumption choices. A number of participants challenged the notion that eating healthily is necessarily expensive and described how buying takeaways would be costly when looking at the perspective of buying every day and for a whole family. However, whilst some participants foregrounded the importance of behaviours such as cooking skills and planning meals ahead, others, through the group discussions, positioned individualised arguments like this against working families' busy lives. They thought that people on a low income were also likely to be 'time poor' and that this would push them towards quicker and easier, but not healthier, 'choices': *'people on low incomes often, a lot of the time they work more hours and they can't afford childcare and stuff so they don't have the time to like prepare meals, which are like really healthy'* (SY2.2). One participant eloquently explained how a lack of time 'forced' parents *'to do—in a way—irrational things, such as constantly sending a fast food order'* (NE2.2).

While in one group some young people initially found it difficult to understand higher rates of obesity among lower socioeconomic groups, through the course of their discussion, they made sense of the apparently counterintuitive link:

Participant A You associate free school meals with poorer families who don't necessarily have obesity, if you get me. So the people who have got the money buy the food and then eat it and then get obese. But for me it's quite interesting that obviously obesity is associated with poorer families.

Participant B Healthier foods tend to be more expensive, like you can get one thing which is like full fat and it'll be like £2 and if you want to get the fat-free version it's like £3.50 or something.

Participant A Yeah, yeah, I was thinking the same as well. Obviously the cheaper stuff's worse, if you get me, and more unhealthy.' (SY1.2)

Young people also highlighted competing priorities for people on a low income (e.g., household bills, activities, clothes), which meant that they could not always 'choose' the healthy option. A salient theme within many food narratives was the shame associated with the inability, or bounded ability, to 'consume correctly': *'When people have to buy cheaper options, sometimes they get ashamed quite a lot, people saying that they're being right cheap or it's bad things or they're being lazy [...]'* (SY1.1). Indeed, some participants highlighted how food banks, designed to attenuate the impacts of poverty, could represent a source of embarrassment and shame for those who used them:

'there's more food banks and stuff opening, which is a good thing, especially in this area but some people might be embarrassed to go to one because they don't want to show that they're in poverty ... people might shame them for it, definitely ... There's like the ideal, you can provide for your family without any help or charity help, and people want to show to be like that and they don't want people to see them as like not working and being lazy, which obviously is not going to be good on the mental health.' (SY2.1)

Such quotes highlight the importance young people attached to the shame associated with poverty, and the use of the word 'lazy' hints at their awareness of deficit discourses of the 'undeserving poor' [47]. In relation to food then, young people demonstrated nuanced understandings of the everyday challenges of life on a low income and described how different factors compounded each other.

3.1.2. Health-Promoting Spaces and Activities

Health-promoting spaces were generally described as places where young people could exercise and/or socialise, and participants related them to both physical and mental health. Opportunities to access and participate in health-promoting spaces and activities were often perceived to be strongly shaped by socioeconomic position. Many young people emphasised the high cost of access to activities and spaces (e.g., gyms, sports clubs), and participants in South Yorkshire and the North East also talked about the prohibitive cost of public transport to different leisure spaces (London participants highlighted that transport was free for young people). Personal accounts described how this played out: *'we did badminton for a while but then they made it £3 a night and barely anyone could afford it [. . .] the whole club fell in on itself and stopped because people couldn't pay to attend it'* (SY1.1). Demonstrating a clear sense of injustice, one participant, talking about meeting at the local snooker hall, argued, *'some places can be unnecessarily expensive, and it's not really fair on them though because like all we's want to do is hang out with friends and we's can't get to it'* (NE2.1). The move from 'them' to 'we' in the course of the short narrative serves to convey how this personally affects the participant and their friends and perhaps hints at how acutely young people experienced the unfairness here. Young people consistently contrasted expensive or inaccessible activities with their local youth groups which were perceived as providing a nearby safe, welcoming and affordable space to relax and socialise: *'[the youth group] is good for our health 'cos we get to hang out with our friends and play out back'* (NE2.1). Youth groups then were depicted as attenuating the impacts of poverty and socioeconomic disadvantage.

A small number of participants voiced a belief that, irrespective of income levels, young people could always use outdoor spaces for exercise. However, across all groups participants spoke of how perceptions of safety in their local areas were key inhibitors to accessing public spaces. Participants frequently described high levels of crime within their local areas compared to other places:

> *'So, when there are a lot of like stabbings going on in the area, people, like their parents won't let them go outside [. . .] so I think if crime could reduce in the area maybe people would have more access to these mental health spaces that are available.'* (L1.1)

The phrase 'these mental health spaces' highlights young people's emphasis on the potential for social spaces to positively impact upon their health and wellbeing. Parks were particularly singled out as places that young people could not enjoy to their full potential due to safety concerns: *'I live near a skate park and sometimes I get intimidated when I'm walking past because a lot of the time they're doing like drugs, drinking. On a night time I wouldn't want to be like round there'* (SY2.2). Narratives about risk (crime and safety) were particularly common among female and LGBTQ+ participants across the different areas. While official supervision (e.g., security, police) was noted in some cases to help young people feel safer and support the use of such spaces, such supervision seemed to be rare. Indeed, for many participants, concerns about public anti-social behaviour, and especially the substance use of other people, was noted to shape perceptions and use of space. There was, however, an acknowledgement from some that 'risky behaviours' were also related to exclusion or a lack of activities for young people to engage in: *'if there's nothing to do then we're going to get ourselves into trouble'* (SY1.1). The movement between describing 'others' in narratives about drug use in the local area and the 'we' and 'ourselves' in this extract affords a pertinent example of how participants moved between individualising, othering narratives to a more collective sense of the importance of socioeconomic circumstances in limiting opportunities.

3.1.3. The Relationship between Poor Housing and Poor Health

Young people highlighted the relationship between poor housing and poor health, particularly mental health:

'I feel like the housing is very cramped in the area, like it's very cramped, like it's very overcrowded and I feel like that also does have a big impact on mental health as well. Because it's so overcrowded you don't have any time to yourself, any time to think, literally with people around.' (L1.1)

Echoing the perceived shame associated with not eating 'correctly', participants described the shame related to living in the 'wrong' kind of housing: *'I've seen people who've felt embarrassed over it, not wanting to like invite friends over and then they're just kind of feeling alone'* (SY1.1). In this way, young people emphasised how poor housing had a significant impact on their social and emotional wellbeing—through everyday stress, embarrassment and reduced opportunities to socialise in one's own home. Although much less salient in their narratives, they also discussed the relationship between housing and physical health. This was articulated particularly in relation to the COVID-19 lockdown measures, which meant people had to stay at home more than usual. Some described how 'richer' families could afford to purchase home exercise machines and contrasted this with poor people who had neither the financial resources nor space to do so: *'So obviously some people might be in a small flat or whatever, no garden, they might not have the space to exercise either indoors or outdoors as such'* (SY1.2).

3.2. Patterning and Pathways in Socioeconomic Inequalities in Health

As well as highlighting specific factors linking socioeconomic position and health, young people voiced their understandings of how inequalities were patterned. They described both geographical (regional and localised) and intergenerational patterns of socioeconomic inequality. They also directly and indirectly emphasised the interrelationships between factors affecting health and the complexity of pathways between socioeconomic position and health outcomes.

3.2.1. Regional and Localised Inequalities

Regional inequalities were seen by the participants as underlying socioeconomic inequalities in health. Young people across all groups described a North–South divide in terms of wealth. The government was perceived to be responsible for creating and perpetuating this inequality through uneven investment, as articulated here by one of the London participants:

'I know that in north England [people] are not as wealthy as the south of England, kind of thing. Because obviously, like, the government, well, over the recent years the government's basically just been focusing on the south of England because of, yeah, that's where the capital is and it's a bit more, the economy in the south of England's a lot better than the north. So I guess, the pandemic has highlighted the fact that they've been, the government has, kind of, been putting the north on the side and just, like, yeah, not paying attention to their needs as much . . . I feel like as, like, as, like, as a whole that the south of England has just got more investment than the north of England.' (L2.2)

Young people vividly articulated how differences in local economies and labour markets between the North and South created tangible differences in everyday working and living conditions: *'Well there's obviously more technical industries in London, so like engineering or ICT work. There isn't those jobs in [South Yorkshire town]'* (SY2.2). Local labour markets in the North were perceived to revolve around hospitality and service sector employment, which many associated with low pay, insecurity and low job satisfaction: *'the more like boring [jobs]'* (SY2.1).

Focus group discussions often contained references to much more local-level inequalities too. In the following narrative, reference is made to a 'clear split' in wealth distribution between different areas:

'There's certain parts of town where you can, they're just known for people being either real poor there or they're barely scraping by and there's also bits where basically people who are wealthy live and it's like quite a clear split. So all those people who live in the, I

wouldn't say dodgy areas but like with poorer people, they haven't got as good quality of diet and stuff because they're probably living off more cheaper meals that are just packed full of like chemicals or sugars and stuff.' (SY2.2)

The participant appears to show some awareness that people and places can be stigmatised and that lack of money and place-level disadvantage are barriers to healthy lifestyles. Hence the participant expresses unease about using the word 'dodgy' and appears to be avoiding individualistic, victim-blaming discourses. Some of the young people in London travelled to schools outside their local area, and this seemed to heighten their awareness of localised inequalities:

'The schools I have been to have generally been in wealthier areas than the area I live in and I've noticed that they definitely have a lot more green space and like generally just a lot more space within school to do sports and stuff as well, yeah . . . in like less like affluent places like there's more like residential spaces and that's, like people would say like [Name of location] has like an overcrowding like housing issue. And like I think like the main reason why is because in wealthier places like people are more spread out like the sort of like, on, like well people who are more affluent tend to have less children, people who are more affluent tend to like live out, more spaced out from each other . . . you can get stuck in a cycle because it's so expensive in Central London so then because it's so expensive you're spending your money on other stuff you won't be able to afford to move out to a wealthier area, where there's like potentially, I don't know more green space and less air pollution. So you can, yeah, you can just kind of get stuck in the, that cycle yeah.' (L2.1)

Here, however, the narrative moves from emphasizing environmental factors (access to green space and better housing) to behavioural factors (affluent families have fewer children) and then back to environmental factors (expensive housing, green space, air pollution). The narrative echoes the interplay and pull between different factors and exemplifies young people's willingness to engage in complex understandings of causal pathways. Further, through their discussions, young people demonstrated an awareness of individualised discourses around blaming. They also consistently highlighted the injustice of the inequality that they perceived: 'It's actually unfair. The facts are right there in front of your eyes, because if you're born quite a poor person, then most people would expect you to stay poor and vulnerable to a lot of diseases' (NE2.2).

Many participants also discussed how substance use (tobacco smoking and drugs) was more prevalent in their area than other, more affluent areas. There was a suggestion that 'other' young people surrounded by drug taking and drinking would go on to engage in these behaviours themselves: 'Like round my area it's quite bad for drugs and stuff like that . . . they see other people doing it, it'll make them want to try it and then they'll probably end up getting addicted and stuff like that' (SY1.1). However, the participants positioned themselves as avoiding the inevitability of this. Thus, they acknowledged structural issues and suggested deterministic outcomes for 'other' young people due to place-based disadvantage but discussed exercising their own agency to avoid this: 'Around my area it's like the teens who are similar to my age have all gone mad with nights out and like drugs and that, so I won't walk out. I see gangs and I'm like no, you're not getting me' (SY1.1).

3.2.2. Intergenerational Patterns of Inequality

Young people repeatedly articulated the interactions between regional and intergenerational patterns of inequality and frequently commented on the presence and transfer of health-damaging practices through families and within communities. In the following narrative, one young person eloquently describes intergenerational continuity in practices and intergenerational cycles of poverty but also the inextricable link between the two:

'If they're in a poor area, it's much worse because their mum and dad might just give them a quid and tell them to go and buy their tea, instead of having like a home-cooked meal that's full of good stuff. If that happens in one place, then it'll start spreading in a *way so more people will be getting poor because, like—let's say one family, if they have two sons and those two sons have sons and they're all like staying in the same area, it multiplies and then there's like these areas where there's shops and stuff and it's all corner shops where they sell like ready meals and stuff and they all live off that and then they don't have as good a diet, which isn't their fault in the first place, it's just where they were born and put into the world.'* (SY2.2)

Highlighting the permeation of adverse health practices, there was an explanation of how health practices, such as diet, were shaped by experiences and exposure to parents' and peers' behaviours in a sociocultural context, which were described as 'normalising' such practices:

'Like we were discussing earlier about, your personal life, your friends and family, and you might adapt to how they are. So if a parent is eating fast food almost every day, then the child might say, "Actually, do you know what? That's OK because my dad is doing it.' (NE2.2)

However, again this needs to be understood alongside young people's foregrounding of the influence of economic and environmental factors on health practices, particularly in relation to food.

3.2.3. Interrelationships between Factors Linking Socioeconomic Position and Health

Young people's discussions consistently highlighted the interrelationships between factors linking socioeconomic circumstance and health. The complex aetiology of health inequalities was both directly and indirectly acknowledged with understandings rooted in experience. Highlighting their focus on the interrelationship between different factors and the pathways through which inequalities were created and perpetuated, they articulated pathways between root causes (such as local labour market precarity) and secondary factors (such as not being able to afford to eat healthily):

'I think obviously because there's high rates of unemployment and that links to not having money and then not like spending loads, that all links into like buying the cheapest food, which is not naturally healthy. So it all kind of links really.' (SY1.1)

The phrase 'it all kind of links really' encapsulates young people's emphasis on the interwoven nature of inequalities. However, they consistently foregrounded poverty as the root cause of socioeconomic patterned inequalities in health: *'if you don't have a very good income then you can't really live in a very good house. It can affect your health as it is and can cause like, it can cause stress which can cause other things'* (SY1.2). The bounding and constraining impacts of stretched financial resources upon health practices and outcomes were clearly highlighted: *'I feel like money is one of the biggest factors for nearly everything, diet, mental health'* (SY1.3). However, while in general young people's narratives demonstrated their awareness of the socioeconomically disadvantaged nature of their local area, at times their discussions hinted that they associated poverty with others rather than themselves. In particular, one participant from one of the North East groups, the most socioeconomically disadvantaged area we worked in, noted: *'The less fortunate could actually find it harder . . . they're not as privileged as we are in terms of money and wealth.'* (NE2.3).

Whether they explicitly made the link or not themselves, young people's narratives illuminated the importance they attached to the impact of poverty on mental health, typically the everyday, chronic stress and strain of living in poverty. They highlighted particular pinch points where limited financial resources were acutely stressful: *'I think there's a certain level of stress if you go knowing that you've maybe not got as much money and there's going to be certain times of the month where you have to really mind what you're spending'* (NE1.2). Mental health was perceived to be a consistent 'link' within a causal cycle of inequality—linked both to a decreased likelihood of engaging in healthful behaviours (such as eating well, engaging in exercise and labour market engagement) and an increased likelihood of engaging in risky behaviours (such as drinking and taking drugs):

'mental health is, like, connected to so many other things ... like, reducing physical activities, and diet, and stuff like that. So mental health is, kind of, like, it could be, like, a major cause for the other things to happen so, like, comfort foods, for example, eating when you're, like, depressed or something, or not getting out of bed due to, like, lack of food, like, due to depression so physical activity is just lower.' (L2.3)

4. Discussion

4.1. Social Determinants Shaping Health: Interacting Factors and Complex Pathways

Through the course of their discussions, participants in our study often demonstrated nuanced understandings of how socioeconomic circumstances shaped health outcomes. Young people's narratives showed how they were making sense of inequalities in health as they talked—at times echoing but, crucially, moving away from more populist individualised, neoliberal explanations for inequalities. Understandings of the relationship between socioeconomic circumstance and health, then, were not fixed and static but rather malleable and dynamic [17]. Overall, their narratives demonstrated a subtle appreciation of the ways in which the SDH get 'under the skin to shape health' through 'interacting material, psychological and behavioural pathways' (Raphael's (2011) Discourse Level Three) [12] (p. 226).

4.1.1. Material Pathways

Young people demonstrated an acute awareness of how differential access to material resources shaped opportunities to eat healthily, access health-promoting spaces and activities and enjoy good housing. Poverty was perceived to be all-pervasive, and young people consistently emphasised limited financial resources as a major barrier to health [48]. However, they also emphasised how this was exacerbated by other factors such as local infrastructures and perceived safety [49]. They also highlighted the uneven socioeconomic patterning of time—a finding not foregrounded by previous research exploring public perspectives of socioeconomic circumstances and health [17]. Their descriptions of the everyday stresses for low-income parents managing unsociable hours and caring responsibilities, particularly in relation to providing healthy food, resonate strongly with Strazdin et al.'s (2016) call to consider time as a social determinant of health as it has the potential to affect so many opportunities for good health—including time to engage in health-promoting activities, rest and care for each other [50]. The participants' emphasis on time perhaps also hints at a weakness in the SDH framework which deals with social 'domains' and determining factors, rather than the mechanisms through which inequalities are sustained.

4.1.2. Psychosocial Pathways

Young people consistently highlighted the importance of psychosocial mechanisms linking socioeconomic circumstance and health inequalities. They discussed the importance of mental health as a critical element in understanding the pervasive, complex influence of socioeconomic circumstance on health behaviours, experiences and outcomes (Discourse Level Three) [12]. Echoing previous studies with mostly adult participants this was particularly poignant in relation to housing [39,51–54]. Young people described both acute and chronic stress of living in inadequate housing, including the associated shame and stigma [39], offering poor housing as an important reason for higher rates of mental ill health among lower socioeconomic groups (Discourse Level Three) [12]. Participants' discussions regarding socioeconomic inequalities in access to safe, green spaces and the 'complex mix of spatial and social intertwinings' also highlighted the impact on mental wellbeing [55] (p. 8). Such understandings contrast with findings from the recent Frameworks Institute project where participants foregrounded a 'mentalism' model in which 'mental health issues such as depression and anxiety [. . .] were seen as being determined by an individual's mindset' (their self-discipline and willpower) [18] (p. 7).

4.1.3. Behavioural Pathways

At times, and particularly early on in discussions, young people emphasised the uneven patterning of risky health behaviours between socioeconomic groups, particularly in relation to substance use, smoking and alcohol (Discourse Level Two) [12]. This resonates with survey-based data with adults [18,53,56], and some qualitative work with both adults and young people [18,26]. Importantly, however, in the context of their discussions, young people's narratives in our study frequently shifted towards a subtler appreciation of the role of the SDH, emphasising material and environmental factors as underpinning health behaviours. This finding differs markedly from recent UK-based research which characterises public understandings as focusing on personal responsibility and contrasts this with expert opinion (among those working in the field of social determinants) that behaviours are the very 'endpoint in a long chain of causes and consequences that produce health outcomes' [18] (p. 7). The young people's accounts in our study resonate much more closely with the 'expert' understandings. They also echo the 'integrated explanations for socioeconomically patterned inequalities' evident among the mainly adult participants in Smith and Anderson's (2018) meta-ethnography [17]. Importantly, however, both the participants in our study and the majority of those in the studies in Smith and Anderson's (2018) review lived in socioeconomically disadvantaged areas and thus had personal experience of how inequalities played out in everyday life [17]. This may well explain the divergence.

4.2. The Role of Public Policy Decisions (and Their Underlying Ideologies)

While young people did not explicitly discuss the intersection between material living circumstances and gender or race (and only rarely referred directly to 'class' (Discourse Level Four) [12]), young people's narratives sometimes demonstrated a critical consciousness of the role of public policy decisions and their underlying political philosophies in creating and sustaining inequity (Discourse Levels Five and Six) [12]. However, this was only really evident in their discussions regarding uneven geographic labour market precarity and the absence of regeneration investment [57]. A lack of political will to invest in the North (and vested interests in ensuring the success of the South) and underinvestment in certain local areas were directly blamed for reducing opportunities for good work and living conditions and, ultimately, good health [58,59]. The narratives echo previous research in which adult participants perceived some policies to be more favourable to some groups than others [14,51,60]. Our participants were also acutely aware of the unequal impact of the economic fallout of the COVID-19 pandemic on already disadvantaged young people [61], echoing research showing that young people suffer disproportionate impacts upon their employment trajectories and wages when exposed to economic uncertainty [62]. Young people's emphasis on the unacceptability of poverty and scale of inequality contrasts with earlier studies (e.g., Shildrick and MacDonald's 2013 study [47]). But reflects broader shifts in societal attitudes with 'both phenomena being more widely regarded as prevalent and unacceptable than in the past' [63] (p. 164). However, in general, there was much less evidence that participants spoke to Raphael's Discourse Level Seven—about the power imbalances that underpin the uneven distribution of the SDH [12]. Health inequalities were described in relation to slightly abstract or faceless phenomena such as unemployment, poverty and regional inequality, but there was very little discussion about who has the power and how it is used to privilege some and marginalise others.

Determinants of Health Inequalities?

While young people's narratives offered apparently little space to disrupt the pathways between socioeconomic insecurity and health inequality, somewhat paradoxically, young people at times positioned themselves as avoiding the inevitability of this. Area fatalism and individual agency to resist risky health behaviours, for example, sat side by side. This was particularly evident in relation to (avoiding) substance use. Their emphasis on 'room for agency' to some extent echoes concerns about the language of social 'determinants'.

McMahon (2021) highlights that such a framing can perpetuate a reductionist approach to health inequalities [64]. Taken to its logical endpoint, this reduces individual people to 'puppets on a string' [65] (p. 475) and loses sight of the interaction between individuals, services, materiality and health [22]. The tension, however, was much less evident in relation to eating healthily and engaging in health-promoting activities where young people were more likely to share personal stories of the barriers they themselves faced [66]. This perhaps links to a greater acknowledgment of the bounding influence on poverty in relation to the food and exercise within public discourses more broadly. Indeed, at the time of the focus groups, a campaign for free school meals, led by Marcus Rashford, a prominent English football player, was the centre of much media attention [67], and the unequal impact of COVID-19 on people's everyday living and working situations was very much in the spotlight [68].

Further, our analysis of young people's emphasis on the interrelationships between pathways to inequalities also supports calls to move away from depicting discrete categories of determinants in relation to health inequalities [69]. Indeed, Dahlgren and Whitehead (2021) highlight that their rainbow model was only ever meant to depict determinants of health, not determinants of health *inequalities* [70]. To fully understand the root causes of health inequalities, they argue, we need to 'take a further conceptual leap and focus on the pathways and mechanisms by which [. . .] determinants [. . .] bring about social gradients in health' [70] (p. 22). Focusing on pathways and mechanisms in this way may also help to address the thorny issue of adequately articulating how health-relevant practices are constrained by people's social and economic environment without inadvertently disempowering and further stigmatising underserved communities [64].

4.3. Study Limitations and Strengths

Our sample of young people from socioeconomically deprived areas may limit the relevance of our findings for young people from more affluent areas. It also plays into a wider critique that by focusing on areas of socioeconomic deprivation such areas are perceived as the only communities in which inequality matters [17]. Further, while our sample as a whole is ethnically diverse, all participants in our North East and South Yorkshire groups were White British.

Our decision to prioritise participant confidentiality also means that we have not provided individual participant demographic information alongside quotes. While this limits our ability to explore the extent to which individual participants held different views and the ways in which their understandings may have developed in the course of the discussions, we believe our commitment to confidentiality helped to facilitate young people's engagement and openness during data generation. We were guided by a desire to ensure young people felt able to talk as freely as possible in the focus group setting. Indeed, we appreciated the limits of confidentiality in group discussions and therefore framed our questions in ways that ensured participants did not have to disclose personal information if they did not wish to and encouraged them to talk generally about people in their areas in light of this. This often resulted in discussions about their experiences and perspectives framed around '(some) young people'.

It is also important to acknowledge the potential limitations of recruitment through existing youth organisations. Many youth organisations undertake work around health; therefore participants may have had more awareness about health inequalities than other groups of young people. Nevertheless, working closely with youth groups afforded many benefits. Youth workers helped to refine our topic guides and facilitate participant engagement, and they provided an invaluable source of trusted support for participants (see Woodrow et al., 2021 [31]).

Our approach of using three interlinked focus groups provided an opportunity to develop rapport, sense check and build on ideas over the sessions. The supportive atmosphere of the focus group in which young people were surrounded by peers and youth workers they knew, as well as research team members experienced in working with young people, perhaps helped to foster a more critical take and to enable participants to challenge each other. The context afforded young people a forum in which to develop understandings rather than being solely a means of extracting ideas. This highlights the importance of giving young people time and space to discuss and reflect on their perspectives on health inequalities [71,72]. Perhaps most importantly, we received consistently positive feedback from both participants and youth leaders across the three areas. Indeed, the retention of our participants over the series of three focus groups, which involved young people actively joining to participate in their free time (both whilst at home and during their youth groups sessions), demonstrates their engagement with and commitment to the project.

Generating data during the COVID-19 pandemic also afforded a unique lens through which the young people viewed and subsequently discussed inequalities in health. Indeed, many young people recognised the unequal impact of the pandemic on health and were, to some extent, aware of the way existing inequalities have been exposed by the pandemic [11]. Therefore, this may help explain some of our findings around young people's nuanced appreciations of the links between socioeconomic position and health.

4.4. Priorities for Future Research

More research exploring young people's perspectives on the relationships between socioeconomic circumstances, inequality and health is needed to address the current paucity. In particular, work with marginalised groups (such as looked-after children, care leavers, homeless young people, young people not in education, employment or training) who may be more likely to experience adverse social determinants of health would be beneficial [73]. Conversely, work with young people from more affluent contexts would provide interesting comparison and help counter a more general focus in the literature on areas of socioeconomic deprivation [17]. Further, research with groups not recruited through youth organisations would help explore if the perspectives found in our work were shaped by the participants' involvement in youth organisations. Finally, it would be beneficial to explore ways to more effectively discuss, describe and teach topics of health inequality and look at ways to explore such topics in ways that are not stigmatising or fatalistic but that encourage positive social change [71].

4.5. Policy and Practice Implications

Our study highlights an ongoing need for policies that address young people's everyday socioeconomic realities and experiences. First and foremost, young people's emphasis on the all-pervasive impact of poverty on their opportunities to enjoy good health underscores the importance of pro-equity policies to end poverty. Their foregrounding of the uneven socioeconomic patterning of time and its impact on health and wellbeing highlights a need to tackle long (and often unsociable) working hours for people living in the most deprived neighbourhoods [74]. Further, there is an ongoing need for policies that address the conditions and impacts of unsuitable housing and that make it easier for young people, particularly those in socioeconomically disadvantaged areas, to eat more healthily and access health-promoting activities and spaces.

While local authorities have responsibility to implement important practical changes here (e.g., enhancing green spaces and parks, making streets safer and establishing cycle lanes), this needs to be enabled by funding. The public health grant awarded to local authorities is currently one billion pounds lower (in real terms per capita) than it was in 2015/16 [24], and reductions in funding allocations have been higher in the poorest areas of the country [75]. In particular, young people in this study highlighted that youth clubs afford a safe space to socialise with peers, access information and advice and form trusting relationships with professionals. Yet, policy decisions have resulted in significant drops in funding for youth services with, for example, 750 youth centres forced to close between 2010/11 and 2018/19 [76]. This worrying trend has been exacerbated by increased funding pressures during COVID-19 [77]. Further, while on the one hand our study points to the importance of cross-sectoral action across a range of policy areas [46,78], we are wary here of falling into the trap of 'shifting from a social inequality to a health inequality frame' [79] (p. 653), and focusing our attention on the lower rather than the higher levels of Raphael's (2011) seven discourses [12]. Such a framing, Lynch (2017) argues, can serve to make tackling inequalities seem like an insurmountable problem and divert attention away from policies (such as taxation, redistribution and labour market regulation) that we know will impact upon socioeconomic inequalities and, in doing so, health inequalities [79,80].

5. Conclusions

Our study affords an important contribution to the dearth of exploration around young people's perspectives on inequalities in health [17,27,28]. Our focus on areas of high deprivation provides important insights and contributes to the limited body of work exploring the perspectives of people living on a low income in socio-epidemiological research more broadly [22,81] and calls for policy to tackle inequalities to be 'grounded in the realities of people living in poverty' [82] (para.2). Our study demonstrates that young people understand that health inequalities are generated by social determinants of health, which in turn influence behaviours. They highlight a complex interweaving of pathways between social determinants and health outcomes. However, they do not tend to think in terms of the SDH and their distribution as resulting from the power and influence of those who create and benefit from health and social inequalities. It may be that they are unused to thinking in this way or that they have understandings that we have not fully appreciated. An informed understanding of the causes of health inequalities, influenced by their own unique generational experiences, is important to help young people achieve greater equity in the future than they perceive at the present.

Supplementary Materials: The following supporting information can be downloaded at: https://www.mdpi.com/article/10.3390/ijerph19063679/s1, Supplementary File S1: Topic guides; Supplementary File S2: Participatory map; Supplementary File S3: Coding framework.

Author Contributions: Conceptualisation, H.F., C.D.-R., M.E., K.L., S.S., C.S. and E.G.; Data curation, H.F., N.W., M.C., E.H., N.G., V.E., P.K. and C.D.-R.; Formal analysis, H.F., N.W., M.C., E.H., N.G., V.E. and P.K.; Investigation, H.F., N.W., M.C., E.H., N.G. and V.E.; Methodology, H.F., N.W., M.C., E.H., N.G., V.E., M.E., K.L., E.R., S.S., C.S. and E.G.; Project administration, H.F., N.W., M.C., E.H., N.G., V.E., P.K., C.D.-R., E.R., C.S. and E.G.; Resources, H.F., C.S. and E.G.; Supervision, H.F., C.D.-R., M.E., K.L., S.S., C.S. and E.G.; Writing—original draft, H.F., N.W., M.E., R.M. and E.R.; Writing—review and editing, M.C., E.H., N.G., V.E., P.K., C.D.-R., M.E., K.L., R.M., E.R., S.S., C.S. and E.G. All authors have read and agreed to the published version of the manuscript.

Funding: This project is funded by the National Institute for Health Research (NIHR) School for Public Health Research (SPHR) (grant reference PD-SPH-2015). The views expressed are those of the authors and not necessarily those of the NIHR or the Department of Health and Social Care.

Institutional Review Board Statement: The study was approved by the School of Health and Related Research (ScHARR) ethics committee at the University of Sheffield. Date of approval: 25 November 2020. Ethics form reference number: 037145. All methods were carried out in accordance with relevant guidelines and regulations.

Informed Consent Statement: Informed consent was obtained from all subjects involved in the study. Written informed consent included consent for publication of the findings and the use of anonymised quotations in publications.

Data Availability Statement: Data available on request due to restrictions. The data presented in this study are available on reasonable request from the corresponding author. The data are not publicly available due to privacy reasons.

Acknowledgments: The authors would like to thank the members of our stakeholder steering group for their support and input throughout the project. We thank members of the youth organisations who piloted and provided feedback on our data generation tools and methods and Naoimh McMahon for commenting on an earlier draft of the manuscript. Finally, we thank the young people and youth organisations that took part in the research for their contributions, insights and enthusiasm.

Conflicts of Interest: The authors do not have any conflict of interest. The funders had no role in the design of the study; in the collection, analyses or interpretation of data; in the writing of the manuscript or in the decision to publish the results.

References

1. Marmot, M.; Allen, J.; Boyce, T.; Goldblatt, P.; Morrison, J. *Health Equity in England: The Marmot Review 10 Years On*; Health Foundation: London, UK, 2020. Available online: https://www.health.org.uk/publications/reports/the-marmot-review-10-years-on (accessed on 6 January 2022).
2. Tinson, A. *Living in Poverty Was Bad for Your Health Long before COVID-19*; The Health Foundation: London, UK, 2020. Available online: https://www.health.org.uk/publications/long-reads/living-in-poverty-was-bad-for-your-health-long-before-COVID-19 (accessed on 6 January 2022).
3. Garthwaite, K.; Bambra, C. "How the other half live": Lay perspectives on health inequalities in an age of austerity. *Soc. Sci. Med.* **2017**, *187*, 268–275. [CrossRef] [PubMed]
4. Shah, R.; Hagell, A.; Cheung, R. *International Comparisons of Health and Wellbeing in Adolescence and Early Adulthood*; The Nuffield Trust: London, UK, 2019. Available online: https://www.nuffieldtrust.org.uk/research/international-comparisons-of-health-and-wellbeing-in-adolescence-and-early-adulthood (accessed on 6 January 2022).
5. Corna, L. A life course perspective on socioeconomic inequalities in health: A critical review of conceptual frameworks. *Adv. Life Course Res.* **2013**, *18*, 150–159. [CrossRef] [PubMed]
6. Kivimäki, M.; Batty, G.; Pentti, J.; Shipley, M.; Sipilä, P.; Nyberg, S.; Suominen, S.; Oksanen, T.; Stenholm, S.; Virtanen, M.; et al. Association between socioeconomic status and the development of mental and physical health conditions in adulthood: A multi-cohort study. *Lancet Public Health* **2020**, *5*, e140–e149. [CrossRef]
7. World Health Organisation. *Closing the Gap in a Generation: Health Equity through Action on the Social Determinants of Health*; World Health Organisation: Geneva, Switzerland, 2008. Available online: https://www.who.int/social_determinants/final_report/csdh_finalreport_2008_execsumm.pdf (accessed on 6 January 2022).
8. Beatty, C.; Fothergill, S. *The Uneven Impact of Welfare Reform: The Financial Losses to Places and People*; Sheffield Hallam University: Sheffield, UK, 2016. Available online: http://shura.shu.ac.uk/15883/1/welfare-reform-2016.pdf (accessed on 6 January 2022).
9. Rashid, T.; Bennett, J.; Paciorek, C.; Doyle, Y.; Pearson-Stuttard, J.; Flaxman, S.; Fecht, D.; Toledano, M.; Li, G.; Daby, H.; et al. Life expectancy and risk of death in 6791 communities in England from 2002 to 2019: High-resolution spatiotemporal analysis of civil registration data. *Lancet Public Health* **2021**, *6*, e805–e816. [CrossRef]
10. N8 Research Partnership. The Child of the North: Building a Fairer Future after COVID-19. N8 Research Partnership: Manchester, UK, 2021. Available online: https://www.n8research.org.uk/report-paints-a-stark-picture-of-inequality-for-children-growing-up-in-the-north/ (accessed on 6 January 2022).
11. Bambra, C.; Riordan, R.; Ford, J.; Matthews, F. The COVID-19 pandemic and health inequalities. *J. Epidemiol. Commun. Health* **2020**, *74*, 648–964. [CrossRef]
12. Raphael, D. A discourse analysis of the social determinants of health. *Crit. Public Health* **2011**, *21*, 221–236. [CrossRef]
13. Babbel, B.; Mackenzie, M.; Hastings, A.; Watt, G. How do general practitioners understand health inequalities and do their professional roles offer scope for mitigation? Constructions derived from the deep end of primary care. *Crit. Public Health* **2019**, *29*, 168–180. [CrossRef]
14. Mackenzie, M.; Collins, C.; Connolly, J.; Doyle, M.; McCartney, G. Working-class discourses of politics, policy and health: 'I don't smoke; I don't drink. The only thing wrong with me is my health'. *Policy Politics* **2017**, *45*, 231–249. [CrossRef]
15. Herrick, C.; Bell, K. Concepts, disciplines and politics: On 'structural violence' and the 'social determinants of health'. *Crit. Public Health* **2020**, *30*, 1–14. [CrossRef]
16. Scott-Samuel, A.; Smith, K. Fantasy paradigms of health inequalities: Utopian thinking? *Soc. Theory Health* **2015**, *13*, 418–436. [CrossRef]
17. Smith, K.; Anderson, R. Understanding lay perspectives on socioeconomic health inequalities in Britain: A meta-ethnography. *Sociol. Health Illn.* **2018**, *40*, 146–170. [CrossRef] [PubMed]
18. Elwell-Sutton, T.; Marshall, L.; Bibby, J.; Volmert, A. *Reframing the Conversation on the Social Determinants of Health*; The Health Foundation: London, UK, 2019. Available online: https://www.health.org.uk/publications/reports/reframing-the-conversation-on-the-social-determinants-of-health?gclid=EAIaIQobChMIu_iUtvvu5wIVwbHtCh2T9ARqEAAYASAAEgJfF_D_BwE (accessed on 6 January 2022).
19. McHugh, N. Eliciting public values on health inequalities: Missing evidence for policy windows? *Evid. Policy J. Res. Debate Pract.* **2021**. [CrossRef]
20. Garthwaite, K.; Smith, K.; Bambra, C.; Pearce, J. Desperately Seeking Reductions in Health Inequalities: Perspectives of UK Researchers on Past, Present and Future Directions in Health Inequalities Research. *Sociol. Health Illn.* **2016**, *38*, 459–478. [CrossRef]
21. Smith, K. Institutional filters: The translation and re-circulation of ideas about health inequalities within policy. *Policy Politics* **2013**, *41*, 81–100. [CrossRef]
22. Dijkstra, I.; Horstman, K. 'Known to be unhealthy': Exploring how social epidemiological research constructs the category of low socioeconomic status. *Soc. Sci. Med.* **2021**, *285*. [CrossRef] [PubMed]

23. Greszczuk, C. *Making Messages Work*; The Health Foundation: London, UK, 2020. Available online: https://www.health.org.uk/thinking-differently-about-health/making-messages-work (accessed on 6 January 2022).
24. The King's Fund. *Public Health: Our Position*; King's Fund: London, UK, 2021. Available online: https://www.kingsfund.org.uk/projects/positions/public-health (accessed on 6 January 2022).
25. Backett-Milburn, K.; Cunningham-Burley, S.; Davis, J. Contrasting lives, contrasting views? Understandings of health inequalities from children in differing social circumstances. *Soc. Sci. Med.* **2003**, *57*, 613–623. [CrossRef]
26. Woodgate, R.; Leach, J. Youth's perspectives on the determinants of health. *Qual. Health Res.* **2010**, *20*, 1173–1182. [CrossRef]
27. Sawyer, S.; Afifi, R.; Bearinger, L.; Blakemore, S.; Dick, B.; Ezeh, A.; Patton, G. Adolescence: A foundation for future health. *Lancet* **2012**, *379*, 1630–1640. [CrossRef]
28. Fergie, G. *Developing a Participatory Approach for Exploring Young People's Perspectives on Health Inequalities*; UK Research and Innovation: Swindon, UK, 2019. Available online: https://gtr.ukri.org/projects?ref=ES%2FS001913%2F1 (accessed on 6 January 2022).
29. O'brien, K.; Selboe, E.; Hayward, B. Exploring youth activism on climate change. *Ecol. Soc.* **2018**, *23*, 42–55. [CrossRef]
30. Institute for Government. *Timeline of UK Government Coronavirus Lockdowns*; Institute for Government: London, UK, 2021. Available online: https://www.instituteforgovernment.org.uk/charts/uk-government-coronavirus-lockdowns (accessed on 6 January 2022).
31. Woodrow, N.; Fairbrother, H.; Crowder, M.; Goyder, E.; Griffin, N.; Holding, E.; Quirk, H. Exploring inequalities in health with young people through online focus groups: Navigating the methodological and ethical challenges. *Qual. Res. J.* **2021**. [CrossRef]
32. Mason, J. *Qualitative Researching*, 3rd ed.; SAGE: Los Angeles, CA, USA, 2018.
33. Furlong, A.; Cartmel, F. *Young People and Social Change: New Perspectives*, 2nd ed.; McGraw-Hill/Open University Press: Maidenhead, UK, 2007.
34. Sawyer, S.M.; Azzopardi, P.S.; Wickremarathne, D.; Patton, G.C. The age of adolescence. *Lancet Child Adolesc. Health* **2018**, *2*, 223–228. [CrossRef]
35. Braun, V.; Clarke, V. To saturate or not to saturate? Questioning data saturation as a useful concept for thematic analysis and sample-size rationales. *Qual. Res. Sport Exerc. Health* **2021**, *13*, 201–216. [CrossRef]
36. Farthing, R. What's Wrong with Being Poor? The Problems of Poverty, as Young People Describe them. *Child. Soc.* **2016**, *30*, 107–119. [CrossRef]
37. Sutton, L. 'They'd only call you a scally if you are poor': The impact of socio-economic status on children's identities. *Child. Geogr.* **2009**, *7*, 277–290. [CrossRef]
38. Bryman, A. *Social Research Methods*, 5th ed.; Oxford University Press: Oxford, UK, 2016.
39. Davidson, R.; Mitchell, R.; Hunt, K. Location, location, location: The role of experience of disadvantage in lay perceptions of area inequalities in health. *Health Place* **2008**, *14*, 167–181. [CrossRef]
40. Jessiman, P.; Powell, K.; Williams, P.; Fairbrother, H.; Crowder, M.; Williams, J.; Kipping, R. A systems map of the determinants of child health inequalities in England at the local level. *PLoS ONE* **2021**, *16*, e0245577. [CrossRef] [PubMed]
41. Braun, V.; Clarke, V. Using thematic analysis in psychology. *Qual. Res. Psychol.* **2006**, *3*, 77–101. [CrossRef]
42. Braun, V.; Clarke, V. One size fits all? What counts as quality practice in (reflexive) thematic analysis? *Qual. Res. Psychol.* **2020**, *18*, 328–352. [CrossRef]
43. Goldfeld, S.; Villanueva, K.; Lee, J.; Robinson, R.; Moriarty, A.; Peel, D.; Katz, I. *Foundational Community Factors (FCFs) for Early Childhood Development: A Report on the Kids in Communities Study*; KiCS: Melbourne, Australia, 2018. Available online: https://www.rch.org.au/uploadedFiles/Main/Content/ccch/CCCH-KICS-Final-Report-April-2018.pdf (accessed on 6 January 2022).
44. Hagell, A.; Shah, R.; Viner, R.; Hargreaves, D.; Varnes, L.; Heys, M. *The Social Determinants of Young People's Health: Identifying the Key Issues and Assessing How Young People Are Doing in the 2010s*; Health Foundation: London, UK, 2018. Available online: https://www.health.org.uk/publications/the-social-determinants-of-young-people%E2%80%99s-health (accessed on 6 January 2022).
45. Pearce, A.; Dundas, R.; Whitehead, M.; Taylor-Robinson, D. Pathways to inequalities in child health. *Arch. Dis. Child.* **2019**, *104*, 998–1003. [CrossRef]
46. Royal College of Paediatrics and Child Health. *State of Child Health*; RCPCH: London, UK, 2020.
47. Shildrick, T.; Macdonald, R. Poverty Talk: How People Experiencing Poverty Deny Their Poverty and Why They Blame 'The Poor'. *Sociol. Rev.* **2013**, *61*, 285–303. [CrossRef]
48. Ridge, T. The everyday costs of poverty in childhood: A review of qualitative research exploring the lives and experiences of low-income children in the UK. *Child. Soc.* **2011**, *25*, 73–84. [CrossRef]
49. Forbes, J.; Sime, D.; McCartney, E.; Graham, A.; Valyo, A.; Weiner, G. *Poverty and Children's Access to Services and Social Participation*; Scottish Universities Insight Institute: Glasgow, UK, 2015. Available online: https://strathprints.strath.ac.uk/55385/1/Forbes_etal_SUII_2015_poverty_and_childrens_access_to_services_and_social_participation.pdf (accessed on 6 January 2022).
50. Strazdins, L.; Welsh, J.; Korda, R.; Broom, D.; Paolucci, F. Not all hours are equal: Could time be a social determinant of health? *Sociol Health Illn.* **2016**, *38*, 21–42. [CrossRef] [PubMed]
51. Garnham, L. Understanding the impacts of industrial change and area-based deprivation on health inequalities, using Swidler's concepts of cultured capacities and strategies of action. *Soc. Theory Health* **2015**, *13*, 308–339. [CrossRef]
52. Parry, J.; Mathers, J.; Laburn-Peart, C.; Orford, J.; Dalton, S. Improving health in deprived communities: What can residents teach us? *Crit. Public Health* **2017**, *17*, 123–136. [CrossRef]

53. Popay, J.; Bennett, S.; Thomas, C.; Williams, G.; Gatrell, A.; Bostock, L. Beyond 'beer, fags, egg and chips'? Exploring lay understandings of social inequalities in health. *Sociol. Health Illn.* **2003**, *25*, 1–23. [CrossRef]
54. Watson, M.; Douglas, F. It's making us look disgusting . . . and it makes me feel like a mink . . . it makes me feel depressed!: Using photovoice to help 'see' and understand the perspectives of disadvantaged young people about the neighbourhood determinants of their mental well–being. *Int. J. Health Promot. Educ.* **2012**, *50*, 278–295. [CrossRef]
55. Birch, J.; Rishbeth, C.; Payne, S. Nature doesn't judge you—How urban nature supports young people's mental health and wellbeing in a diverse UK city. *Health Place* **2020**, *62*, 102296. [CrossRef]
56. Popay, J.; Thomas, C.; Williams, G.; Bennett, S.; Gatrell, A.; Bostock, L. A proper place to live: Health inequalities, agency and the normative dimensions of space. *Soc. Sci. Med.* **2003**, *57*, 55–69. [CrossRef]
57. Agrawal, S.; Phillips, D. *Catching up or Falling behind? Geographical Inequalities in the UK and How They Have Changed in Recent Years*; The Institute for Fiscal Studies: London, UK, 2020. Available online: https://ifs.org.uk/uploads/Geographical-inequalities-in-the-UK-how-they-have-changed.pdf (accessed on 6 January 2022).
58. Vancea, M.; Utzet, M. How unemployment and precarious employment affect the health of young people: A scoping study on social determinants. *Scand. J. Public Health* **2017**, *45*, 73–84. [CrossRef]
59. Minh, A.; O'Campo, P.; Guhn, M.; McLeod, C. Out of the labour force and out of school: A population-representative study of youth labour force attachment and mental health. *J. Youth Stud.* **2020**, *23*, 853–868. [CrossRef]
60. Rind, E.; Jones, A. 'I used to be as fit as a linnet'—Beliefs, attitudes, and environmental supportiveness for physical activity in former mining areas in the North-East of England. *Soc. Sci. Med.* **2015**, *126*, 110–118. [CrossRef] [PubMed]
61. Major, L.; Eyles, A.; Machin, S. *Generation COVID: Emerging Work and Education Inequalities. A CEP COVID-19 Analysis*; Centre for Economic Performance, London School of Economics and Political Science: London, UK, 2020. Available online: https://cep.lse.ac.uk/pubs/download/cepcovid-19-011.pdf?utm_source=miragenews&utm_medium=miragenews&utm_campaign=news (accessed on 6 January 2022).
62. Henehan, K. *Class of 2020: Education Leavers in the Current Crisis*; Resolution Foundation: London, UK, 2020. Available online: https://dera.ioe.ac.uk//35542/1/Class-of-2020.pdf (accessed on 6 January 2022).
63. Curtice, J.; Clery, E.; Perry, J.; Phillips, M.; Rahim, N. (Eds.) *British Social Attitudes: The 36th Report*; The National Centre for Social Research: London, UK, 2019. Available online: https://www.bsa.natcen.ac.uk/media/39363/bsa_36.pdf (accessed on 6 January 2022).
64. McMahon, N. Framing action to reduce health inequalities: What is argued for through use of the 'upstream–downstream' metaphor? *J. Public Health* **2021**, *1*, 1–8. [CrossRef] [PubMed]
65. Lundberg, O. Next steps in the development of the social determinants of health approach: The need for a new narrative. *Scand. J. Public Health* **2020**, *48*, 473–479. [CrossRef] [PubMed]
66. Willis, M.; Sime, D.; Lerpiniere, J. *Poverty and Children's Health and Well-Being*; Scottish Universities Institute: Glasgow, UK, 2015. Available online: https://strathprints.strath.ac.uk/57330/1/Willis_etal_2015_Poverty_and_children_s_health_and_well_being.pdf (accessed on 6 January 2022).
67. Lalli, G. A review of the English school meal: 'Progress or a recipe for disaster'? *Camb. J. Educ.* **2021**, *51*, 627–639. [CrossRef]
68. Bibby, J.; Everest, G.; Abbs, I. *Will COVID-19 Be a Watershed Moment for Health Inequalities?* Health Foundation: London, UK, 2020. Available online: https://www.health.org.uk/publications/long-reads/will-covid-19-be-a-watershed-moment-for-health-inequalities?gclid=CjwKCAiAqIKNBhAIEiwAu_ZLDgrrsiAcvuRs2GaoIsU61gDNknu9Shr07svsUjm2awVD3aM-KNbV3BoCBq4QAvD_BwE (accessed on 6 January 2022).
69. McMahon, N.E. What shapes local health system actors' thinking and action on social inequalities in health? A meta-ethnography. *Soc. Theory Health* **2022**, *20*, 1–21. [CrossRef]
70. Dahlgren, G.; Whitehead, M. The Dahlgren-Whitehead model of health determinants: 30 years on and still chasing rainbows. *Public Health* **2021**, *199*, 20–24. [CrossRef]
71. Mogford, E.; Gould, L.; Devoght, A. Teaching critical health literacy in the US as a means to action on the social determinants of health. *Health Promot. Int.* **2011**, *26*, 4–13. [CrossRef]
72. Smith, K.; Macintyre, A.; Weakley, S.; Hill, S.; Escobar, O.; Fergie, G. Public understandings of potential policy responses to health inequalities: Evidence from a UK national survey and citizens' juries in three UK cities. *Soc. Sci. Med.* **2021**, *291*, 114458. [CrossRef]
73. Patton, G.; Sawyer, S.; Santelli, J.; Ross, D.; Afifi, R.; Allen, N.; Arora, M.; Azzopardi, P.; Baldwin, W.; Bonell, C.; et al. Our future: A Lancet commission on adolescent health and wellbeing. *Lancet* **2016**, *387*, 2423–2478. [CrossRef]
74. Munford, L.; Mott, L.; Davies, H.; McGowan, V.; Bambra, C. *Overcoming Health Inequalities in 'Left behind' Neighbourhoods*; Northern Health Science Alliance and the APPG for 'Left behind' Neighbourhoods: London, UK, 2022. Available online: https://www.thenhsa.co.uk/app/uploads/2022/01/Overcoming-Health-Inequalities-Final.pdf (accessed on 6 January 2022).
75. Finch, D.; Marshall, L.; Bunbury, S. *Why Greater Investment in the Public Health Grant Should Be a Priority*; The Health Foundation: London, UK, 2021. Available online: https://www.health.org.uk/news-and-comment/charts-and-infographics/why-greater-investment-in-the-public-health-grant-should-be-a-priority (accessed on 6 January 2022).
76. YMCA. *Out of Service: A Report Examining Local Authority Expenditure on Youth Services in England & Wales*; YMCA: London, UK, 2020. Available online: https://www.ymca.org.uk/wp-content/uploads/2020/01/YMCA-Out-of-Service-report.pdf (accessed on 6 January 2022).

77. UK Youth. *The Impact of CVOID-19 on Young People & the Youth Sector*; UK Youth: London, UK, 2021. Available online: https://www.ukyouth.org/wp-content/uploads/2021/01/UK-Youth-Covid-19-Impact-Report-.pdf (accessed on 6 January 2022).
78. Inequalities in Health Alliance. In *Inequalities in Health Alliance*; RCP: London, UK, 2022. Available online: https://www.rcplondon.ac.uk/projects/inequalities-health-alliance (accessed on 11 January 2022).
79. Lynch, J. Reframing inequality? The health inequalities turn as a dangerous frame shift. *J. Public Health* **2017**, *39*, 653–660. [CrossRef]
80. Sayer, R.A.; Richard, W. *Why We Can't Afford the Rich Bristol, England*; Polity Press: Chicago, IL, USA, 2015.
81. Lister, R. A politics of recognition and respect: Involving people with experience of poverty in decision-making that affects their lives. In *The Politics of Inclusion and Empowerment*; Andersen, J., Siim, B., Eds.; Palgrave Macmillan: London, UK; pp. 116–138.
82. Wincup, E. *What Matters in Participatory Research on Poverty?* Joseph Rowntree Foundation: York, UK, 2021. Available online: https://medium.com/inside-jrf/what-matters-in-participatory-research-on-poverty-665e7cdf1d47 (accessed on 6 January 2022).

Article

Household Tenure and Its Associations with Multiple Long-Term Conditions amongst Working-Age Adults in East London: A Cross-Sectional Analysis Using Linked Primary Care and Local Government Records

Elizabeth Ingram [1,*], Manuel Gomes [1], Sue Hogarth [2], Helen I. McDonald [3], David Osborn [4,5] and Jessica Sheringham [1]

1. Department of Applied Health Research, University College London, London WC1E 7HB, UK; m.gomes@ucl.ac.uk (M.G.); j.sheringham@ucl.ac.uk (J.S.)
2. London Boroughs of Camden and Islington, London N1 1XR, UK; sue.hogarth@islington.gov.uk
3. London School of Hygiene and Tropical Medicine, London WC1E 7HT, UK; helen.mcdonald@lshtm.ac.uk
4. Division of Psychiatry, University College London, London W1T 7BN, UK; d.osborn@ucl.ac.uk
5. Camden and Islington NHS Foundation Trust, London NW1 0PE, UK
* Correspondence: e.ingram.17@ucl.ac.uk

Abstract: Multiple long-term conditions (MLTCs) are influenced in extent and nature by social determinants of health. Few studies have explored associations between household tenure and different definitions of MLTCs. This study aimed to examine associations between household tenure and MLTCs amongst working-age adults (16 to 64 years old, inclusive). This cross-sectional study used the 2019–2020 wave of an innovative dataset that links administrative data across health and local government for residents of a deprived borough in East London. Three definitions of MLTCs were operationalised based on a list of 38 conditions. Multilevel logistic regression models were built for each outcome and adjusted for a range of health and sociodemographic factors. Compared to working-age owner-occupiers, odds of basic MLTCs were 36% higher for social housing tenants and 19% lower for private renters (OR 1.36; 95% CI 1.30–1.42; $p < 0.001$ and OR 0.81, 95% CI 0.77–0.84, $p < 0.001$, respectively). Results were consistent across different definitions of MLTCs, although associations were stronger for social housing tenants with physical-mental MLTCs. This study finds strong evidence that household tenure is associated with MLTCs, emphasising the importance of understanding household-level determinants of health. Resources to prevent and tackle MLTCs among working-age adults could be differentially targeted by tenure type.

Keywords: multimorbidity; multiple long-term conditions; comorbidity; social determinants of health; housing; household tenure; data linkage

1. Introduction

The co-occurrence of multiple long-term conditions (MLTCs) within a single individual is a major public health challenge both globally and in the UK. The nature and extent of MLTCs is influenced by social determinants of health (SDoH) [1]. The role of individual- and area-level social determinants has been widely reported—prevalence and incidence of MLTCs are greater with increasing age, for women, for ethnic minorities, and those living with greater socioeconomic deprivation [1–6]. Yet recent evidence suggests that household-level SDoH (such as household tenure) are often overlooked as determinants of MLTCs despite comparatively large effect sizes for household compared to area-level SDoH [7]. In their landmark report, the Academy of Medical Sciences (AMS) concluded that most evidence focuses on "population or individual-level" determinants and that "it will be valuable to consider whether factors that operate at the household-level can also influence MLTCs" [1]. In addition, exploring these relationships amongst working-age adults has received little attention [1,7,8]. This is despite recent evidence that suggests the median age of onset of MLTCs decreased from 56 years in 2004 to 46 years in 2019 [9].

Household tenure—whether someone privately rents their home, rents from social housing, or owner-occupies—is widely considered a SDoH [10]. In recent years, home-ownership in England has increased amongst older adults and decreased in mid-life, with the private rental market increasingly housing working-age adults [11]. First introduced in 1980, the UK Government's Right to Buy policy and its future iterations enabled some more wealthier social housing tenants to legally buy their properties at a discount, resulting in tenure types more segregated by economic status and social class [12]. Different tenure types are thought to influence health through differences in exposure to various household- and area-level stressors, such as household overcrowding and access to green space [13–15]. However, studies examining associations between household tenure and MLTCs report mixed results, have not explored associations in the English context and have not examined interactions between tenure and other household-level sociodemographic circumstances [7]. This is important as evidence suggests that context-specific factors such as degree of homeownership, and supply and conditions of rented housing may profoundly influence the meaning associated with residing in different tenures across geographies and over time [7,14,16,17].

Using an innovative dataset linking data from local government, health and social care, this study aimed to examine and quantify associations between household tenure and MLTCs amongst working-age adults residing in a deprived borough of East London.

2. Materials and Methods

2.1. Study Design, Data Source and Participants

This cross-sectional study uses the Care City Cohort, which links administrative health and social data across local government services, health providers, and health commissioners for residents of Barking and Dagenham (LBBD) [18]. Data are linked at both individual and household levels. LBBD is a deprived, outer borough of East London, with approximately 211,988 residents and a younger and more ethnically diverse population compared to the rest of England [19]. See Appendix A for an overview of the dataset and data linkage steps. This manuscript was prepared following the RECORD checklist [20].

This study used a cross-section of the primary care and local government data taken on 1st April 2019. Individuals were included if they were of working age (between 16 and 64 years old, inclusive) [21], identified as residents of the borough by Mayhew and Harper's Residents' Matrix [22], and were not living in a residential home.

2.2. Outcome Measures: MLTCs

MLTCs status was determined based on the presence or absence of 38 long-term conditions recorded in a participant's primary care record. Flags of these conditions were derived using publicly available code lists [23].

This study operationalised three definitions of MLTCs in consultation with patients and clinicians:

1. Basic MLTCs, the co-occurrence of two or more long-term conditions within a single individual;
2. Physical-mental MLTCs, the co-occurrence of two or more long-term conditions within a single individual, one of which must be depression or anxiety and one of which must be a physical condition;
3. Complex MLTCs, the co-occurrence of three or more long-term conditions affecting three or more different bodily systems within a single individual [24].

The third definition was operationalised as conditions originating from different bodily systems are thought to be harder to treat due to different origins and/or treatment plans [1,24]. See Table A2 for the 38 conditions, how these conditions were grouped by bodily system and their distribution across the study cohort. Binary variables were created to indicate the presence or absence of each MLTCs outcome for each participant.

2.3. Main Exposure: Household Tenure

Individuals were defined as "owner-occupiers" if living in an owner-occupied household (outright or with a mortgage), "private renters" if living in a privately rented property, or "social housing tenants" if living in a socially rented household (from local government or a housing association). A fourth "unknown" category was created to account for missing data. Data on tenure were extracted from the council's housing data systems.

2.4. Covariates

Data on age and sex were extracted from primary care records. Eight categories were created to code individuals' ages in years (<16, 16–29, 30–44, 45–54, 55–64, 65–74, 75–84, and 85+). Sex was coded as male or female. Data on ethnicity were extracted from council records and coded into five categories: "White", "Black", "Asian", "Other" and "Unknown". Data on BMI and smoking status were extracted from primary care records. BMI was coded into five categories defined by the NHS as follows: underweight (below 18.5), healthy (between 18.5 and 24.9), overweight (between 25 and 29.9), obese (between 30 and 39.9) and morbidly obese (over 40), with a sixth "unknown" category to account for missing data. Smoking status data were coded into four categories: non-smoker, smoker, ex-smoker, or "unknown".

Data on household welfare benefits, occupancy and household type were extracted from council housing records. Households receiving welfare benefits to support rental payments ('housing benefit') were classified by whether eligibility was based on receipt of other welfare benefits and, if so, the type: Employment Support and Allowance (ESA), Pension Credit, Income Support or Job Seeker's Allowance (JSA). Two further categories reflecting households solely in receipt of housing benefit or in receipt of no benefits were created. Occupancy data were recorded into four categories to reflect 1–2, 3–5, 6–10 and 11 or more people within a household. Data on household type captured households as six types: adults with children, adults with no children, single adult with children, single adult, older adults with no children, and three generations.

To provide a marker of overall deprivation in each participants' residential area relative to other areas in the borough, borough-specific Index of Multiple Deprivation (IMD) quintiles were calculated for each small geographical area (Lower Super Output Area; LSOA) using 2019 IMD scores [25]. Each LSOA comprised a maximum of 3000 residents and 1200 households [26].

2.5. Main Data Analysis

Multilevel logistic regression modelling was used to explore associations between household tenure and MLTCs prevalence amongst working-age residents with complete data (see Table 1 and Figure A1). To assess the relative impact of adjusting for individual compared to household-level covariates on the association between tenure and MLTCs prevalence, we built three distinct models for each outcome. First, an unadjusted model with no covariates included. Second, a model adjusted for individual-level sociodemographic characteristics available in the dataset and found to be associated with both MLTCs prevalence and household tenure in previous literature [17,27–29]. These covariates were age, sex, ethnicity, BMI and smoking. The third and final model for each outcome additionally adjusted for household benefits receipt, occupancy and type to control for potential household-level factors correlated with both household tenure and MLTCs (see covariates above). We chose to adjust for household benefits receipt as it was the best proxy measure available in the dataset for other important covariates such as employment. We chose to adjust for household occupancy and type as a previous systematic review examining household- and area-level social determinants of MLTCs found these factors were associated with MLTCs prevalence in some contexts [7]. Model fit was assessed using Akaike's Information Criteria (AIC). We considered multilevel models to account for the potential clustering of individuals within geographical areas, as individuals are likely to be more similar in terms of individual, household- and area-level factors if residing in the same areas than if residing in different areas. All models included random effects at the Lower Layer Output Area (LSOA) level to account for clustering within areas. Models were estimated using the lme4 package in R, using restricted maximum likelihood [30]. The 95% confidence intervals were calculated using the Wald test [31].

Table 1. Characteristics of study participants (N = 132,296).

	Total Sample (N = 132,296)	Basic MLTCs (N = 23,683)		Physical-Mental MLTCs (N = 6269)		Complex MLTCs (N = 7931)	
	N (%)	N (%)	Odds Ratio (95% CI)	N (%)	Odds Ratio (95% CI)	N (%)	Odds Ratio (95% CI)
Individual-level variables							
Age							
16–29	37,486 (28.3)	2502 (10.6)	1 (baseline)	578 (9.22)	1 (baseline)	329 (4.15)	1 (baseline)
30–44	49,284 (37.3)	5689 (24.0)	1.82 (1.74–1.92)	1669 (26.6)	2.24 (2.04–2.46)	1274 (16.1)	3.00 (2.66–3.39)
45–54	26,560 (20.1)	7021 (29.6)	5.02 (4.79–5.28)	1898 (30.3)	4.91 (4.47–5.41)	2372 (29.9)	11.1 (9.87–12.5)
55–65	18,966 (14.3)	8471 (35.8)	11.3 (10.7–11.9)	2124 (33.9)	8.05 (7.34–8.85)	3956 (49.9)	29.8 (26.6–33.4)
Sex							
Female	68,004 (51.4)	13,298 (56.1)	1 (baseline)	4112 (65.6)	1 (baseline)	4628 (58.4)	1 (baseline)
Male	64,292 (48.6)	10,385 (43.9)	0.79 (0.77–0.82)	2157 (34.4)	0.54 (0.51–0.57)	3303 (41.6)	0.74 (0.71–0.78)
Ethnicity							
White	69,611 (52.6)	14,472 (61.1)	1 (baseline)	4755 (75.8)	1 (baseline)	5181 (65.3)	1 (baseline)
Black	28,335 (21.4)	4178 (17.6)	0.66 (0.63–0.68)	617 (9.84)	0.30 (0.28–0.33)	1174 (14.8)	0.54 (0.50–0.57)
Asian	31,879 (24.1)	4822 (20.4)	0.68 (0.66–0.70)	852 (13.6)	0.37 (0.35–0.40)	1524 (19.2)	0.62 (0.59–0.66)
Other	1957 (1.48)	175 (0.74)	0.37 (0.32–0.44)	40 (0.64)	0.28 (0.20–0.38)	40 (0.50)	0.26 (0.19–0.35)
Unknown	514 (0.39)	36 (0.15)	0.29 (0.20–0.40)	5 (0.08)	0.13 (0.05–0.29)	12 (0.15)	0.30 (0.16–0.50)
BMI categories							
Underweight	4332 (3.27)	522 (2.20)	0.85 (0.77–0.94)	144 (2.30)	0.89 (0.74–1.05)	119 (1.50)	0.72 (0.60–0.87)
Healthy weight	33,918 (25.6)	4707 (19.9)	1 (baseline)	1264 (20.2)	1 (baseline)	1274 (16.1)	1 (baseline)
Overweight	35,870 (27.1)	6854 (28.9)	1.47 (1.41–1.53)	1677 (26.8)	1.27 (1.18–1.37)	2143 (27.0)	1.63 (1.52–1.75)
Obese	27,941 (21.1)	7893 (33.3)	2.44 (2.35–2.54)	2142 (34.2)	2.14 (2.00–2.30)	3045 (38.4)	3.13 (2.93–3.35)
Morbidly obese	4820 (3.64)	2106 (8.90)	4.82 (4.51–5.14)	709 (11.3)	4.46 (4.04–4.91)	1001 (12.6)	6.72 (6.14–7.34)
Unknown	25,415 (19.2)	1601 (6.76)	0.42 (0.39–0.44)	333 (5.31)	0.34 (0.30–0.39)	349 (4.40)	0.36 (0.32–0.40)
Smoking status							
Non-smoker	77,913 (58.9)	12,972 (54.8)	1 (baseline)	2851 (45.5)	1 (baseline)	4117 (51.9)	1 (baseline)
Ex-smoker	15,834 (12.0)	4536 (19.2)	2.01 (1.93–2.09)	1366 (21.8)	2.49 (2.32–2.66)	1806 (22.8)	2.32 (2.18–2.45)
Smoker	25,495 (19.3)	5849 (24.7)	1.49 (1.44–1.54)	2013 (32.1)	2.26 (2.13–2.39)	1987 (25.1)	1.52 (1.43–1.60)
Unknown	13,054 (9.87)	326 (1.38)	0.13 (0.11–0.14)	39 (0.62)	0.08 (0.06–0.11)	21 (0.26)	0.03 (0.02–0.04)
Household-level variables							
Tenure							
Owner-occupied	54,324 (41.1)	9278 (39.2)	1 (baseline)	1801 (28.7)	1 (baseline)	2853 (36.0)	1 (baseline)
Privately rented	39,885 (30.1)	5143 (21.7)	0.72 (0.69–0.75)	1328 (21.2)	1.00 (0.93–1.08)	1554 (19.6)	0.73 (0.69–0.78)
Social housing	35,776 (27.0)	9004 (38.0)	1.63 (1.58–1.69)	3085 (49.3)	2.75 (2.59–2.92)	3450 (43.5)	1.93 (1.83–2.03)
Unknown	2311 (1.75)	258 (1.09)	0.61 (0.53–0.69)	55 (0.88)	0.71 (0.54–0.92)	74 (0.93)	0.60 (0.47–0.75)
Benefit receipt							
None	116,306 (87.9)	18,615 (78.6)	1 (baseline)	4184 (66.7)	1 (baseline)	4569 (57.6)	1 (baseline)
ESA	5636 (4.26)	2926 (12.4)	6.02 (5.69–6.36)	1499 (23.9)	11.3 (10.5–12.1)	1652 (20.8)	9.09 (8.52–9.69)
Pension	1842 (1.39)	489 (2.06)	2.01 (1.81–2.23)	130 (2.07)	2.36 (1.96–2.82)	183 (2.31)	2.42 (2.06–2.82)
Income support	2491 (1.88)	758 (3.20)	2.44 (2.23–2.66)	243 (3.88)	3.36 (2.92–3.84)	300 (3.78)	3.00 (2.65–3.39)
JSA	638 (0.48)	168 (0.71)	1.99 (1.66–2.37)	597 (0.65)	2.13 (1.53–2.90)	63 (0.79)	2.40 (1.83–3.09)
Housing benefit only	5383 (4.07)	727 (3.07)	1.40 (1.34–1.46)	172 (2.74)	2.14 (1.99–2.29)	1164 (14.7)	1.61 (1.51–1.72)
Occupancy (number of people in household)							
1–2	29,082 (22.0)	7878 (33.3)	1 (baseline)	2557 (40.8)	1 (baseline)	3117 (39.3)	1 (baseline)
3–5	76,291 (57.7)	12,438 (52.5)	0.52 (0.51–0.54)	3040 (48.5)	0.43 (0.41–0.45)	3855 (48.6)	0.44 (0.42–0.47)
6–10	25,251 (19.1)	3205 (13.5)	0.39 (0.37–0.41)	639 (10.2)	0.27 (0.25–0.29)	913 (11.5)	0.31 (0.29–0.34)
11+	1672 (1.26)	162 (0.68)	0.29 (0.24–0.34)	33 (0.53)	0.21 (0.14–0.29)	46 (0.58)	0.24 (0.17–0.31)

Table 1. Cont.

	Total Sample (N = 132,296)	Basic MLTCs (N = 23,683)		Physical-Mental MLTCs (N = 6269)		Complex MLTCs (N = 7931)	
	N (%)	N (%)	Odds Ratio (95% CI)	N (%)	Odds Ratio (95% CI)	N (%)	Odds Ratio (95% CI)
Household type							
Adults with children	60,648 (45.8)	7715 (32.6)	1 (baseline)	1767 (28.2)	1 (baseline)	2110 (26.6)	1 (baseline)
Adults with no children	41,974 (31.7)	9023 (38.1)	1.88 (1.82–1.94)	2344 (37.4)	1.97 (1.85–2.10)	3269 (41.2)	2.34 (2.22–2.48)
Single adult with children	7274 (5.50)	1103 (4.66)	1.23 (1.14–1.31)	355 (5.66)	1.71 (1.52–1.92)	254 (3.20)	1.00 (0.88–1.14)
Single adult	10,675 (8.07)	3341 (14.1)	3.13 (2.98–3.28)	1212 (19.3)	4.27 (3.95–4.61)	1405 (17.7)	4.20 (3.92–4.51)
Older cohabiting adults	7226 (5.46)	1865 (7.87)	2.39 (2.25–2.53)	467 (7.45)	2.30 (2.07–2.55)	695 (8.76)	2.95 (2.70–3.23)
Three generations	4499 (3.40)	636 (2.69)	1.13 (1.03–1.23)	124 (1.98)	0.94 (0.78–1.13)	198 (2.50)	1.28 (1.10–1.48)
Area-level variables							
Index of Multiple Deprivation Quintiles *							
1 (least deprived)	27,305 (20.6)	4538 (19.2)	1 (baseline)	1017 (16.2)	1 (baseline)	1467 (18.5)	1 (baseline)
2	26,338 (19.9)	4401 (18.6)	1.01 (0.96–1.05)	1068 (17.0)	1.09 (1.00–1.19)	1374 (17.3)	0.97 (0.90–1.05)
3	26,556 (20.1)	4718 (19.9)	1.08 (1.04–1.13)	1271 (20.3)	1.30 (1.19–1.41)	1589 (20.0)	1.12 (1.04–1.21)
4	25,868 (19.6)	4778 (20.2)	1.14 (1.09–1.19)	1328 (19.5)	1.40 (1.29–1.52)	1617 (20.4)	1.17 (1.09–1.26)
5 (most deprived)	26,229 (19.8)	5248 (22.2)	1.25 (1.20–1.31)	1585 (19.6)	1.66 (1.53–1.80)	1884 (23.8)	1.36 (1.27–1.46)

Note: the denominator for all characteristics (individual and household) is the number of individuals. OR = odds ratio; 95% CI = 95% confidence interval; ESA = Employment Support and Allowance, and JSA = Job Seeker's Allowance. * Calculated for Barking and Dagenham based on raw Index of Multiple Deprivation scores (2019) [25].

2.6. Subgroup and Sensitivity Analyses

Three interaction terms were separately added to the final model for each outcome to evaluate potential interactions between household tenure and other household factors. We assessed interactions with receipt of benefits, household occupancy and type (see covariates above) as these are most likely to modify the association between housing tenure and MLTCs, and they also act at the household-level. Any differences in these household-level characteristics by tenure type can be found in Table A3.

3. Results

3.1. Participant Characteristics

Of the 232,671 participants whose primary care and local government records were successfully linked, 132,296 participants were eligible for inclusion in this study. A total of 78,379 records (33.7%) were excluded as individuals were not of working age, 21,847 records (9.39%) were excluded due to unconfirmed resident status and 95 were excluded due to living in a residential home (0.04%) (see Figure A1).

The 132,296 study participants resided in 59,535 households and 110 LSOAs. Table 1 gives an overview of the study participants. A total of 86,770 participants (65.6%) were between the ages of 16 and 44 years old and 68,004 (51.4%) were female. A total of 69,611 (52.6%) were of White ethnicity and 68,631 (51.8%) were overweight, obese or morbidly obese. A total of 54,324 participants (41.1%) were owner-occupiers, 39,885 (30.1%) were private renters and 35,776 (27.0%) were social housing tenants. Crude prevalence of basic, physical-mental, and complex MLTCs was 17.9% (23,683/132,296), 4.7% (6269/132,296) and 6.0% (7931/132,296), respectively.

The number of participants with missing data on tenure, ethnicity, BMI, and smoking status were 2311 (1.75%), 514 (0.39%), 25,415 (19.2%) and 13,054 (9.87%), respectively. A total of 102,430 participants had complete data across all variables and were included in analyses (see Figure A1).

3.2. Household Tenure and MLTCs

After adjusting for individual-level characteristics (age, sex, ethnicity, BMI, and smoking), social housing tenants were more likely to have basic MLTCs (OR 1.90; 95% CI 1.83–1.98), physical-mental MLTCs (OR 2.60, 95% CI 2.43–2.79,) and complex MLTCs (OR

2.23, 95% CI 2.10–2.37) when compared to owner-occupiers (Table 2). For private renters, there was no evidence of a difference in the odds of basic MLTCs compared to owner-occupiers ($p = 0.630$). Conversely, private renters were more likely to have physical-mental and complex MLTCs when compared to owner-occupiers (physical-mental MLTCs: OR 1.29, 95% CI 1.19–1.40; complex MLTCs: OR 1.16, 95% CI 1.08–1.25).

Table 2. Estimated odds ratios of multiple long-term conditions (MLTCs) with household tenure for working-age adult residents with complete data (N = 102,430).

	MLTCs Prevalence N (%)	Model 1 [a] Unadjusted OR (95% CI)	p Value	Model 2 [b] Adjusted OR (95% CI)	p Value	Model 3 [c] Adjusted OR (95% CI)	p Value
Basic MLTCs							
Household tenure							
OOC * (ref)	8645 (39.8)	-		-		-	
Social housing	8269 (38.1)	1.82 (1.76–1.89)	<0.001	1.90 (1.83–1.98)	<0.001	1.36 (1.30–1.42)	<0.001
Privately rented	4805 (22.1)	0.76 (0.73–0.79)	<0.001	1.01 (0.97–1.05)	0.630	0.81 (0.77–0.84)	<0.001
Variance Partition Coefficient (%)		2.96		1.42		1.14	
Physical-mental MLTCs							
Household tenure							
OOC * (ref)	1705 (29.1)	-		-		-	
Social housing	2894 (49.4)	3.03 (2.83–3.23)	<0.001	2.60 (2.43–2.79)	<0.001	1.46 (1.35–1.58)	<0.001
Privately rented	1261 (21.5)	1.08 (1.00–1.17)	0.042	1.29 (1.19–1.40)	<0.001	0.85 (0.78–0.93)	<0.001
Variance Partition Coefficient (%)		6.05		1.98		1.31	
Complex MLTCs							
Household tenure							
OOC * (ref)	2740 (36.6)	-		-		-	
Social housing	3276 (43.7)	2.12 (2.00–2.25)	<0.001	2.23 (2.10–2.37)	<0.001	1.34 (1.25–1.44)	<0.001
Privately rented	1479 (19.7)	0.77 (0.72–0.83)	<0.001	1.16 (1.08–1.25)	<0.001	0.81 (0.74–0.87)	<0.001
Variance Partition Coefficient (%)		4.11		1.36		0.88	

Complex MLTCs = the co-occurrence of three or more long-term conditions affecting three or more different body systems within a single individual. * OOC = owner-occupied. [a] Model 1—an unadjusted model with no covariates. [b] Model 2—model adjusted for individual-level covariates: age, sex, ethnicity, BMI and smoking status. [c] Model 3—model adjusted for model 2 covariates plus household benefits receipt, household occupancy and household type.

After additional adjustment for household-level characteristics (benefits receipt, occupancy, and household type), social housing tenants were still more likely to have MLTCs compared to owner-occupiers, but associations were weaker for all three definitions of MLTCs (basic MLTCs: OR 1.36, 1.30–1.42; physical-mental MLTCs: OR 1.46, 95% CI 1.35–1.58; complex MLTCs: OR 1.34; 95% CI 1.25–1.44). On the other hand, private renters were less likely to have basic MLTCs (OR 0.81, 95% CI 0.77–0.84), physical-mental MLTCs (OR 0.85, 95% CI 0.78–0.93) and complex MLTCs (OR 0.81, 95% CI 0.74–0.87) (Table 2). IMD quintiles were not included in final models for the three MLTCs outcomes as adding these resulted in poorer model fit.

3.3. Subgroup Analyses

Our subgroup analyses suggest subgroup effects according to household benefits receipt, occupancy and household type (see Tables A4–A6). The odds of MLTCs for private renters (compared to owner-occupiers) were considerably stronger for households in receipt of benefits compared to those not receiving benefits. For example, odds of basic MLTCs were 76% greater for privately rented households where someone was in receipt of ESA compared to households not receiving ESA (OR 1.76, 95% CI 1.35–2.29). There was no evidence of an interaction between living in social housing and household benefits receipt (see Table A4). The odds of MLTCs for both social housing tenants and private renters (compared to owner-occupiers) were higher for single-adult households compared to households with adults and children. For example, the odds of basic MLTCs for social housing tenants compared to owner-occupiers were 31% greater for single-adult households (OR 1.31, 95% CI 1.15–1.50). Evidence for subgroup effects for other household types were weaker, with most interactions not statistically significant (see Table A6).

4. Discussion

4.1. Summary of Study Findings

Risk of MLTCs amongst working-age residents of a deprived East London borough was greater for social housing tenants and lower for privately renters, when compared to owner-occupiers. These associations remained significant after adjusting for a range of individual- and household-level characteristics and were consistent across different definitions of MLTCs. Other household-level variables—household benefits receipt, occupancy, and type—were important modifying factors, with associations between tenure and MLTCs greater for individuals in single-adult households and households in receipt of certain benefits.

4.2. Comparisons with Existing Literature

Our prevalence estimates are in keeping with previous estimates for this age group [6,9,32,33]. Prevalence of MLTCs was greater with increasing age and for females, consistent with previous literature [1,6]. However, prevalence was lower for ethnic minority compared with White participants, which contradicts many studies and may be an age-related effect [1,27,32]. In this study, participants lived in a deprived borough in East London where older and younger individuals tend to be White and ethnic minorities, respectively.

We found that social housing tenants exhibited greater risk of MLTCs compared to owner-occupiers, aligning with findings from Northern Ireland yet contradicting those from a Hong Kong-based study [34,35]. This supports the idea that associations between household-level SDoH and MLTCs may be context specific, influenced by housing policy, supply and conditions of social housing, stigma and other household circumstances such as benefits receipt (see Table A3) [7]. In the UK specifically, social housing tenants may be exposed to various "hard" (material) and "soft" (psychological) factors that interact to cause or exacerbate MLTCs [14]. Evidence suggests social housing tenants in the UK have higher levels of C-reactive protein, a biomarker of inflammation associated with various long-term conditions [17,36]. In addition, social housing tenants have less control over the condition of their property and their built environment, and are less able to leave their property, whilst owner-occupying affords ontological security—the sense of security and control afforded when owning your home [37,38]. On top of this, the UK Housing Act (1998) requires social housing to be allocated based on certain criteria, one of which is ill health. As such, MLTCs may be a qualifying characteristic for eligibility for social housing, which may explain our estimated associations.

The lower risk of MLTCs found for private renters compared to owner-occupiers contradicts previous research from the US and Northern Ireland [32,35]. Our analyses adjusted for variables not adjusted for in these studies—household benefits receipt, occupancy, and household type. Our findings suggest these were important explanatory factors for the association between tenure and MLTCs, but they did not explain all of the additional risk experienced by social housing tenants, nor the decreased risk for private renters. In the UK, the private rental market is expanding considerably, and private renters are an increasingly heterogenous group in terms of their demographic, social and economic circumstances [11]. As such, more longitudinal, causal analyses are needed to unpick the complex relationships between different tenure types and MLTCs, taking into account the influence of other household characteristics.

We found that the association between tenure and MLTCs was greater for individuals in single-adult households and households with one or two occupants when compared to higher numbers of occupants. However, previous research examining associations between living alone and MLTC prevalence presents mixed results [7]. In our context, a deprived borough of East London, single-adult households may have less social support and be more financially uncertain than households with multiple occupants, increasing their vulnerability to any adverse effects imposed by their tenure [39]. We also found that the association between tenure and MLTCs was greater for individuals in households where someone was in receipt of certain benefits. Only one previous study has explored subgroup effects in the relationship between tenure and MLTCs and they similarly found that household financial burden mediated this relationship, albeit with a small effect [34]. Our findings support this work, and, again, suggest further research should capture data on, and account for, other household-level characteristics when examining relationships between tenure and MLTCs.

Differences in the risk of MLTCs with tenure type were not explained by commonly used area-level deprivation measures as most areas in our study are amongst the most deprived nationally [7]. These findings further demonstrate the importance of capturing data on, and understanding, household-level SDoH as this information could support service planning when area-level deprivation measures are unable to capture enough variation to model socioeconomic inequalities in MLTCs. In addition, our findings were consistent across different definitions of MLTCs, illustrating the importance of household tenure as a risk factor for MLTCs.

4.3. Strengths and Limitations

This is the first study to explore associations between household tenure and MLTCs in England. Our findings add to the current literature, and our analyses would not have been possible without the innovative linkage of primary care and local government data. We operationalised three definitions of MLTCs that captured different types of MLTCs with different degrees of complexity. We used publicly available code lists to determine the presence of each condition.

Our study was conducted in one deprived borough in East London and, whilst our findings could be generalisable to other urban areas, they may not hold in contexts that are less deprived, more rural and have different tenure profiles [7,40]. We restricted our analyses to complete cases, which assumes that any differences between individuals with missing and complete data are explained by differences in observed individual and household characteristics included in the regression models. We recognise that there may be other variables associated with the missing data that we have not adjusted for. However, this is unlikely to have significantly changed the results due to the limited role that BMI and smoking status have in the association between tenure and MLTCs prevalence [41]. We did not account for disease severity or symptom burden on the patient, or other dimensions of MLTCs such as frailty. We may have misclassified households where owner-occupiers privately rented rooms, which may have biased estimates towards the null if private renters who co-resided with their owner-occupying landlords differed systematically in their health compared to private renters who did not. In addition, our measure of household benefits receipt did not capture eligibility for benefits, and we could not adjust for other important factors such as education. The cross-sectional study design did not allow us to explore temporal relationships between tenure and MLTCs. We adjusted for household benefits receipt, occupancy, and household type as potential confounders, but also demonstrated important subgroup effects according to some of these characteristics. It is possible these variables may modify the relationship between tenure and MLTCs. More longitudinal analyses are needed to determine how these factors interact over time to impact MLTCs.

4.4. Implications for Practice and Policy

Most interventions for MLTCs focus on retired, older adults, yet our findings indicate that working-age adults are an important population to consider when aiming to address MLTCs. There is currently a gap in models of care or interventions aimed at working-age adults, for whom there may be greater opportunity for prevention of MLTCs through addressing SDoH than amongst older adults [1]. Initiatives that target preventative resources at working-age adults with MLTCs who live in social housing could slow the progression of MLTCs and improve health outcomes, ultimately saving future costs [8].

5. Conclusions

This study finds strong evidence that risk of MLTCs amongst working-age residents of a deprived East London borough was greater for social housing tenants and lower for privately renters when compared to owner-occupiers. Associations were consistent across different definitions of MLTCs, which emphasises the importance of understanding and addressing household-level determinants of health. Our findings suggest that resources to prevent and tackle MLTCs could be differentially targeted by tenure type and that working-age adults are an important population to consider in preventative strategies. Further research should employ longitudinal research methods to assess temporal relationships between household social determinants and MLTCs.

Author Contributions: Conceptualisation, E.I., M.G., S.H., H.I.M., D.O. and J.S.; data curation, E.I.; formal analysis, E.I.; funding acquisition, J.S.; investigation, E.I.; methodology, E.I., M.G., H.I.M. and D.O.; project administration, E.I.; software, E.I.; supervision, M.G., S.H., H.I.M., D.O. and J.S.; writing—original draft, E.I.; writing—review and editing, E.I., M.G., S.H., H.I.M., D.O. and J.S. All authors have read and agreed to the published version of the manuscript.

Funding: This study is independent research funded by the National Institute for Health Research School for Public Health Research (Grant Reference Number PD-SPH -2015-10025) and the National Institute for Health Research Applied Research Collaboration (ARC) North Thames. The views expressed in this publication are those of the authors and not necessarily those of the National Institute for Health Research or the Department of Health and Social Care. The APC was funded by the National Institute for Health Research School for Public Health Research. DO is also supported by the National Institute for Health Research (NIHR) Biomedical Research Centre (BRC) at University College London Hospitals (UCLH).

Institutional Review Board Statement: This study was conducted in accordance with the Declaration of Helsinki. The study protocol was approved on 13th March 2020 by Care City's formal process for data access (no project identification code provided).

Informed Consent Statement: Patient consent was waived as this work uses data provided by patients and collected by the NHS as part of their care and support. Only anonymised data were released.

Data Availability Statement: Restrictions apply to the availability of these data. Data were obtained from Care City and no applicable data are available without their permission. The study protocol is available on request.

Acknowledgments: The authors would like to thank Jenny Shand, Simon Lam and Phil Canham for their support with data access and their help with understanding the origins of the data. We would also like to thank Melvyn Jones, the Care City Community Board and the NIHR ARC North Thames Research Advisory Panel for their advice and expertise when developing our definitions of multiple long-term conditions.

Conflicts of Interest: The authors declare conflict of interest. The funders had no role in the design of the study; in the collection, analyses, or interpretation of data; in the writing of the manuscript, or in the decision to publish the results.

Appendix A. Overview of the Care City Cohort and Data Linkage Steps

In 2017, the leaders of Barking and Dagenham Council, North East London NHS Foundation Trust (NELFT) and Barking and Dagenham, Havering and Redbridge Clinical Commissioning Group (BHR CCG), and their Caldicott guardians (a senior person within each organisation who is responsible for protecting the confidentiality of people's health and care information and making sure it is used properly), signed data sharing agreements to create a dataset that linked administrative data for the population of Barking and Dagenham (B&D) between 1st April 2011 and 31st March 2017. Since its creation, the dataset has been updated on an annual basis. It is hosted in the Barking and Dagenham, Havering, and Redbridge NHS Accredited Data Safe Haven, with governance and oversight provided by the Barking and Dagenham, Havering, and Redbridge Information Governance Steering Committee.

The dataset was created as part a larger research programme of work [18]. It contains routinely collected administrative health and social data across local government services, health providers, and health commissioners. Data are linked at the individual and household levels using linkage keys (replacing NHS numbers and Unique Property Reference Numbers; UPRNs). The data are pseudonymised and include information on sociodemographic characteristics, health variables, household variables and data on health and social care service utilisation. Data on all sociodemographic and health variables for each cross-section are taken as a snapshot on 1st April 2019 to account for in-year changes in variables. The dataset is not currently publicly available but was made available to the wider research community in Autumn 2020.

More information on the dataset can be found here [42] and here [43]. More information on the codes and algorithms used to classify variables as part of the creation of the Care City Cohort can be found at this reference [18].

This study used data from the 2019/20 cross-section of the Care City Cohort. We requested access to pseudonymised sociodemographic and health variables extracted from primary care data, and resident data extracted from local government data. We did not have access to other data available within the Care City Cohort, such as data on health and care service utilisation.

Data were provided unlinked with linkage keys, i.e., with the identification codes generated to replace NHS numbers and UPRNs. We used these to link the data at the individual and household levels. First, we linked the individual- and household-level local government data on Household_ID (the household-level identification code created by Care City to replace UPRNs). Second, we linked the individual-level primary care data to the linked local government data on Patient_ID (the individual-level identification code created by Care City to replace NHS numbers). Third, we linked a fourth dataset provided by Care City that detailed care homes in Barking and Dagenham and their Household_IDs. We linked this to the cohort data on Household_ID. Finally, we linked a fifth dataset from ONS that contained area-level deprivation data from 2019. We linked this dataset to the data on LSOA code (a unique number identifying each small area/LSOA in England). All linkages were conducted in R software using the merge function from the R base package. Figure A1 illustrates the results of the linkages of the separate primary care and local government datasets. A total of 232,671 individuals were linked across primary care and local government datasets (84.0% of the original primary care records).

To assess whether there were any potential selection biases in the linkage results, we calculated standardised differences in key variables for matched and unmatched primary care records [44]. Standardised differences of 0.2, 0.5, and 0.8 indicate small, medium and large effect sizes, respectively [44]. We were not able to assess potential biases in social variables extracted from local government records (i.e., in the household tenure variable and other household variables) as, by definition, unmatched primary care records did not have corresponding local government data. However, the number of unmatched local government records was considerably low (N = 369). Table A1 presents the results of analyses conducted to assess potential biases in the linkage results for matched and unmatched primary care records. These results indicate that selection biases were not introduced in selected variables originating from primary care records as a result of the success of data linkages, which is in keeping with previous analyses of this data [18].

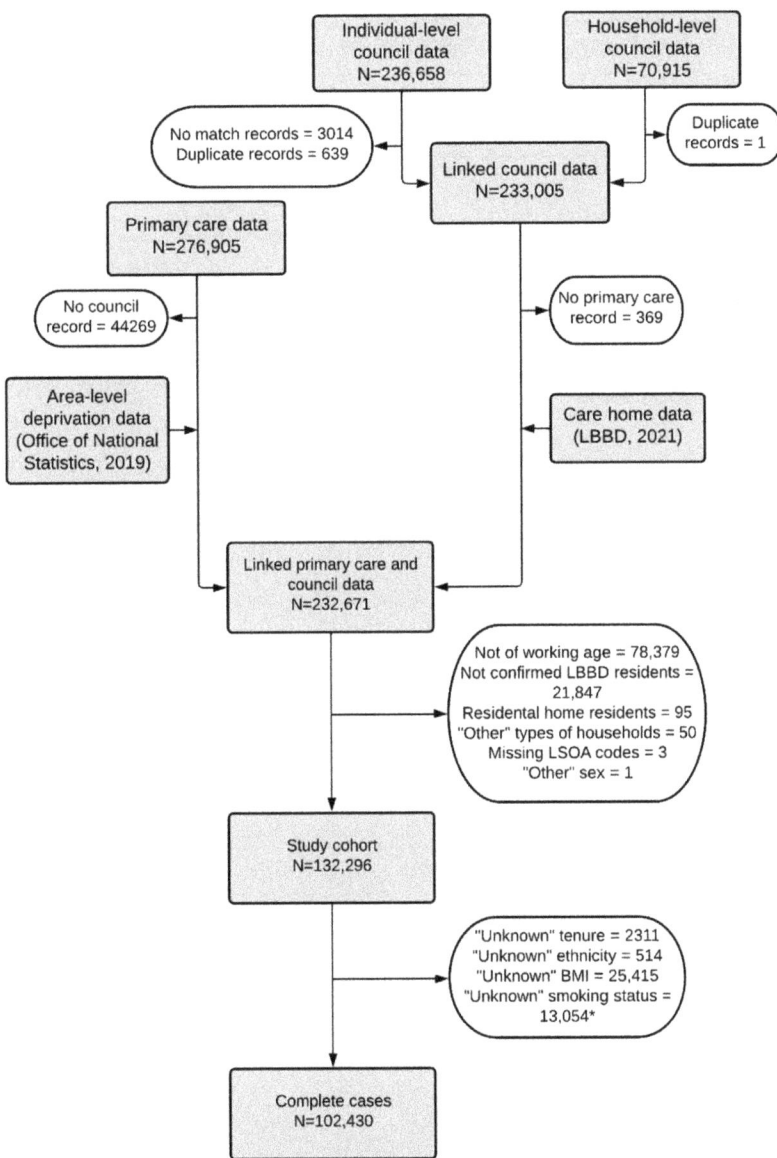

Figure A1. Results of data linkages. * Number of participants with missing data on each variable sum to greater than 29,866 (132,296 minus 102,430) as some participants had missing data across more than one variable.

Table A1. Results of analyses to assess potential biases in the linkage results for matched (N = 232,671) and unmatched (N = 44,269) primary care records.

	Primary Care Matched Records N = 232,671	Primary Care Unmatched Records N = 44,269	Standardised Difference
Age: N (%)			
<16	57,402 (24.7)	8877 (20.1)	0.150
16–29	42,325 (18.2)	8593 (19.4)	
30–44	59,891 (25.7)	11,942 (27.0)	
45–54	30,738 (13.2)	5679 (12.8)	
55–64	21,338 (9.17)	4101 (9.26)	
65–74	11,602 (4.99)	2461 (5.56)	
75–84	6366 (2.74)	1414 (3.19)	
85+	3009 (1.29)	1202 (2.72)	
Sex: N (%)			
Female	116,186 (49.9)	21,787 (49.2)	0.025
Male	116,484 (50.1)	22,472 (50.8)	
Other/Missing	1 (0.00)	10 (0.00)	
Ethnicity *: N (%)			
White	76,524 (32.9)	13,633 (31.4)	0.128
Black	32,708 (14.1)	5029 (11.4)	
Asian	42,222 (18.1)	9710 (21.9)	
Mixed	6285 (2.70)	1137 (2.57)	
Other	4309 (1.85)	831 (1.88)	
Unknown	67,493 (29.0)	13,629 (30.8)	
Basic MLTCs: N (%)			
Present	41,329 (17.8)	7931 (17.9)	0.004
Absent	191,342 (82.2)	36,338 (82.1)	
Physical-mental MLTCs: N (%)			
Present	9077 (3.90)	1542 (3.48)	0.022
Absent	223,594 (96.1)	42,727 (96.5)	
Complex MLTCs N (%):			
Present	17,721 (7.65)	3562 (8.09)	0.016
Absent	214,950 (92.4)	40,707 (91.6)	
BMI categories: N (%)			
Underweight	11,645 (5.00)	2115 (4.78)	0.077
Healthy weight	48,101 (20.7)	10,355 (23.4)	
Overweight	49,180 (21.1)	9493 (21.4)	
Obese	37,566 (16.1)	6612 (14.9)	
Morbidly obese	6077 (2.61)	934 (2.11)	
Unknown	80,102 (34.4)	14,760 (33.3)	
Smoking status: N (%)			
Non-smoker	107,326 (46.1)	21,247 (48.0)	0.043
Ex-smoker	24,385 (10.5)	4620 (10.4)	
Smoker	33,722 (14.5)	6372 (14.4)	
Unknown	67,238 (28.9)	12,030 (27.2)	

MLTCs = multiple long-term conditions. * Variable taken from primary care records, unlike in the study analyses.

Table A2. The 38 long-term conditions grouped by 10 bodily systems and their distribution across the study cohort (N = 132,296).

Respiratory	N (%)
Asthma (currently treated)	6551 (4.95)
Bronchiectasis	143 (0.11)
Chronic obstructive pulmonary disorder	1325 (1.00)
Sensory	
Blindness and low vision	905 (0.68)
Chronic sinusitis	1617 (1.22)
Hearing loss	4726 (3.57)
Psoriasis or eczema	812 (0.61)
Cardiovascular	
Atrial fibrillation	451 (0.34)
Coronary heart disease	1446 (1.09)
Heart failure	302 (0.23)
Hypertension	14,518 (11.0)
Peripheral vascular disease	169 (0.13)
Endocrine	
Diabetes	8728 (6.60)
Thyroid disorders	4403 (3.33)
Cancer	
Cancer (in last 5 years)	1157 (0.87)
Musculoskeletal	
Painful conditions	7417 (5.61)
Rheumatoid arthritis (or other inflammatory polyarthropathies and systematic connective tissue disorders)	2871 (2.17)
Mental health	
Alcohol problems	1170 (0.88)
Anorexia and bulimia	820 (0.62)
Anxiety (and other neurotic, stress-related and somatoform disorders)	3935 (2.97)
Depression	9055 (6.84)
Dementia	58 (0.04)
Psychoactive substance misuse	1451 (1.10)
Schizophrenia and bipolar	8624 (6.52)
Neurological	
Epilepsy (currently treated)	750 (0.57)
Learning disability	905 (0.68)
Migraine	331 (0.25)
Stroke and transient ischaemic attack	844 (0.64)
Multiple sclerosis	177 (0.13)
Parkinson's disease	54 (0.04)
Genitourinary	
Chronic kidney disease	444 (0.34)
Prostate disorders	666 (0.50)
Gastrointestinal	
Chronic liver disease and viral hepatitis	1341 (1.01)
Constipation (treated)	741 (0.56)
Diverticular disease of intestine	893 (0.68)
Irritable bowel syndrome	3914 (2.96)
Inflammatory bowel disease	718 (0.54)
Peptic ulcer disease	760 (0.57)

Table A3. Household benefits receipt, occupancy, and household type, by tenure for complete cases (N = 102,430).

	Owner-Occupied N = 43,444	Social Housing N = 27,766	Privately Rented N = 31,220
Household benefits receipt: N (%)			
None	41,670 (95.9)	18,140 (65.3)	21,337 (68.3)
ESA	374 (0.86)	2883 (10.4)	1294 (4.14)
Pension	405 (0.93)	676 (2.43)	419 (1.34)
Income Support	135 (0.31)	1143 (4.12)	612 (1.96)
JSA	32 (0.07)	309 (1.11)	134 (0.43)
Housing benefit only	828 (1.91)	4615 (16.6)	7424 (23.8)
Household occupancy: N (%)			
1–2	9044 (20.8)	8668 (31.2)	6423 (20.6)
3–5	26,458 (60.9)	15,316 (55.2)	16,978 (54.4)
6–10	7531 (17.3)	3668 (13.2)	7153 (22.9)
11+	411 (0.95)	114 (0.41)	666 (2.13)
Household type: N (%)			
Adults with children	17,749 (40.9)	10,884 (39.2)	17,313 (55.5)
Adults with no children	15,888 (36.6)	8917 (32.1)	7164 (22.9)
Single adult with children	1179 (2.71)	2176 (7.84)	2827 (9.06)
Single adult	2948 (6.79)	3593 (12.9)	2380 (7.62)
Older cohabiting adults	3615 (8.32)	1602 (5.77)	660 (2.11)
Three generations	2065 (4.75)	594 (2.14)	876 (2.81)

Note: the denominator for all variables is the number of individuals rather than households. +ESA = Employment Support and Allowance; JSA = Job Seeker's Allowance.

Table A4. Estimated odds ratios of basic, physical-mental, and complex MLTCs with household tenure when the final models tested for interactions between tenure and household benefits receipt for working-age adults residing in B&D in 2019/20 (N = 102,430).

Independent Variables		Basic MLTCs		Physical-Mental MLTCs		Complex MLTCs	
		OR (95% CI)	*p* Value	OR (95% CI)	*p* Value	OR (95% CI)	*p* Value
Tenure	OOC	-	-	-	-	-	-
	Privately rented	0.78 (0.74–0.82)	<0.001	0.77 (0.69–0.86)	<0.001	0.77 (0.70–0.84)	<0.001
	Social housing	1.38 (1.32–1.45)	<0.001	1.54 (1.41–1.68)	<0.001	1.34 (1.24–1.45)	<0.001
Household benefits receipt	No benefits	-	-	-	-	-	-
	ESA	4.21 (3.35–5.28)	<0.001	7.83 (6.04–10.1)	<0.001	6.85 (5.33–8.79)	<0.001
	Pension credit	1.52 (1.19–1.94)	<0.001	1.67 (1.08–2.57)	0.021	1.62 (1.14–2.31)	0.008
	Income support	2.78 (1.90–4.06)	<0.001	2.29 (1.24–4.25)	0.008	2.39 (1.44–3.97)	<0.001
	JSA	0.96 (0.41–2.24)	0.924	0.72 (0.10–5.39)	0.752	1.60 (0.53–4.79)	0.401
	Housing benefit only	1.92 (1.63–2.26)	<0.001	2.45 (1.89–3.17)	<0.001	1.92 (1.52–2.43)	<0.001
Tenure*Household benefitsreceipt	Privately rented*no benefits	-	-	-	-	-	-
	Privately rented*ESA	1.76 (1.35–2.29)	<0.001	1.42 (1.05–1.93)	0.024	1.36 (1.01–1.83)	0.043
	Privately rented*pension credit	1.40 (1.00–1.96)	0.052	1.86 (1.05–3.31)	0.034	1.57 (0.96–2.58)	0.073
	Privately rented*income support	1.08 (0.71–1.66)	0.711	1.47 (0.73–2.93)	0.279	1.57 (0.87–2.84)	0.137
	Privately rented*JSA	2.31 (0.90–5.90)	0.080	1.97 (0.22–17.4)	0.541	1.53 (0.44–5.36)	0.509
	Privately rented*housing benefit only	0.92 (0.78–1.10)	0.356	0.95 (0.71–1.28)	0.752	1.03 (0.79–1.36)	0.807

Table A4. Cont.

Independent Variables		Basic MLTCs		Physical-Mental MLTCs		Complex MLTCs	
		OR (95% CI)	p Value	OR (95% CI)	p Value	OR (95% CI)	p Value
Tenure*Household benefits receipt (continued)	Social housing*no benefits	-	-	-	-	-	-
	Social housing*ESA	1.12 (0.88–1.43)	0.359	0.74 (0.56–0.99)	0.039	0.95 (0.72–1.25)	0.708
	Social housing*pension credit	1.01 (0.75–1.36)	0.956	0.93 (0.57–1.54)	0.784	0.93 (0.60–1.42)	0.724
	Social housing*income support	0.93 (0.62–1.39)	0.714	1.14 (0.60–2.18)	0.683	1.56 (0.91–2.68)	0.106
	Social housing*JSA	1.59 (0.66–3.86)	0.303	1.96 (0.25–15.1)	0.519	1.08 (0.34–3.42)	0.895
	Social housing*housing benefit only	0.96 (0.80–1.15)	0.681	1.01 (0.76–1.33)	0.966	1.21 (0.94–1.57)	0.142

Table A5. Estimated odds ratios of basic, physical-mental, and complex MLTCs with household tenure when the final models tested for interactions between tenure and household occupancy for working-age adults residing in B&D in 2019/20 (N = 102,430).

Independent Variables		Basic MLTCs		Physical-Mental MLTCs		Complex MLTCs	
		OR (95% CI)	p Value	OR (95% CI)	p Value	OR (95% CI)	p Value
Tenure	OOC	-	-	-	-	-	-
	Privately rented	0.99 (0.91–1.08)	0.800	1.04 (0.90–1.20)	0.564	1.02 (0.89–1.16)	0.782
	Social housing	1.54 (1.43–1.66)	<0.001	1.57 (1.40–1.77)	<0.001	1.61 (1.45–1.79)	<0.001
Occupancy categories	1–2 occupants	-	-	-	-	-	-
	3–5 occupants	1.03 (0.96–1.10)	0.415	0.98 (0.87–1.11)	0.781	1.04 (0.94–1.15)	0.464
	6–10 occupants	1.02 (0.93–1.13)	0.611	0.82 (0.67–0.99)	0.041	1.12 (0.96–1.31)	0.141
	11+ occupants	0.95 (0.70–1.28)	0.727	0.68 (0.32–1.47)	0.326	1.29 (0.80–2.08)	0.291
Tenure*Occupancy	Privately rented*1–2 occupants	-	-	-	-	-	-
	Privately rented*3–5 occupants	0.77 (0.70–0.85)	<0.001	0.73 (0.61–0.87)	<0.001	0.74 (0.63–0.87)	<0.001
	Privately rented*6–10 occupants	0.73 (0.64–0.83)	<0.001	0.80 (0.62–1.03)	0.089	0.66 (0.53–0.81)	<0.001
	Privately rented*11+ occupants	0.69 (0.46–1.03)	0.072	0.88 (0.35–2.21)	0.791	0.37 (0.18–0.75)	0.006
	Social housing*1–2 occupants	-	-	-	-	-	-
	Social housing*3–5 occupants	0.84 (0.77–0.92)	<0.001	0.88 (0.77–1.02)	0.093	0.78 (0.69–0.89)	<0.001
	Social housing*6–10 occupants	0.86 (0.75–0.97)	0.019	0.97 (0.76–1.23)	0.794	0.63 (0.51–0.78)	<0.001
	Social housing*11+ occupants	0.42 (0.22–0.78)	0.007	0.86 (0.29–2.55)	0.785	0.42 (0.17–1.04)	0.060

Table A6. Estimated odds ratios of basic, physical-mental, and complex MLTCs with household tenure when the final models tested for interactions between tenure and household type for working-age adults residing in B&D in 2019/20 (N = 102,430).

Independent Variables		Basic MLTCs		Physical-Mental MLTCs		Complex MLTCs	
		OR (95% CI)	p Value	OR (95% CI)	p Value	OR (95% CI)	p Value
Tenure	OOC	-	-	-	-	-	-
	Privately rented	0.75 (0.70–0.81)	<0.001	0.81 (0.70–0.92)	<0.001	0.67 (0.59–0.75)	<0.001
	Social housing	1.40 (1.30–1.50)	<0.001	1.54 (1.35–1.75)	<0.001	1.22 (1.09–1.38)	<0.001

Table A6. Cont.

Independent Variables		Basic MLTCs		Physical-Mental MLTCs		Complex MLTCs	
		OR (95% CI)	p Value	OR (95% CI)	p Value	OR (95% CI)	p Value
Household type	Adults with children	-	-	-	-	-	-
	Adults with no children	1.27 (1.19–1.35)	<0.001	1.28 (1.13–1.46)	<0.001	1.17 (1.05–1.30)	0.003
	Single adult with children	0.92 (0.76–1.11)	0.364	0.78 (0.53–1.17)	0.233	0.72 (0.49–1.07)	0.103
	Single adult	1.16 (1.04–1.30)	0.009	1.46 (1.20–1.78)	<0.001	1.01 (0.85–1.21)	0.892
	Older cohabiting adults	1.47 (1.34–1.62)	<0.001	1.35 (1.12–1.62)	0.001	1.38 (1.19–1.60)	<0.001
	Three generations	1.06 (0.93–1.21)	0.405	1.08 (0.81–1.43)	0.592	1.14 (0.91–1.42)	0.259
Tenure*Household type	Privately rented*adults with children	-	-	-	-	-	-
	Privately rented*adults with no children	1.09 (0.98–1.20)	0.105	1.03 (0.85–1.24)	0.788	1.25 (1.06–1.48)	0.009
	Privately rented*single adult with children	1.17 (0.93–1.46)	0.179	1.29 (0.82–2.04)	0.267	1.18 (0.74–1.88)	0.480
Tenure*Household type (continued)	Privately rented*single adult	1.57 (1.34–1.82)	<0.001	1.39 (1.08–1.79)	0.011	1.85 (1.46–2.35)	<0.001
	Privately rented*older cohabiting adults	1.24 (1.00–1.53)	0.052	1.37 (0.97–1.95)	0.076	1.72 (1.28–2.32)	<0.001
	Privately rented*three generations	0.96 (0.75–1.23)	0.774	0.91 (0.56–1.49)	0.720	1.15 (0.77–1.72)	0.494
	Social housing*adults with children	-	-	-	-	-	-
	Social housing*adults with no children	0.90 (0.82–0.99)	0.029	0.88 (0.74–1.04)	0.132	1.11 (0.96–1.28)	0.170
	Social housing*single adult with children	1.22 (0.98–1.52)	0.079	1.38 (0.90–2.14)	0.142	1.49 (0.97–2.30)	0.070
	Social housing*single adult	1.31 (1.15–1.50)	<0.001	1.07 (0.86–1.33)	0.557	1.48 (1.21–1.81)	<0.001
	Social housing*older cohabiting adults	0.76 (0.65–0.89)	<.001	0.88 (0.68–1.13)	0.315	0.87 (0.69–1.10)	0.244
	Social housing*three generations	0.91 (0.70–1.17)	0.451	0.79 (0.49–1.23)	0.318	0.93 (0.61–1.41)	0.728

References

1. The Academy of Medical Sciences. *Multimorbidity: A Priority for Global Health Research*; Academy of Medical Sciences: London, UK, 2018; pp. 1–127.
2. Marengoni, A.; Angleman, S.; Melis, R.; Mangialasche, F.; Karp, A.; Garmen, A.; Meinow, B.; Fratiglioni, L. Aging with multimorbidity: A systematic review of the literature. *Ageing Res. Rev.* **2011**, *10*, 430–439. [CrossRef]
3. Violán, C.; Foguet-Boreu, Q.; Flores-Mateo, G.; Salisbury, C.; Blom, J.; Freitag, M.; Glynn, L.; Muth, C.; Valderas, J.M. Prevalence, determinants and patterns of multimorbidity in primary care: A systematic review of observational studies. *PLoS ONE* **2014**, *9*, e102149. [CrossRef] [PubMed]
4. Salisbury, C.; Johnson, L.; Purdy, S.; Valderas, J.M.; Montgomery, A. Epidemiology and impact of multimorbidity in primary care: A retrospective cohort study. *Br. J. Gen. Pract.* **2011**, *61*, 12–21. [CrossRef] [PubMed]
5. Khanolkar, A.R.; Chaturvedi, N.; Kuan, V.; Davis, D.; Hughes, A.; Richards, M.; Bann, D.; Patalay, P. Socioeconomic inequalities in prevalence and development of multimorbidity across adulthood: A longitudinal analysis of the MRC 1946 National Survey of Health and Development in the UK. *PLoS Med.* **2021**, *18*, e1003775. [CrossRef]
6. Barnett, K.; Mercer, S.W.; Norbury, M.; Watt, G.; Wyke, S.; Guthrie, B. Epidemiology of multimorbidity and implications for health care, research, and medical education: A cross-sectional study. *Lancet* **2012**, *380*, 37–43. [CrossRef]
7. Ingram, E.; Ledden, S.; Beardon, S.; Gomes, M.; Hogarth, S.; McDonald, H.; Osborn, D.P.; Sheringham, J. Household and area-level social determinants of multimorbidity: A systematic review. *J. Epidemiol. Community Health* **2021**, *75*, 232–241. [CrossRef] [PubMed]
8. Head, A.; Fleming, K.; Kypridemos, C.; Pearson-Stuttard, J.; O'Flaherty, M. Multimorbidity: The case for prevention. *J. Epidemiol. Community Health* **2021**, *75*, 242–244. [CrossRef]

9. Head, A.; Fleming, K.; Kypridemos, C.; Schofield, P.; Pearson-Stuttard, J.; O'Flaherty, M. I Inequalities in incident and prevalent multimorbidity in England, 2004–2019: A population-based, descriptive study. *Lancet Healthy Longev.* **2021**, *2*, e489–e497. [CrossRef]
10. Solar, O.; Irwin, A. *A Conceptual Framework for Action on the Social Determinants of Health*; WHO Document Production Services: Geneva, Switzerland, 2010. [CrossRef]
11. Office for National Statistics. Living longer: Changes in Housing Tenure Over Time 2020. Available online: https://www.ons.gov.uk/releases/livinglongerchangesinhousingtenureovertime (accessed on 27 October 2021).
12. Office for National Statistics. English Housing Survey 2019 to 2020: Headline Report 2020. Available online: https://www.gov.uk/government/statistics/english-housing-survey-2019-to-2020-headline-report (accessed on 27 October 2021).
13. Ellaway, A.; Macintyre, S. Does housing tenure predict health in the UK because it exposes people to different levels of housing related hazards in the home or its surroundings? *Health Place* **1998**, *4*, 141–150. [CrossRef]
14. Shaw, M. Housing and public health. *Annu. Rev. Public Health* **2004**, *25*, 397–418. [CrossRef]
15. Macintyre, S.; Ellaway, A.; Hiscock, R.; Kearns, A.; Der, G.; McKay, L. What features of the home and the area might help to explain observed relationships between housing tenure and health? Evidence from the west of Scotland. *Health Place* **2003**, *9*, 207–218. [CrossRef]
16. Reeves, A.; Clair, A.; McKee, M.; Stuckler, D. Reductions in the United Kingdom's Government Housing Benefit and Symptoms of Depression in Low-Income Households. *Am. J. Epidemiol.* **2016**, *184*, 421–429. [CrossRef]
17. Clair, A.; Hughes, A. Housing and health: New evidence using biomarker data. *J. Epidemiol. Community Health* **2019**, *73*, 256–262. [CrossRef] [PubMed]
18. Shand, J. Towards Integrated Care: Using Linked Data to Explore Health and Social Care Utilisation for Adult Residents of Barking and Dagenham in 2016/17. Ph.D. Thesis, University College London (UCL), London, UK, 2020.
19. London Borough of Barking and Dagenham. Joint Strategic Needs Assessment. 2018. Available online: https://www.lbbd.gov.uk/joint-strategic-needs-assessment-jsna (accessed on 7 November 2019).
20. Benchimol, E.I.; Smeeth, L.; Guttmann, A.; Harron, K.; Moher, D.; Petersen, I.; Sørensen, H.T.; von Elm, E.; Langan, S.M.; RECORD Working Committee. The REporting of studies Conducted using Observational Routinely-collected health Data (RECORD) Statement. *PLoS Med.* **2015**, *12*, e1001885. [CrossRef] [PubMed]
21. Office for National Statistics. Working Age Population. 2020. Available online: https://www.ethnicity-facts-figures.service.gov.uk/uk-population-by-ethnicity/demographics/working-age-population/latest (accessed on 21 March 2022).
22. Harper, G.; Mayhew, L. Using Administrative Data to Count an Local Applications. *Appl. Spat. Anal. Policy* **2012**, *5*, 97–122. [CrossRef]
23. Cambridge C@. Codes Lists Version 1.1—October 2018—Primary Care Unit. 2018. Available online: https://www.phpc.cam.ac.uk/pcu/cprd_cam/codelists/v11/ (accessed on 6 November 2019).
24. Harrison, C.; Britt, H.; Miller, G.; Henderson, J. Examining different measures of multimorbidity, using a large prospective cross-sectional study in Australian general practice. *BMJ Open* **2014**, *4*, e004694. [CrossRef] [PubMed]
25. Office for National Statistics. National Statistics—English Indices of Deprivation 2019. 2019. Available online: https://www.gov.uk/government/statistics/english-indices-of-deprivation-2019 (accessed on 13 September 2021).
26. Office for National Statistics. Census Geography. 2011. Available online: https://www.ons.gov.uk/methodology/geography/ukgeographies/censusgeography (accessed on 13 September 2021).
27. Bobo, W.V.; Yawn, B.P.; St. Sauver, J.L.; Grossardt, B.R.; Boyd, C.M.; Rocca, W.A. Prevalence of Combined Somatic and Mental Health Multimorbidity: Patterns by Age, Sex, and Race/Ethnicity. *J. Gerontol. A Biol. Sci. Med. Sci.* **2016**, *71*, 1483–1491. [CrossRef]
28. Office for National Statistics. Home Ownership—Ethnicity Facts and Figures. 2020. Available online: https://www.ethnicity-facts-figures.service.gov.uk/housing/owning-and-renting/home-ownership/latest (accessed on 20 September 2021).
29. Katikireddi, S.V.; Skivington, K.; Leyland, A.H.; Hunt, K.; Mercer, S.W. The contribution of risk factors to socioeconomic inequalities in multimorbidity across the lifecourse: A longitudinal analysis of the Twenty-07 cohort. *BMC Med.* **2017**, *15*, 152. [CrossRef]
30. Bates, D.; Mächler, M.; Bolker, B.; Walker, S. Fitting linear mixed-effects models using lme4. *J. Stat. Softw.* **2015**, *67*, 48. [CrossRef]
31. Doerken, S.; Avalos, M.; Lagarde, E.; Schumacher, M. Penalized logistic regression with low prevalence exposures beyond high dimensional settings. *PLoS ONE* **2019**, *14*, e0217057. [CrossRef]
32. Johnson-Lawrence, V.; Zajacova, A.; Sneed, R. Education, race/ethnicity, and multimorbidity among adults aged 30–64 in the National Health Interview Survey. *SSM—Popul. Health* **2017**, *3*, 366–372. [CrossRef] [PubMed]
33. Taylor, A.W.; Price, K.; Gill, T.K.; Adams, R.; Pilkington, R.; Carrangis, N.; Shi, Z.; Wilson, D. Multimorbidity: Not just an older person's issue. Results from an Australian biomedical study. *Soc. Psychiatry Psychiatr. Epidemiol.* **2011**, *46*, 351. [CrossRef]
34. Chung, R.Y.; Mercer, S.; Lai, F.T.T.; Yip, B.H.K.; Wong, M.C.S.; Wong, S.Y.S. Socioeconomic determinants of multimorbidity: A population-based household survey of Hong Kong Chinese. *PLoS ONE* **2015**, *10*, e0140040. [CrossRef] [PubMed]
35. Ferry, F.R.; Rosato, M.G.; Curran, E.J.; O'Reilly, D.; Leavey, G. Multimorbidity among persons aged 25–64 years: A population-based study of social determinants and all-cause mortality. *J. Public Health* **2020**, *44*, e59–e67. [CrossRef] [PubMed]
36. Ansar, W.; Ghosh, S. C-reactive protein and the biology of disease. *Immunol. Res.* **2013**, *56*, 131–142. [CrossRef] [PubMed]
37. Hiscock, R.; Kearns, A.; MacIntyre, S.; Ellaway, A. Ontological security and psycho-social benefits from the home: Qualitative evidence on issues of tenure. *Hous. Theory Soc.* **2001**, *18*, 50–66. [CrossRef]

38. Scanlon, K.; Kochan, B. Towards a Sustainable Private Rented Sector. The Lessons from Other Countries. 2011. Available online: http://eprints.lse.ac.uk/56070/1/Towards_a_sustainable_private_rented_sector.pdf (accessed on 29 June 2021).
39. Palmer, G. "Single Person Households" Issues That JRF Should Be Thinking about. Joseph Rowntree Found. 2006. Available online: https://www.jrf.org.uk (accessed on 22 December 2021).
40. Zaccai, J.H. How to assess epidemiological studies. *Postgrad. Med. J.* **2004**, *80*, 140–147. [CrossRef]
41. Pigott, T.D. A Review of Methods for Missing Data. *Educ. Res. Eval.* **2001**, *7*, 353–383. [CrossRef]
42. Care City Cohort 2019. Available online: https://www.carecity.london/component/content/article/95-what-we-do/216-care-city-cohort (accessed on 7 February 2022).
43. Shand, J.; Morris, S.; Gomes, M. Understanding health and care expenditure by setting—Who matters to whom? *J. Health Serv. Res. Policy* **2020**, *26*, 77–84. [CrossRef]
44. Harron, K.L.; Doidge, J.; Knight, H.E.; Gilbert, R.; Goldstein, H.; Cromwell, D.A.; Van Der Meulen, J.H. A guide to evaluating linkage quality for the analysis of linked data. *Int. J. Epidemiol.* **2017**, *46*, 1699–1710. [CrossRef] [PubMed]

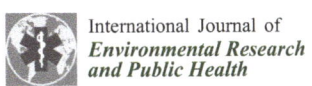

Protocol

A Protocol for a Mixed-Methods Process Evaluation of a Local Population Health Management System to Reduce Inequities in COVID-19 Vaccination Uptake

Georgia Watson [1], Cassie Moore [1], Fiona Aspinal [2], Claudette Boa [3], Vusi Edeki [3], Andrew Hutchings [4], Rosalind Raine [2] and Jessica Sheringham [2,*]

1. London Boroughs of Camden & Islington, London N1 1XR, UK; Georgia.watson@islington.gov.uk (G.W.); cassie.moore@islington.gov.uk (C.M.)
2. Department of Applied Health Research, University College London, London WC1E 7HB, UK; f.aspinal@ucl.ac.uk (F.A.); r.raine@ucl.ac.uk (R.R.)
3. Public Health England, London SE1 8UG, UK; claudette.boa@phe.gov.uk (C.B.); vusi.edeki@phe.gov.uk (V.E.)
4. London School of Hygiene and Tropical Medicine, London WC1E 7HT, UK; andrew.hutchings@lshtm.ac.uk
* Correspondence: j.sheringham@ucl.ac.uk; Tel.: +44-20-7679-8286

Abstract: Population health management is an emerging technique to link and analyse patient data across several organisations in order to identify population needs and plan care. It is increasingly used in England and has become more important as health policy has sought to drive greater integration across health and care organisations. This protocol describes a mixed-methods process evaluation of an innovative population health management system in North Central London, England, serving a population of 1.5 million. It focuses on how staff have used a specific tool within North Central London's population health management system designed to reduce inequities in COVID-19 vaccination. The COVID-19 vaccination Dashboard was first deployed from December 2020 and enables staff in North London to view variations in the uptake of COVID-19 vaccinations by population characteristics in near real-time. The evaluation will combine interviews with clinical and non-clinical staff with staff usage analytics, including the volume and frequency of staff Dashboard views, to describe the tool's reach and identify possible mechanisms of impact. While seeking to provide timely insights to optimise the design of population health management tools in North Central London, it also seeks to provide longer term transferable learning on methods to evaluate population health management systems.

Keywords: population health management; data linkage; population health; inequalities; inequities; process evaluation; protocol

1. Introduction

In many countries, health policy has moved towards greater integration between different organisations that plan, commission, and deliver health and care [1]. In the latest stage of policy reforms in England, for example, all areas were statutorily required to form integrated care systems (ICSs) by April 2021 that include hospital, mental health, and community trust healthcare providers; primary care providers; clinical commissioning groups; and local authorities, which have a lead role for public health [2].

Sharing patient information across organisations is recognised as a key part of health system integration. An evaluation of four international integrated care systems conducted by the Nuffield Trust describes 'informational integrative processes' as one of the six key factors in the success of, or difficulties in, these programs. The challenges of data sharing across organisations, both in the United Kingdom and internationally, have been well documented [3]. However, a number of data sharing systems are now being developed and deployed. For example, the Whole Systems Integrated Care (WSIC) system in North

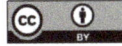

West London, England was set up in part to facilitate the journey towards integrated care systems [4].

It is increasingly accepted that data sharing in itself is not sufficient to drive integration, and in turn improve population health outcomes [5]. As Scott et al. argue, 'data alone does not save lives. It is knowledge derived from data analysis and applied in practice that saves lives' [6]. Population health management (PHM) is an emerging technique used by local health and care partnerships in England. It uses data to help practitioners to understand their population, and then to use this understanding to inform practice [7]. It involves linking and analysing health and care data from different organisations to understand the health of a local population and their current service need, and to predict what local people will need in the future. In a PHM approach, this information is then used to inform decisions on the design and delivery of services in order to improve the health and wellbeing of the population and reduce inequities [8].

There is a lack of evidence about how (or whether) PHM can achieve its aims. There is some evidence that the use of data sharing platforms could influence patient care, but this is mainly from case studies, where evaluation has often been conducted in-house [9,10]. Before considering evaluating the effectiveness of such tools on population health, we need to know more about how PHM data sharing platforms may enable a population health management approach, i.e., to inform decisions to improve the health and wellbeing of their population and reduce inequities. This information is needed to optimise the design of PHM platforms and programs and inform impact evaluations in the future.

Process evaluations—which seek to describe how, and why, a program or intervention works—are often used alongside impact evaluations [11]. For emerging interventions, they can also serve a useful purpose to understand key aspects of delivery of an intervention under development. This protocol describes a process evaluation of a population health management system in London, England using quantitative and qualitative methods. It has dual aims:

- To understand how staff use a specific population health management system tool to inform decisions and ways of working that reduce inequities in order to help the local area further develop their system;
- To develop the capacity for wider evaluation of PHM systems.

1.1. Context: The Population Health Management Innovation

This evaluation is centred on North Central London's Integrated Care System (North London Partners, NLP), which provides care to 1.5 million people across five boroughs of London. North Central London is comparatively well advanced in its deployment of a near real-time population health management tool that integrates health and care data from across the system.

NLP uses HealtheIntent, a PHM platform developed by the digital provider, Cerner, which combines data across the 28 local authorities and health and care organisations in the integrated care system. It links and standardises data from across the health and social care system (such as general practices and hospitals) and re-presents these data—as 'registries' and 'dashboards'—to staff based in the constituent organisations. An aim of NLP's PHM program is to identify and reduce health inequities and, consequently, elements of HealtheIntent are specifically designed to assist users to identify segments of the population with unequal access to care to inform the development of targeted responses [7]. The design of the tools is underpinned by several core principles, including the relevance of intersectionality (i.e., recognising that social characteristics, such as ethnicity, gender, and socioeconomic circumstances, are interconnected and can create distinct, and sometimes amplified, experiences of disadvantage), the conceptualisation of health inequities as existing on a gradient rather than as a binary (present or absent), and the roots of inequities being in material and psychosocial factors upheld by political and economic structures.

One of the first HealtheIntent tools used in NLP was a COVID-19 vaccination dashboard. Nationally, COVID-19 vaccinations were rolled out in phases. In the first phase, starting from 8 December 2020, the target was for all adults over 65 years of age, those in care homes, NHS and care staff, and clinically vulnerable people to have been offered a first vaccine dose by 15 February 2021 [12]. The second phase of the vaccination rollout, from 13 April 2021, covered the population aged 18–64 years and maintained priority by age and clinical risk [13]. As with many vaccination programs, there was concern that inequalities in uptake would result in inequalities in the risk of COVID-19 infections and serious sequelae. The Scientific Advisory Group for Emergencies (SAGE) reported that, in previous roll outs of national vaccine programs, there was lower uptake in minority ethnic populations [14]. Given the ethnic inequities in COVID-19 death rates, there were specific concerns about ethnic inequities in COVID-19 vaccine uptake [15].

The HealtheIntent COVID-19 vaccination Dashboard (referred to in the rest of the paper as the Dashboard) was developed at the end of 2020 (Figure 1). It sought to enable staff to view variations in COVID-19 vaccination uptake almost in real time. It became available to end users (NLP staff) in December 2020 and continues to be developed, updated, and improved in response to changing requirements. This has led to many iterations of the Dashboard, but, at the time of this evaluation, the Dashboard contained an overview page, a page describing uptake by eligibility cohorts, several demographic and equalities pages, data quality pages, a case-finding tool, and a user guide.

Users have access to different versions of the Dashboard depending on their staff role and type. All users, including non-clinical staff, can see anonymised, aggregated data, but only those with permission, such as primary care staff, can access individual patient data. An Overview page describes overall vaccination uptake. An Equalities and Demographics page segments (i.e., enables users to stratify) the population by gender, ethnicity, IMD quintile, first language spoken, age, and geography. An example of segmentation is by the level of deprivation experienced. The Dashboard stratifies the population into five deprivation quintiles, in line with evidence about health inequalities existing on a gradient [16]. While this design cannot guarantee that users of the tool focus on the middle quintiles as well as the lowest quintile, it does provide users with the capability to do so and respond to findings.

The Dashboard tool also allows users to tailor what they view by providing filters (i.e., restricting the view to specific sub-populations). The Dashboard's many filters include the user view (where users can limit what they see to their own care team type or organisation), COVID-19 information (vaccination eligible cohort, number of doses received, vaccine manufacturer), and health and care information (carer status, known to adult social care, long term conditions, number of long term conditions, mental health conditions, homelessness, bedbound and housebound status). The demographic variables displayed in charts on the Demographics and Equalities pages can also be used to filter data. The system is designed to prevent presenting data in numbers so small that identification might be (theoretically) possible to those without permission to access identifiable data.

1.2. Objectives

In order to address our first aim of understanding how a population health management system is used, we have proposed two objectives:

- To describe how (or whether) staff report using evidence of inequities in uptake available in the HealtheIntent COVID-19 Vaccination Dashboard to address inequities;
- To describe staff usage of the HealtheIntent COVID-19 Vaccination Dashboard, particularly those parts of the Dashboard that display evidence of inequities in uptake.

To address our second aim of building capacity for wider evaluation of PHM systems, there are two objectives to equip public health practitioners, working as embedded researchers in NLP, with the skills to undertake with supervision both the qualitative and the quantitative arms of the study.

To reflect on the suitability of our methods, in particular we work closely with and train locally embedded researchers to determine the extent to which this model is a workable model for future evaluations of population health management.

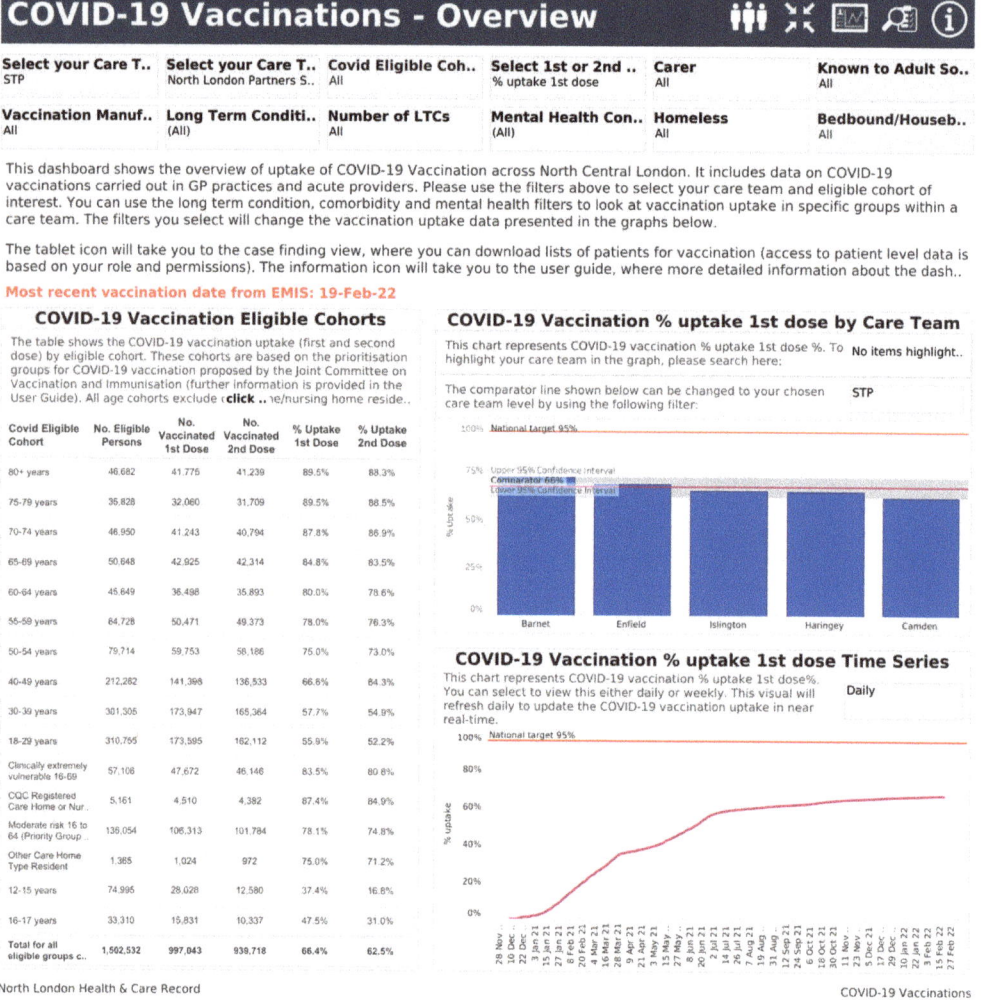

Figure 1. Illustrative screenshot of the HealtheIntent COVID-19 Vaccination Dashboard. Copyright: North London Partners.

2. Materials and Methods

This study will combine qualitative methods to identify potential mechanisms of impact of the Dashboard and quantitative analysis of Dashboard usage and reach.

To support part of the study's capacity building aim, university researchers will be working in collaboration with public health practitioners who are seconded part-time to a research role, funded by a grant intended to build capacity for public health research in local authorities. The seconded practitioners' main public health roles are within public health teams in local and regional government. The practitioners will gain transferable skills in research and evaluation through access to specific courses and seminars (e.g., in evaluation methods) and through undertaking all stages of the research process, from submission for ethical review to dissemination of findings, with supervision and guidance from university researchers. If this objective is fulfilled, it will equip the seconded practitioners with the experience and skills to undertake evaluation of NLP's PHM tools in the future. It will also advance our understanding of how such collaborations could be used to conduct evaluations of other PHM systems.

The evaluation is designed to be relatively rapid (i.e., completed within 6–12 months) to ensure the findings are timely enough to influence future local population health management innovations. Therefore, we will incorporate the following elements of rapid evaluation approaches: multiple researchers collecting data concurrently; and sharing interim findings with stakeholders to shape interpretation and analysis, and to sustain their involvement and support [17].

The study was granted approval by UCL Ethics Committee, ref: 2037/005. We started activities for the evaluation in September 2021. We envisage completing most stages of the evaluation by the end of June 2022, though further analysis of the dataset may be undertaken after this date.

2.1. Proposed Qualitative Data Collection and Analysis

We will undertake semi-structured interviews ($n \approx 20$) online using MS Teams with a purposive sample of staff who have responsibility for an aspect of COVID-19 vaccination planning or delivery.

Study population: We will interview staff at different levels of seniority, in clinical, strategic, commissioning, and analytical roles across different organisations in NLP (primary care, hospital or mental health providers, social care, public health), and will seek to ensure we capture experiences across all five North Central London boroughs. The sample size is approximate because some individuals will have more than one role, and thus will be able to cover more than one of our desired attributes.

Interviews will explore staff experiences of using the Dashboard and how variations in vaccination uptake shown in the Dashboard informed their actions to address inequities. We have developed a topic guide (an example provided as Supplementary Data) informed by normalisation process theory, which provides guidance for exploring the perceptions of staff and the actions that staff take when a new product or innovation is introduced into an organization [18]. In line with normalisation process theory, the interviews will explore the following:

- Motivation to use the Dashboard;
- Specific features of the Dashboard and their advantages or limitations for the user;
- Contextual enablers or barriers to using the Dashboard;
- How the participants considered that usage of the Dashboard influenced ways of working and decisions, e.g., about COVID-19 vaccination planning or delivery.

To develop the guides and to develop consistency between interviewers, an exercise of 'concept mapping' was undertaken by the lead interviewer (G.W.) with supervision from F.A., whereby, for each topic covered by the guide, a short 'concept' description was developed to guide interviewers on what the question was seeking to obtain. This led to revisions of the interview schedule and enabled each interviewer to tailor their own guide to their own language and style. The guide was initially 'soft' pilot tested with a colleague and then, after refinements, was piloted with three staff working in North Central London. No significant changes were made to the guide at this point, so these interviews will be included in the final dataset.

Interviews will be conducted by several individuals (G.W., C.M., V.E., C.B.) working within and external to NLP, to expedite data collection. All interviewees will be asked to sign a consent form before being interviewed. Participants' names and roles will not be disclosed and all data will be anonymised to minimise the risk of identifying participants. All interviews will be recorded and transcribed in full by a transcription service. The transcribers will remove any identifiers such as names and organizations before securely returning transcripts to the researchers. Researchers will read and further redact transcripts if any potentially identifiable information remains in the text. To expedite analysis, interviewers will note key points from their interviews immediately after conducting them.

Transcripts will be analysed using the Framework Method using Excel by G.W. and C.M. with reading of selected transcripts by J.S. and F.A [19]. A preliminary coding framework drawn from the topic guide was developed by G.W. and C.M. in discussion with J.S. and F.A. to expedite initial descriptive analysis. Further codes and overarching themes and refinements to the analytical strategy will be generated inductively. Discussions with the wider team will take place to discuss emerging findings and resolve discrepancies in coding and interpretation of the data.

Documents and correspondence about the Dashboard, including descriptions of the rollout of vaccination in NLP and iterations of the Dashboard, will be examined to provide contextual evidence for the interviews and to build a timeline of key events in the program to inform both qualitative and quantitative analysis (see Combining Qualitative and Quantitative Data).

2.2. Proposed Quantitative Data Extraction and Analysis

The proposed quantitative data collation and analysis part of the study will use anonymised staff usage data already stored within HealtheIntent to describe variations in usage of the COVID-19 vaccination Dashboard since its launch in December 2020. It seeks to capitalise on the extensive data automatically generated about usage whenever these population health management tools are used. A request for anonymised data has been submitted to the HealtheIntent service desk. This request includes the numbers of staff by organization and over time that are registered to use the Dashboard. It also includes a request for figures on the actual use of the Dashboard, both in terms of logins and activities while on the Dashboard.

Initial descriptive analysis of usage will be undertaken in Stata and will involve two components [20]. First, the analysis will seek to enumerate the denominator population (i.e., the number of accounts of individuals that were registered to use the COVID-19 Dashboard) and its characteristics (e.g., organisation and geographical area). Second, the proportion of those using the Dashboard among those registered will be generated in key time periods (informed by the timeline constructed, see Proposed Qualitative Data Collection and Analysis section). Usage will be examined for any part of the Dashboard. Where possible, usage will be examined for specific equalities pages of the Dashboard and among specific groups of users, defined by organisation, staff role type, and geographical area.

2.3. Combining Qualitative and Quantitative Data: Proposed Approach

As described above, we have planned to use the qualitative and documentary data to construct a timeline of key events that will inform the intervals for the quantitative analysis. Interim findings from the qualitative and quantitative data will be shared within the study team at regular intervals, to inform the interpretation of findings from each method, and potentially to prompt further analysis. For example, interview data that reports barriers to, or motivations for, usage may be used to support interpretation of quantitative data showing variations in usage patterns. The extent to which it is possible to combine qualitative and quantitative findings will depend on the data obtained. We will seek to use both qualitative and quantitative findings to support the development of candidate program theories by which population health management could achieve its intended outcomes that could be used in future impact evaluations.

3. Discussion

This protocol describes a process evaluation of a specific population health management tool within one geographical area of England. It will combine qualitative and quantitative methods to describe staff usage of a specific tool, the COVID-19 vaccination uptake Dashboard, and how it informs their decisions and ways of working to reduce inequities in vaccine uptake. Working with colleagues based in North Central London means that any learning gained even in the earliest stages of the process evaluation can be rapidly fed back to inform continuing Dashboard development and new population health management tool development and rollouts. The findings from the study also have the potential to have wider significance in advancing methods for evaluating population health management, and thus could build capacity for further evaluations of population health management programs.

Strengths and Limitations

A key strength of this evaluation is the collaboration between academia, local public health, health care, and regional public health teams. The use of embedded local researchers combined with senior sponsorship promises to ensure the evaluation remains grounded in local service priorities and serves to build local evaluation capacity. The timeliness of the evaluation, and sharing of preliminary findings, aligns with the principle of continuous learning and improvement underlying NLP's PHM program and, more specifically, its use of linked data to support health and care providers addressing inequities. Regional public health input has brought a wider policy perspective and academic input brings independence and objectivity to the evaluation and provides methodological rigour.

The evaluation is subject to some important limitations or challenges. It is taking place in 2021 and 2022, at a time of considerable uncertainty owing to the COVID-19 pandemic. Therefore, it is possible this will affect access to interview participants and access to quantitative data. Strategic input from internal project sponsors will be sought to address barriers and encourage participation to reduce the risk of the project stalling due to other priorities. In the ongoing qualitative data collection and analysis, rapid evaluation approaches were chosen to enable timely findings and feedback to NLP and will also be subject to further in-depth analysis.

We anticipate two major challenges in the quantitative aspect of the evaluation. Access to data held within the population health management system by an external partner, such as a university-employed researcher, would require extensive information governance procedures, reducing the timeliness of the evaluation. However, all organisations within NLP contribute data to the system and are designated data controllers. This designation enables all partners access to non-identifiable data, which makes internal evaluation a possibility. To make use of the opportunity for internal analysis, a local analyst in a funded embedded researcher role will undertake the analysis with the support of external quantitative expertise from ARC North Thames. In addition, the data on staff usage have not previously been subject to evaluation or monitoring. It is thus not well understood what information is feasible to extract from the system, what processes are required to make this information suitable for analysis, or how best to do this. Therefore, the evaluation also seeks to clarify the range of data available, the processes for data extraction, and management before analysis. We will also iterate what data we request and develop a more detailed analysis plan as our understanding of the data evolves.

4. Conclusions

This protocol describes an evaluation that seeks to understand how staff use a specific population health management system tool to inform decisions and ways of working that reduce inequities in vaccine uptake. In the short term, achieving this aim should serve the local health and care system by providing useful insights to inform future population health management activities. The evaluation also aims to develop the capacity for wider evaluation of PHM systems. We will have met this aim if our evaluation equips local practitioners with the skills to conduct further evaluation and if it generates transferable learning about the methods for evaluating such programs in collaboration with local health and care professionals in the future.

Supplementary Materials: The following supporting information can be downloaded at https://www.mdpi.com/article/10.3390/ijerph19084588/s1, S1: topic guide for interviews.

Author Contributions: Conceptualization, G.W., C.M., F.A., A.H. and J.S.; methodology, G.W., C.M., F.A., A.H. and J.S.; investigation, G.W., C.M., V.E. and C.B.; writing—original draft preparation, G.W., C.M. and J.S.; writing—review and editing, A.H., F.A. and R.R.; funding acquisition, J.S. and R.R. All authors have read and agreed to the published version of the manuscript.

Funding: This report is independent research funded by the National Institute for Health Research ARC North Thames (NIHR200163), Clinical Research Network North Thames capacity building for public health, and Agile Workforce Funding (UCL004). The views expressed in this publication are those of the author(s) and not necessarily those of the National Institute for Health Research or the Department of Health and Social Care.

Institutional Review Board Statement: The study was granted approval by UCL Ethics Committee, ref: 2037/005.

Informed Consent Statement: Informed consent was obtained from all subjects involved in the study.

Data Availability Statement: Not applicable.

Acknowledgments: The authors would like to Amy Bowen, Director of System Improvement, North London Partners in Health and Care, and Sarah Dougan, Director of Population Health Management, North London Partners in Health and Care & Consultant in Public Health, London Boroughs of Camden & Islington, for their vital shaping of the study design and ongoing sponsorship of the evaluation. The authors would also like to thank Fola Tayo and Nira Shah, and other members of the ARC North Thames Research Advisory Panel for their advice on the study design and on communicating population health management to a lay audience.

Conflicts of Interest: The authors declare no conflict of interest. The funders had no role in the design of the study; in the collection, analyses, or interpretation of data; in the writing of the manuscript; or in the decision to publish the results.

References

1. NHS England. NHS Long Term Plan. 2019. Available online: https://www.longtermplan.nhs.uk/ (accessed on 28 February 2022).
2. Department of Health and Social Care. Integration and Innovation: Working Together to Improve Health and Social Care for All. 2021. Available online: https://www.gov.uk/government/publications/working-together-to-improve-health-and-social-care-for-all (accessed on 28 February 2022).
3. Rosen, R.; Mountford, J.; Lewis, G.; Lewis, R.; Shand, J.; Shaw, S. Integration in Action: Four International Case Studies The Nuffield Trust: London, UK. 2011. Available online: https://www.nuffieldtrust.org.uk/research/integration-in-action-four-international-case-studies (accessed on 28 February 2022).
4. Bottle, A.; Cohen, C.; Lucas, A.; Saravanakumar, K.; Ul-Haq, Z.; Smith, W.; Majeed, A.; Aylin, P. How an electronic health record became a real-world research resource: Comparison between London's Whole Systems Integrated Care database and the Clinical Practice Research Datalink. *BMC Med. Inform. Decis. Mak.* **2020**, *20*, 71. [CrossRef] [PubMed]
5. Ingram, E.; Cooper, S.; Beardon, S.; Körner, K.; McDonald, H.I.; Hogarth, S.; Gomes, M.; Sheringham, J. Barriers and facilitators of use of analytics for strategic health and care decision-making: A qualitative study of senior health and care leaders' perspectives. *BMJ Open* **2022**, *12*, e055504. [CrossRef] [PubMed]
6. Scott, P.; Emerson, K.; Henderson-Reay, T. Data saves lives. *BMJ* **2021**, *374*, n1694. [CrossRef] [PubMed]
7. Bhuiya, A.D.; Hajimirsadeghi, S.O.; North, H. When Population Health Meets General Practice—A Brief Introduction to Dashboards and Registries BJGP Life [Online]. 2022. Available online: https://bjgplife.com/when-population-health-meets-general-practice-a-brief-introduction-to-dashboards-and-registries/ (accessed on 28 February 2022).
8. NHS England. Population Health and the Population Health Management Programme. Available online: https://www.england.nhs.uk/integratedcare/what-is-integrated-care/phm/ (accessed on 28 February 2022).
9. MICO Consultancy. The Leeds Care Record: Benefits Review & Evaluation. Available online: https://www.leedscarerecord.org/content/uploads/2020/04/Leeds-Care-Record-Benefits-19-20.pdf (accessed on 28 February 2022).
10. Alam, R.; Cheraghi-Sohi, S.; Panagioti, M.; Esmail, A.; Campbell, S.; Panagopoulou, E. Managing diagnostic uncertainty in primary care: A systematic critical review. *BMC Fam. Pract.* **2017**, *18*, 79. [CrossRef] [PubMed]
11. Moore, G.F.; Audrey, S.; Barker, M.; Bond, L.; Bonell, C.; Hardeman, W.; Moore, L.; O'Cathain, A.; Tinati, T.; Wight, D.; et al. Process evaluation of complex interventions: Medical Research Council guidance. *BMJ* **2015**, *350*, h1258. [CrossRef] [PubMed]
12. Department of Health and Social Care. Priority Groups for Coronavirus (COVID-19) Vaccination: Advice from the JCVI, 30 December 2020. Available online: https://www.gov.uk/government/publications/priority-groups-for-coronavirus-covid-19-vaccination-advice-from-the-jcvi-30-december-2020 (accessed on 7 January 2022).

13. Department of Health and Social Care. JCVI Final Statement on Phase 2 of the COVID-19 Vaccination Programme: 13 April 2021. Available online: https://www.gov.uk/government/publications/priority-groups-for-phase-2-of-the-coronavirus-covid-19-vaccination-programme-advice-from-the-jcvi/jcvi-final-statement-on-phase-2-of-the-covid-19-vaccination-programme-13-april-2021 (accessed on 6 January 2022).
14. The Scientific Advisory Group for Emergencies (SAGE). *Factors Influencing COVID-19 Vaccine Uptake among Minority Ethnic Groups*; DHSC: London, UK, 2021. Available online: https://assets.publishing.service.gov.uk/government/uploads/system/uploads/attachment_data/file/952716/s0979-factors-influencing-vaccine-uptake-minority-ethnic-groups.pdf (accessed on 28 February 2022).
15. Williamson, E.J.; Walker, A.J.; Bhaskaran, K.; Bacon, S.; Bates, C.; Morton, C.E.; Curtis, H.J.; Mehrkar, A.; Evans, D.; Inglesby, P.; et al. Factors associated with COVID-19-related death using OpenSAFELY. *Nature* **2020**, *584*, 430–436. [CrossRef] [PubMed]
16. Smith, K.B.; Hill, C.S.E. Background and Introduction: UK Experiences of Health Inequalities. In *Health Inequalities: Critical Perspectives*; Smith, K.B., Hill, C.S.E., Eds.; Oxford Scholarship Online: Online, 2016.
17. Vindrola-Padros, C.; Johnson, G.A. Rapid Techniques in Qualitative Research: A Critical Review of the Literature. *Qual. Health Res.* **2020**, *30*, 1596–1604. [CrossRef] [PubMed]
18. May, C.; Finch, T. Implementing, Embedding, and Integrating Practices: An Outline of Normalization Process Theory. *Sociology* **2009**, *43*, 535–554. [CrossRef]
19. Gale, N.K.; Heath, G.; Cameron, E.; Rashid, S.; Redwood, S. Using the framework method for the analysis of qualitative data in multi-disciplinary health research. *BMC Med. Res. Methodol.* **2013**, *13*, 117. [CrossRef] [PubMed]
20. *StataCorp Stata Statistical Software: Release 16*; StataCorp LP: College Station, TX, USA, 2016.

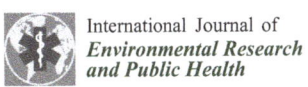

International Journal of
Environmental Research and Public Health

Article

Development of Public Health Core Outcome Sets for Systems-Wide Promotion of Early Life Health and Wellbeing

Liina Mansukoski [1,*], Alexandra Albert [2], Yassaman Vafai [1,3], Chris Cartwright [3], Aamnah Rahman [3], Jessica Sheringham [4], Bridget Lockyer [3], Tiffany C. Yang [3], Philip Garnett [5] and Maria Bryant [1,6,*]

1. Department of Health Sciences, University of York, York YO10 5DD, UK; yassaman.vafai@york.ac.uk
2. Thomas Coram Research Unit, University College London (UCL), London WC1H 0AL, UK; a.albert@ucl.ac.uk
3. Bradford Institute for Health Research, Bradford Teaching Hospitals NHS Foundation Trust, Bradford BD9 6RJ, UK; chris.cartwright@bthft.nhs.uk (C.C.); aamnah.rahman@bthft.nhs.uk (A.R.); bridget.lockyer@bthft.nhs.uk (B.L.); tiffany.yang@bthft.nhs.uk (T.C.Y.)
4. Department of Applied Health Research, University College London (UCL), London WC1E 6BT, UK; j.sheringham@ucl.ac.uk
5. School of Management, University of York, York YO10 5DD, UK; philip.garnett@york.ac.uk
6. Hull York Medical School, University of York, York YO10 5DD, UK
* Correspondence: liina.mansukoski@york.ac.uk (L.M.); maria.bryant@york.ac.uk (M.B.)

Abstract: We aimed to develop a core outcome set (COS) for systems-wide public health interventions seeking to promote early life health and wellbeing. Research was embedded within the existing systems-based intervention research programme 'ActEarly', located in two different areas with high rates of child poverty, Bradford (West Yorkshire) and the Borough of Tower Hamlets (London). 168 potential outcomes were derived from five local government outcome frameworks, a community-led survey and an ActEarly consortium workshop. Two rounds of a Delphi study (Round 1: 37 participants; Round 2: 56 participants) reduced the number of outcomes to 64. 199 members of the community then took part in consultations across ActEarly sites, resulting in a final COS for systems-based public health interventions of 40 outcomes. These were grouped into the domains of: Development & education (N = 6); Physical health & health behaviors (N = 6); Mental health (N = 5); Social environment (N = 4); Physical environment (N = 7); and Poverty & inequality (N = 7). This process has led to a COS with outcomes prioritized from the perspectives of local communities. It provides the means to increase standardization and guide the selection of outcome measures for systems-based evaluation of public health programmes and supports evaluation of individual interventions within system change approaches.

Keywords: early life health; core outcome set; public health interventions; systems approach

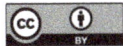

1. Introduction

1.1. Background and Objectives

Core outcome sets (COS) are "an agreed standardized collection of outcomes" used in evaluations of intervention research [1]. The use of COS has been promoted to harmonize the outcomes used and to ensure that key stakeholders are consulted on the relevance of what is being measured in evaluations [2]. No existing core outcome set has been adapted specifically for the systems-wide promotion of early life health and wellbeing in public health research in the UK, two widely used outcomes frameworks are the Public Health Outcomes Framework (PHOF) and the NHS Outcomes Framework [3,4]. Though an important resource to highlight key indicators to measure the success of some early life interventions, the most widely used existing framework for public health, the PHOF, was not developed to ensure the use of a minimum set of outcomes to be used across studies to facilitate comparisons. Most COS in the pediatric literature, on the other hand, focus on a specific illness or disease, not on public health outcomes [5].

We sought a COS to support the evaluation of a UKPRP-funded programme of research called ActEarly. ActEarly is a large research consortium aimed at promoting health and wellbeing in early life in two different areas with high rates of child poverty: Bradford in West Yorkshire and the Borough of Tower Hamlets in London [6]. Living in an area with high levels of child poverty often coincides with exposure to other economic, physical, cultural, learning, social and service environmental risk factors, which can predispose children and their families to poorer mental and physical health outcomes. In 2019, ActEarly was launched to address these issues with the aim of creating testbeds of upstream interventions within 'whole system city settings' (i.e., understanding and addressing the interconnectedness of distal and proximal determinants) [6,7]. The programme is a partnership between academics, local governments, the NHS, Bradford Institute for Health Research, community and third sector organizations and staff/students at affiliated universities (University of York, Leeds, Bradford, Queen Mary University London, University College London, London School of Hygiene and Tropical Medicine). The ActEarly programme combines interventions with citizen science and the co-production of research with local communities across the two study sites [8,9].

As ActEarly is a system-wide intervention, it necessitates system-wide outcome sets that incorporate multiple aspects of health, well-being and the physical and social environment in which the families and children of Bradford and Tower Hamlets live. The COS was deemed essential, not only to ensure consistency and comparability in what is being measured by planned project evaluations within ActEarly, but to facilitate a system-wide meta-evaluation of the whole ActEarly programme, including planned long-term economic modelling [10]. The lack of an agreed set of core public health outcomes specific to early years and childhood health and well-being that takes a whole-systems perspective was identified as a key gap in our evaluation work in this area. Rather than providing a wider selection of outcomes (i.e., similar to the PHOF framework), the COS presented here was intended to represent the 'minimum' required set of outcomes (though not necessarily excluding the inclusion of other outcomes). Thus, we aimed to develop the public health 'Core Outcome Set for Early Years (COS-EY)'. The specific objectives of this COS development were to:

1. Identify an agreed minimal dataset of potential outcomes from locally relevant frameworks.
2. Achieve expert consensus on the COS through a two-stage Delphi consultation process.
3. Incorporate the perspective of the local communities in which early years and childhood interventions are targeted, in the COS development.
4. Arrive at a final COS-EY.

1.2. Scope

To define the scope of the COS development, we followed the Core Outcome Measures in Effectiveness Trials (COMET) guidance [2]. However, rather than targeting a specific health condition, we extended our scope to include outcomes that would be deemed important across the whole system. Given the intended breadth of this work, we therefore anticipated that we would develop a series of combined COS within domains such as: Social environment, Physical health, Poverty, etc. Thus, although our goal was to develop an overarching systems-based COS, we also anticipated developing domains, and that each of the domains would generate a separate sub-COS consisting of a smaller set of outcomes (~three to seven).

1.3. Interventions

The development of the COS-EY was guided by ActEarly's three themes (Healthy places; Healthy livelihoods; and Healthy learning) and four cross-cutting themes (Food & healthy weight; Play and physical activity; Co-production and Citizen science; and Evaluation). Each theme consists of multiple projects located across the two study sites. Examples of ActEarly projects include an evaluation of the Healthy School Streets programme in both

Bradford and Tower Hamlets; the Join Us: Move. Play (JU:MP) local delivery pilot which aims to test and learn more about what helps children aged 5–14 years to be active; and co-production of the Horton Park regeneration project in Bradford (for further details of these and other ActEarly projects, see [11]). There are no constraints placed on potential study designs and there is a great variety of approaches taken within ActEarly to achieve the overall goal of early promotion of good health and wellbeing. This means the process to develop the COS needed to be flexible and fit for purpose to accommodate different study designs, populations and evaluations.

2. Materials and Methods

Guided by the principles set out in the COMET (Core Outcome Measures in Effectiveness Trials) Handbook [2], we designed a modified Delphi study consisting of two rounds of a consensus survey administered to our panel of experts and stakeholders, followed by a face-to-face public consultation with community members using 'dot voting' (details below). The Delphi method was first developed by the RAND corporation and is commonly used to create consensus by asking participants to answer questions across multiple rounds. After each round, responses are fed back to the participants [2,12]. The decision to start the process with the expert and stakeholder consultation, followed by the community consultation, was taken because of their knowledge of interventions and the whole system changes needed to be seen.

2.1. Registration

The COS development was registered on the COMET website (#1910) and the reporting of the study is in line with the COS-STAR Statement [13,14].

2.2. Participants

The populations that are the targets for the application of the COS-EY in the first instance were children and families living within the ActEarly study areas: Bradford Metropolitan Area in West Yorkshire and the Borough of Tower Hamlets in London (Figure 1).

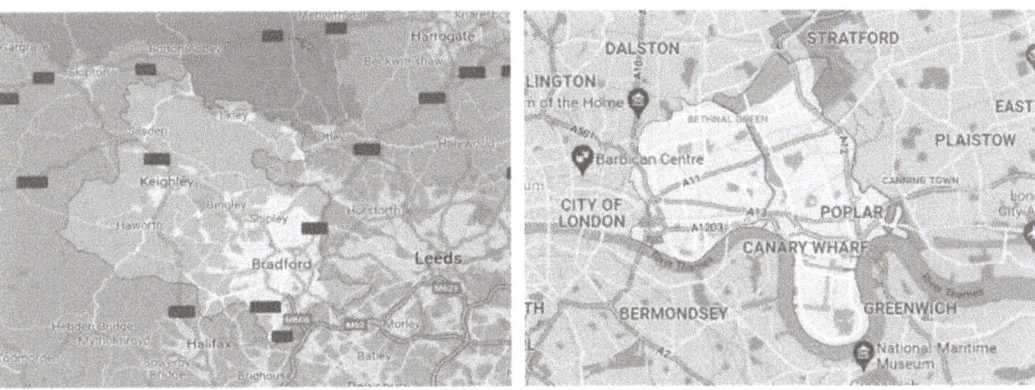

Figure 1. Maps of ActEarly study areas: Bradford Metropolitan District (**left**) and the London Borough of Tower Hamlets (**right**).

Stakeholder groups who were involved in the COS development included: ActEarly researchers, community and council partners and community members in Bradford and Tower Hamlets. This wide consultation allowed us to consider the viewpoints and expertise of academics, as well as affiliated local government and public health professionals. In addition, it was considered vital that the communities in which ActEarly operates were consulted to prioritize the evaluation of changes in factors that were important and meaningful to the families and children living in each local area.

For the first round of the survey, anyone within the immediate or wider ActEarly team, including academics, practitioners, local government, voluntary sector organizations and community representation, was eligible to take part (due to the snowball sampling, it is not possible to provide a precise sample size of how many people were invited to take part in the Delphi surveys but we estimate that the link to the survey may have reached anywhere between 70 to 100 people).

For round two, the eligibility criteria stayed the same, but we extended our promotion and reach in an attempt to get wider participation. At this point, the project had grown in size and reach and we felt it was important to ensure individuals who had newly joined, or newly become collaborators, had the opportunity to contribute to the COS development. Potential participants were identified from the activity logs of the ActEarly projects and by asking ActEarly theme-leads to signpost key collaborators and partners, local government links and members of the communities associated with ActEarly and other related projects.

The eligibility criteria for participation in the community consultations were purposefully left open and included any adult attending any of the events at which the consultations took place. To widen the reach of the consultation, we conducted all three consultations in open, public areas. In Bradford, this included Horton Park and Peel Park. Both parks held free entry events that were visited by local children and families over the summer of 2021. In Horton Park, the event was an Eid celebration aimed at local families. In Peel Park, the event was a council-funded Play Bradford event. We estimate that each event was attended by 100+ local families but do not have exact figures. We did not collect demographic, social or health information from the families but most participants arrived at the events on foot from the surrounding neighborhoods. In Tower Hamlets, the consultation was conducted in collaboration with the Bromley by Bow Centre who identified the Old Ford Road Summer Fun Day event at Butley Court as suitable for the consultation.

2.3. Information Sources (Development of the Minimal Dataset)

The initial list of potential outcomes was derived from existing local sources including: the Bradford Key Indicators set; Tower Hamlets key indicators; Tower Hamlets 'I' statements (publicly derived framework); the Tower Hamlet common outcomes framework; ActEarly community survey codes; and individual suggestions from stakeholders at previous ActEarly workshops (Figure 2). This process involved collating all outcomes from each of these local sources, in which the words and presentation of text were retained. Outcomes which were repeated by more than one source (e.g., childhood obesity) were only included once in the minimal dataset. However, those deemed to be 'similar', but not identical, were retained as separate outcomes (e.g., 'mental health' and 'mental well-being'). The listed outcome sources were developed locally and are regularly updated (thus links cannot be provided).

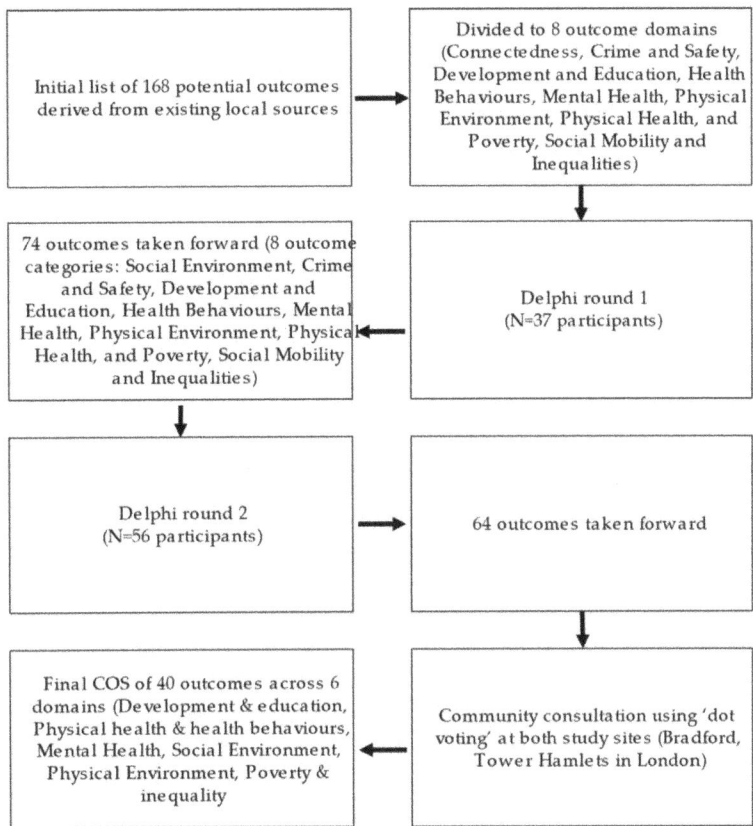

Figure 2. Process to reduce the number of outcomes.

2.4. Consensus Process

2.4.1. Surveys

The outcomes in the surveys were based on a collation of everything gathered from the activities in the 'information sources (development of the minimal dataset)' paragraph. Potential participants in the consensus surveys learnt about the study via email or word of mouth and snowballing of these (e.g., via existing groups/teams). The purpose of the study was summarized to participants on the first page of the survey to give context. The survey was completed using the online survey platform Qualtrics [15]. Invited participants received reminder emails. This survey asked participants to rate the importance of each outcome on a scale of 1–9 (from 1 "Not important at all" to 9 "Very important"). After all outcomes were rated, participants were asked to suggest any new outcomes not yet included. Our Delphi process did not include the collection of identifying information, but survey respondents were asked to state their stakeholder role (i.e., Academic, Clinical academic, Local government, Voluntary sector, Community representative, National/regional government, Commercial sector, Other).

The shortened Round 2 survey was also sent using Qualtrics. As in Round 1, invited participants received email reminders about the survey. In addition to asking participants to rate the importance of each survey, the Round 2 survey presented the group-average results of the first survey and encouraged participants to review these results before re-rating the outcomes. At the end of the Round 2 survey, there was an option to request outcomes that had been excluded after Round 1 to be re-introduced, as well as space to leave any other comments or suggestions.

2.4.2. Community Consultation

The final part of the consensus process was undertaken after the second survey had been analyzed (and the number of outcomes was hence reduced) with community members, that is, local families with children (Figure 3). In consensus methods, consultation with patients, or community members, is recommended when there is no clear consensus among the experts and it can ensure that outcomes are included that are important to community members [2]. The community member consultation was conducted using 'dot voting' and by utilizing principles of the nominal group technique, which facilitates quick, structured decision making [16–18]. In dot voting, participants are given colored dot stickers that they can use to indicate their votes in priority setting and consensus exercises. In addition to the 'dot voting,' we facilitated a play activity that children could engage in, whilst adults were asked to contribute to the core outcome consultation.

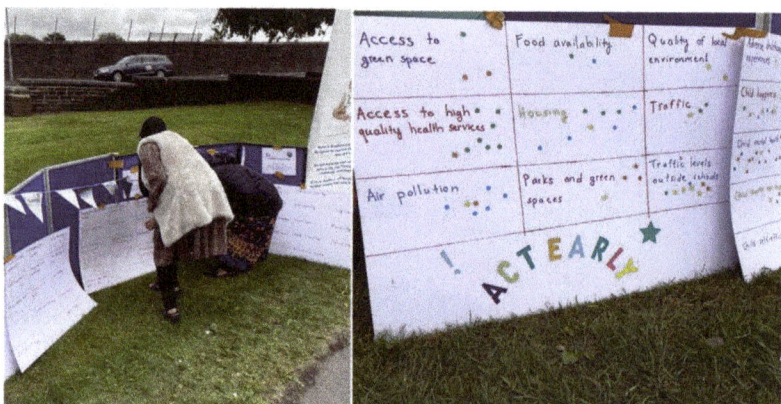

Figure 3. Community consultation in Bradford.

To make the process of voting as easy as possible, participants were asked to select and rank three outcomes they considered to be most important by placing their colored stickers on posters that included all the outcome names (green sticker for most important, yellow for second most important and orange for third most important outcome). The consultation facilitators (researchers) were present to answer any questions that arose and help explain the project and the outcomes that were voted on.

2.5. Analysis

2.5.1. Outcome Scoring/Feedback

Survey items were scored on a 9-point Likert scale (where 1 was "Not important at all" and 9 was "Very important"). Although no definitive recommendation exists on the optimal number of points for a Likert scale in COS development, a 9-point Likert scale has been proposed for use in consensus processes to reduce the number of outcomes, before face-to-face consultations are taken to reach a final consensus [19]. The scores generated from Round 1 and Round 2 of the consensus surveys were analyzed using descriptive statistics (mean and median score, standard deviation, range) and by calculating expert agreement to identify which outcomes participants agreed were less important, outcomes for which there was good agreement for prioritizing and outcomes about which participants were uncertain.

The proportion of experts/stakeholders (details of participants in Table 1) agreeing was calculated as:

$$Proportion\ in\ agreement = \frac{N\ of\ experts\ scoring\ an\ item\ within\ a\ specified\ range}{Total\ N\ of\ experts}$$

Table 1. Participants who took part in the Delphi surveys.

Participant Group	Delphi Round 1 (N Participants)	Delphi Round 2 (N Participants)
Academic	22	31
Clinical academic	3	3
Local government	5	12
Voluntary sector	2	3
Community representative	1	1
National/regional government	0	2
Commercial sector	1	0
Other [1]	3	4
Total	37	56

[1] This category includes people who identified their participant group as being 'Other' and defined it as: regional sport's charity, clinical commissioning group, think tank, research manager and community researcher.

The 'proportion in agreement' is sometimes referred to as the agreement index and multiplying the index by 100 results in the % of experts who agree with a given outcome based on our criteria set above.

All statistical analyses were performed using Stata 16 [20].

2.5.2. Consensus Definition

To define consensus, we used 'proportion within a range'. This definition of agreement is widely used in Delphi studies [21]. Agreement was defined as more than 80% of the panel scoring an item within a specified range on the 9-point Likert scale. Commonly, items scored as 1–3 are considered to indicate the outcome is of limited importance, items scored 4–6 are considered to be important but not critical and items scored 7–9 are deemed to be critical [2].

As recommended by the literature, we selected our agreement threshold of 80% in advance [22,23]. 80% is above the median threshold reported in the literature for the determination of consensus, which is 75% [21]. This slightly stricter threshold was selected due to the relatively large initial number of items in the Round 1 survey (N = 168), which needed to be reduced considerably to arrive at a feasible number of core outcomes. Disagreement was defined as <80% of the panel scoring an item within the specified range.

Thus, our process for keeping or removing outcomes applied the following rules:

1. Automatic inclusion: More than 80% of the participants scored the outcome 7, 8 or 9.
2. Automatic exclusion: More than 80% of the participants scored the outcome 1, 2, or 3.
3. For all remaining outcomes: the decision whether to include or exclude items from the subsequent round (Round 2) of the survey was considered following discussion within the immediate study team (M.B. & L.M.). Key considerations were the distance from the 80% automatic inclusion agreement index cut-off (% of experts ranking outcome 7 or higher); Round 1 median score; the balance of representation of outcomes across the outcome domains; and feedback from the open-ended comments made by participants in the survey. Adaptations to the approach were considered as appropriate based on the outcomes identified for the minimum dataset and how they were constructed, in addition to our need to reduce outcome lists to represent 'core sets' where participants were unable to deprioritize their importance.

This procedure was repeated with the Round 2 data following Round 2 survey implementation; however, we applied a less stringent inclusion cut-off (>70% of experts scoring 7 or higher) at this stage to provide members of the public in both communities with a large range of potential outcomes to consider. Missing observations (where an expert did not score a given outcome) were excluded from analyses.

2.5.3. Community Consultation—Analysis

Following the dot voting process, outcomes were ranked by the number of votes by each study site with the aim of creating a 'top 10' ranking for each site. Each dot was given a score of 1 (dot color was not considered), and these were summed for each outcome. Outcomes ranked in the top 10 for each site were included in the final COS, even if the expert consensus on the given outcome was below the 80% cut-off (>80% of experts scoring the item 7 or higher) to signify the importance of public opinion.

2.6. Ethics

The University of York Department of Health Sciences Research Governance Board approved the study (reference: HSRGC/2021/458/E). Survey participants were asked to consent to take part. Community consultation did not collect any personal or identifiable information about the participants beyond the dot votes, and no informed consent was obtained.

3. Results

3.1. Participants

37 participants completed the Delphi questionnaire in Round 1 and 56 in Round 2. Due to us using snowball sampling when sending out the survey, we could not estimate how many of the people receiving the survey chose to participate in it. Participant stakeholder representation for the Delphi surveys is provided in Table 1, indicating that most respondents were academics or representatives from local government. A total of 199 members of the community took part in consultations (135 in total for the two events held in Bradford and 64 in total for the one event held in Tower Hamlets, London).

3.2. Outcomes Considered at the Start of the Process (Minimal Dataset)

The lists of outcomes from existing sources from both localities were reviewed and presented in our surveys using the same text/format as the original source. Unless they were described using identical terms (e.g., more than one source including 'childhood obesity'), all outcomes were included even if they appeared to be measuring similar constructs (e.g., 'Speech/language/communication' and 'vocabulary'). This resulted in a minimal dataset of N = 168 outcomes (Figure 2; Supplementary Table S1). The outcomes were subsequently grouped into eight draft COS domains by the immediate study team (Connectedness; Crime and safety; Development and education; Health behaviors; Mental health; Physical environment; Physical health; and Poverty, Social mobility and inequalities (Supplementary Table S1).

3.3. Delphi Studies

Following Round 1, 28 out of the 168 outcomes met the 80% threshold for automatic inclusion and were automatically included in Round 2 of the survey. According to our prespecified criteria, no outcomes could be automatically excluded following Round 1 as none had more than 80% of participants who scored 3 points or lower (=considered to be of limited importance). Overall, we noted that all outcomes received relatively high scores and were considered important by our experts (range in mean scores 5.4–8.2). This meant that to reduce the number of outcomes, while also ensuring that there were enough outcomes left across the different domains, we had to adapt our approach to include outcomes that did not meet the automatic inclusion threshold. To achieve this, we decided to include any outcome that achieved higher than 70% agreement (=% of experts giving a score of 7 or higher), rather than 80% agreement, in the second round following discussions within the research team. Additionally, we refined our list, including removing three outcomes representing the same construct as other outcomes provided responses were not dissimilar (e.g., self-confidence, removed due to presence of self-efficacy). One outcome was moved from the Physical environment domain to Development and education (language acquisition), and one outcome label was changed (from maternal physical activity to parental physical activity). These changes were made based on the expert feedback received in Round 1. Finally, one outcome domain name ('Connectedness') was changed to 'Social environment' and included outcomes from the Connectedness category, as well as four outcomes previously included under Physical environment (Figure 2).

Round 2 of the survey included 74 outcomes across 8 outcome domains. 36 outcomes were scored 7 or higher by >80% of the Delphi survey respondents and were automatically included in the community consultation. As in Round 1, no outcomes achieved the threshold for automatic exclusion. There was a discussion within the research team to decide which of the remaining outcomes should be taken forward to the next stage of the consensus process. As in Round 1, it was agreed that outcomes for which there was some consensus, but which did not reach the automatic inclusion threshold, would be included (=agreement > 70%). In addition, we chose to add back in any outcome where three or more stakeholders had suggested re-introducing an outcome that had been deleted following Round 1.

In total, 64 outcomes were taken forward for review within the community consultation. After summing up the community votes for each outcome, we found that several outcomes that ranked highly had the same number of votes. Thus, rather than having our intended 'top 10 community-ranked outcomes', we had 11 in Bradford and 14 in Tower Hamlets. Despite the overall similarity between the sites, some highly ranked outcomes in Tower Hamlets were considered of less importance in Bradford, and vice versa. For instance, participants in Tower Hamlets saw housing, traffic and air quality as key issues, whereas in Bradford, mental health outcomes and access to high-quality health services were brought up by many.

A comparison between the outcomes rated highly by the community and the expert agreement scores revealed that four of the most highly rated outcomes from the community consultations had not achieved 80% agreement from the experts. As planned, these outcomes were included in the final COS-EY (educational attainment, traffic, traffic levels outside schools and child weight). The remaining outcomes that were included in the community top rankings were consistent with those ranked by the experts (all achieved over 80% expert agreement) and therefore met the criteria for automatic inclusion. A total of 24 remaining outcomes that were ranked less frequently by members of the public, and where expert agreement was <80%, were removed.

3.4. Final COS-EY

To formulate the final COS, we once again reviewed the outcome labels and domains for clarity, including considerations of outcome hierarchy, as recommended by some of our stakeholders. An example of this is the outcome called 'traffic', which until this point was separate from another outcome called "traffic levels outside schools". In the final COS-EY, these two are captured by the higher-level outcome label 'traffic'. Overall, this process resulted in five outcomes being combined with an existing outcome, and one outcome being split into two outcomes. We reduced the number of domains from eight to six, to ensure each domain had a balanced number of outcomes (Table 2). The final COS-EY consisted of 40 outcomes, divided into six domains: Development & education; Physical health & health behaviors; Mental health; Social environment; Physical environment; Poverty & inequality (Table 2).

Table 2. Final COS-EY.

Core Outcome Set	Outcome Name
COS-EY 1: Development & education	1.1 Access to education 1.2 Speech, language & communication 1.3 Emotional & social development 1.4 Children get best start in life 1.5 Educational attainment 1.6 Access to books
COS-EY 2: Physical health & health behaviors	2.1 Child physical activity 2.2 Child sedentary behavior 2.3 Healthy eating 2.4 Child weight 2.5 Childhood obesity 2.6 Adult obesity
COS-EY 3: Mental health	3.1 Child happiness 3.2 Child mental health (incl. children's stress and anxiety) 3.3 Child mental well-being 3.4 Parental mental health 3.5 Parental mental well-being
COS-EY 4: Social environment	4.1 Family & social relationships 4.2 Safety at home 4.3 Domestic abuse 4.4 Child social relationships & bullying
COS-EY 5: Physical environment	5.1 Use, quality, and satisfaction with open space 5.2 Parks & green spaces (incl. access to green space) 5.3 Access to high quality health services 5.4 Air pollution 5.5 Food availability 5.6 Quality of local environment 5.7 Traffic (incl. traffic levels outside schools, parking)
COS-EY 6: Poverty & inequality	6.1 Housing (incl. homelessness; house crowding; availability of affordable housing) 6.2 Access to opportunity 6.3 Basic care needs met 6.4 Employment 6.5 Financial stability 6.6 Inequalities 6.7 Poverty

4. Discussion

This study has resulted in the development of a public health COS with six domains which can be used collectively or individually to support the evaluation of system-wide programmes designed to promote health and well-being at a population level. The COS-EY provides a set of outcomes that we recommend other evaluators adapt to align with their stakeholder priorities. We developed the COS using the ActEarly consortium as an exemplar and to support the ActEarly evaluation. There were no published COS available that were suited to our purpose, and overall, there are relatively few COS specifically designed to be used in public health interventions, particularly those delivered across a whole city [5]. There was high stakeholder agreement on the final 40 ActEarly core outcomes and the final decision on which outcomes to include was based on a large community consultation. We recommend that going forward, the COS-EY is considered for adaptation for evaluation research in this area. For ActEarly, the next step is to identify existing data sources and to decide on precise measures to assess each outcome. This work will utilize routine data collected across both study sites and aligns with the ongoing efforts to link different routine data sources [24].

4.1. Comparisons with Existing Outcomes Frameworks and Literature

There is a significant overlap between the COS-EY and the PHOF, which may relate to at least some of the stakeholders being aware of the existing framework; therefore, they may have used it as a point of reference when thinking about core outcomes for public health. It is important to note that, whereas the PHOF is a tool to highlight key indicators to consider, the COS-EY is a minimum set of outcomes to include in the evaluation of system-level interventions in early years and childhood settings. The overlap between the COS-EY and the PHOF means that there are publicly available data for many outcomes, including, for example, parental and child obesity, physical activity, child development, air pollution, (self-reported), well-being and homelessness. Similarly, outcomes that are included in the key indicator frameworks used by the two ActEarly local governments, (the Bradford Metropolitan District Council and the Borough of Tower Hamlets), achieved high expert consensus and are included in the COS-EY. Examples include housing, poverty and employment. Taken together, the six domains that our outcomes are categorized under (Development & education; Physical health & health behaviors; Mental health; Social environment; Physical environment; Poverty & inequality) highlight the system-wide factors that underpin early years health and well-being. The inclusion of outcomes such as 'access to opportunity' and 'children get best start in life' can be considered unique in that as far as we are aware, the existing frameworks do not include them, but both were considered highly important in our consensus work. One of the partners of ActEarly, the Bromley by Bow Centre in Tower Hamlets has further investigated the meaning of the 'children get best start in life' outcome and found that key elements contributing to this outcome for the Tower Hamlets community were: how families inhabit the environment and space around them; the role of play and activities for children; the stability and security needed for a firm family foundation; and the connection and support within families' wider networks [25]. The final point raised by the communities, "connection and support within a family's wider network", can be understood as a systems-level outcome in that no singular measure can be expected to capture it.

There were a few unexpected exclusions that resulted from the consensus process. Breastfeeding, a key indicator in early years health research, and one of the outcomes in the PHOF that is relevant to ActEarly, was not included in the final COS-EY. Similarly, healthy life expectancy at birth, infant mortality and adverse childhood experiences (ACE), were removed. Life expectancy and infant mortality are globally tracked and are reported summary indicators that are thought to capture the overall quality of the early life period [26–28]. These outcomes were removed following the community consultation after failing to reach either a stakeholder consensus that was high enough for automatic inclusion, or a high priority ranking from the community. ACE were also not included in the final COS-EY despite the growing body of evidence that ACE scores are a risk factor for later-life physical and mental health outcomes, and as such, could be thought a key outcome to include in any early life research [29,30]. It is not known to us why the listed outcomes did not achieve the consensus threshold, but it could be that stakeholders felt that the interventions included in ActEarly are unlikely to result in changes in these markers of early life circumstance, or stakeholders were not familiar with the ACE concept. For community members, we think these outcomes may have felt intangible or far removed from their everyday experience—unlike other outcomes that were highly ranked (e.g., traffic). The interactions in the dot voting process are short, which means that there was not time for extensive discussions about each outcome. It is worth highlighting that our outcome sets are the minimum outcomes advocated in this area of research; thus, this does not preclude others from adding in outcomes that are deemed of high relevance even if they are not within the COS-EY.

The development of existing local government or public health outcome frameworks should include interaction with the public, rather than solely consultation with professional bodies, though this is not always done. In our community consultations, we found there was a great interest in providing researchers with feedback on what measures were meaningful to the community. The consultations further highlighted how preconceived notions held by the researchers (e.g., regarding what the most pressing public health issues are) may not reflect the lived experiences of community members. In Bradford, this became evident in the high priority given to wider, structural outcomes such as happiness and mental health, access to high-quality healthcare, employment and poverty, compared to outcomes related to diet, exercise and obesity prevention, which are some of the most pressing national and international public health priorities [31,32]. In addition, safety at home and domestic abuse were of importance for members of the public at one of our study sites and were raised despite the stigma that is commonly associated with discussing these issues [33]. It could be that the anonymity provided by our consultation method may have helped community members feel confident to give their votes to these outcomes, compared to, for example, focus groups or interview methods where the researcher knows the identity of the participant [34].

In Tower Hamlets, an important focus of discussions and responses was around housing and the issue of overcrowding (particularly during lockdown) was mentioned. Another key issue was around traffic, in particular parking and the tensions arising from it. The differences we observed between the two sites suggest that it may be advisable that researchers wishing to use and adapt the COS-EY for their own purposes start with the list of outcomes provided here, followed by some consultation with key local stakeholders to ensure they are fit for purpose.

4.2. Limitations

This study did not aim to achieve consensus on what the best measures or data sources are for each outcome and work needs to be undertaken before the COS-EY can be used in practice. Furthermore, some outcomes are relatively ambiguous and could be understood to mean multiple things, e.g., "access to opportunity". There is also some overlap between different outcomes—it could be argued that diet and physical activity are very closely related to obesity and therefore not all three need to be included separately. On the other hand, obesity is a complex and multifaceted issue which does not only relate to food and physical activity (which in themselves, contribute to many things beyond an individual's weight status), therefore, we chose not to combine these outcomes.

The Delphi process is dependent on the expert knowledge of stakeholders that are consulted [35]. This means that it cannot be considered an objective 'truth'. With our chosen sampling strategy, it was not possible to estimate a response rate for the surveys, and therefore, we do not know who chose not to take part in the consultation and why. This was mitigated by us contacting and identifying researchers and local authority staff who were already involved with ActEarly and have a stake in selecting appropriate and meaningful outcomes. A limitation of the dot voting process was that community members only spent a few moments reading and reviewing the potential outcomes and understanding the voting process before voting and moving on. There was less time and space for more in-depth interactions and conversations with the researcher. This means there was a trade-off between low participant burden (and ease of access to the consultation) and the depth of the information we could collect from the community. In many settings in the UK, an additional barrier to community consultations can be language barriers. We mediated this in Bradford by involving a bilingual researcher in the team that collected the community consultation data. This meant that families and individuals who did not speak fluent English could ask questions about the project and the consultation in their native language. Finally, it is worth highlighting that the exclusion of outcomes from the final COS-EY does not necessarily mean that they are not of value or should not be considered by researchers. Importantly, choosing to employ the public health COS-EY in any intervention evaluation should not be taken to mean that other outcomes should not be considered, and we recommend adapting this COS to the local context wherever appropriate. For instance, if the focus of a future project was more specific than that of ActEarly, e.g., solely around the physical environment, the researchers may wish to explore that specific subset of outcomes in more depth and consult local communities on whether some of the excluded outcomes should be brought 'back in'.

4.3. Next Steps

The COS-EY outcome selection to date has not been driven by what can be measured, which means that for now, we cannot be sure that all the outcomes included in the COS can be reported in a meaningful way. Therefore, and before the COS-EY can be fully implemented, we recommend that further work is undertaken to confirm the definition of each outcome, prior to deciding on the most appropriate measures or data sources. This process may be quite challenging for outcomes that cannot be captured by a single metric, but at this stage in the work, we do not think this should mean the automatic exclusion of such outcomes from the COS. Rather, we encourage further research into the area to tackle the issue of defining measures for outcomes such as 'children get best start in life', as clearly, these are priorities for stakeholders and communities alike. One solution to this may be the development of short lists of outcome measures that would represent each core outcome (with e.g., varying degrees of data collection burden or depending on local data availability, such as long and short versions of a questionnaire; or household vs individual level data). These lists could then be used as a starting point by investigators. While not offering perfect standardization the way a single measure per outcome would do, the process of creating lists of appropriate measures would be a step towards better standardization of public health outcomes across studies. Another avenue for future work would be to explore the relevance of the COS-EY from a policy and practice perspective and consider to what extent this work may be useful outside the research context. For instance, the COS-EY could be used by local authorities when making decisions about routine data collection practices and availability.

5. Conclusions

The public health COS-EY represents an initial attempt at system-wide core outcome sets developed to evaluate interventions that promote early life health and well-being, in consultation with local communities. Our chosen approach resulted in a comprehensive list of 40 outcomes, and highlighted important differences between expert knowledge and lived experience across Bradford and Tower Hamlets. Our aim was to use the COS-EY in the evaluation of the ActEarly research program in the first instance, but the COS could be applied to other settings where there is interest in evaluating early life health and well-being from a 'wider determinants' of health perspective.

Supplementary Materials: The following supporting information can be downloaded at: https://www.mdpi.com/article/10.3390/ijerph19137947/s1, Table S1: Original list of 168 potential outcomes.

Author Contributions: Conceptualization, M.B. and L.M.; methodology, M.B. and L.M.; software, M.B., L.M. and Y.V.; formal analysis, L.M., A.A. and M.B.; investigation, L.M., A.A., A.R. and Y.V.; data curation, L.M., A.A. and Y.V.; writing—original draft preparation, L.M.; writing—review and editing, L.M., A.A., Y.V., C.C., A.R., J.S., B.L., T.C.Y., P.G., M.B.; visualization, L.M.; supervision, M.B. All authors have read and agreed to the published version of the manuscript.

Funding: This research was funded by UK Prevention Research Partnership (UKPRP), grant number MR/S037527/1. Individual projects within ActEarly receive funding from universities and directly from different funding agencies. The funders had no role in the design and planning of the present work. C.C. and A.R. were funded through the National Institute for Health Research under its Applied Research Collaboration Yorkshire and Humber [NIHR200166] and J.S. was part funded by The National Institute for Health Research under its Applied Research Collaboration in North Thames. This report is independent research supported by the National Institute for Health and Care Research ARC. The views expressed in this publication are those of the authors and not necessarily those of the National Institute for Health and Care Research or the Department of Health and Social Care.

Institutional Review Board Statement: The study was conducted in accordance with the Declaration of Helsinki, and approved by the Institutional Review Board (or Ethics Committee) of The University of York Department of Health Sciences Research Governance Board (protocol code HSRGC/2021/458/E, date of approval 9 July 2021).

Informed Consent Statement: Informed consent was obtained from all subjects involved in the study.

Data Availability Statement: The data presented in this study are available on request from the corresponding authors to ensure anonymity of participants.

Acknowledgments: We would like to thank all the participants for their invaluable input to this study.

Conflicts of Interest: The authors declare no conflict of interest. The funders had no role in the design of the study; in the collection, analyses, or interpretation of data; in the writing of the manuscript, or in the decision to publish the results.

References

1. Williamson, P.R.; Altman, D.G.; Blazeby, J.M.; Clarke, M.; Devane, D.; Gargon, E.; Tugwell, P. Developing core outcome sets for clinical trials: Issues to consider. *Trials* **2012**, *13*, 1–8. [CrossRef]
2. Williamson, P.R.; Altman, D.G.; Bagley, H.; Barnes, K.L.; Blazeby, J.M.; Brookes, S.T.; Clarke, M.; Gargon, E.; Gorst, S.; Harman, N.; et al. The COMET Handbook: Version 1.0. *Trials* **2017**, *18*, 1–50. [CrossRef]
3. Public Health England. *Proposed Changes to the Public Health Outcomes Framework from 2019/20: A Consultation about Public Health England*; Public Health England: London, UK, 2019.
4. NHS Outcomes Framework Indicators-August 2021 Release. Available online: https://digital.nhs.uk/data-and-information/publications/statistical/nhs-outcomes-framework/august-2021 (accessed on 22 May 2022).
5. Gargon, E.; Gorst, S.L.; Matvienko-Sikar, K.; Williamson, P.R. Choosing important health outcomes for comparative effectiveness research: 6th annual update to a systematic review of core outcome sets for research. *PLoS ONE* **2021**, *16*, e0244878. [CrossRef]
6. Wright, J.; Hayward, A.C.; West, J.; Pickett, K.; McEachan, R.M.; Mon-Williams, M.; Christie, N.; Vaughan, L.; Sheringham, J.; Haklay, M.; et al. ActEarly: A City Collaboratory approach to early promotion of good health and wellbeing. *Wellcome Open Res.* **2019**, *4*, 156. [CrossRef]
7. Stansfield, J.; South, J.; Mapplethorpe, T. What are the elements of a whole system approach to community-centred public health? A qualitative study with public health leaders in England's local authority areas. *BMJ Open* **2020**, *10*, 1–11. [CrossRef]
8. Lockyer, B.; Islam, S.; Rahman, A.; Dickerson, J.; Pickett, K.; Sheldon, T.; Wright, J.; McEachan, R.; Sheard, L. Understanding COVID-19 misinformation and vaccine hesitancy in context: Findings from a qualitative study involving citizens in Bradford, UK. *Health Expect.* **2021**, *24*, 1158–1167. [CrossRef]
9. McEachan, R.R.C.; Dickerson, J.; Bridges, S.; Bryant, M.; Cartwright, C.; Islam, S.; Lockyer, B.; Rahman, A.; Sheard, L.; West, J.; et al. The Born in Bradford COVID-19 Research Study: Protocol for an adaptive mixed methods research study to gather actionable intelligence on the impact of COVID-19 on health inequalities amongst families living in Bradford. *Wellcome Open Res.* **2020**, *5*, 1–19. [CrossRef]
10. Skarda, I.; Asaria, M.; Cookson, R. (Preprint)LifeSim: A Lifecourse Dynamic Microsimulation Model of the Millennium Birth Cohort in England. *medRxiv* **2021**. [CrossRef]
11. ActEarly. ActEarly [Internet]. 2022. Available online: https://actearly.org.uk/our-projects/ (accessed on 22 May 2022).
12. Brown, B.B. Delphi process: A methodology used for the elicitation of opinions of experts. *ASTME Vectors* **1968**, 1–15.
13. COMET. Development of Public Health Core Outcome Sets for Early Life Health and Wellbeing: ActEarly Consortium [Internet]. COMET Initiative. 2021. Available online: https://comet-initiative.org/Studies/Details/1910 (accessed on 22 May 2022).
14. Kirkham, J.J.; Gorst, S.; Altman, D.G.; Blazeby, J.M.; Clarke, M.; Devane, D.; Gargon, E.; Moher, D.; Schmitt, J.; Tugwell, P.; et al. Core Outcome Set-STAndards for Reporting: The COS-STAR Statement. *PLoS Med.* **2016**, *13*, e1002148. [CrossRef]
15. Qualtrics. Qualtrics: Provo, UT, USA, 2020. Available online: https://www.qualtrics.com/ (accessed on 22 May 2022).
16. Delbecq, A.; Van de Ven, A. A Group Process Model for Problem Identification and Problem Planning. *J. Appl. Behav. Sci.* **1971**, *7*, 466–492. [CrossRef]
17. Fallon, S.; Smith, J.; Morgan, S.; Stoner, M.; Austin, C. "Pizza, patients and points of view": Involving young people in the design of a post registration module entitled the adolescent with cancer. *Nurse Educ. Pract.* **2008**, *8*, 140–147. [CrossRef]
18. Donald, M.; Beanlands, H.; Straus, S.; Ronksley, P.; Tam-Tham, H.; Finlay, J.; Smekal, M.; Elliott, M.J.; Farragher, J.; Herrington, G.; et al. Preferences for a self-management e-health tool for patients with chronic kidney disease: Results of a patient-oriented consensus workshop. *CMAJ Open* **2019**, *7*, E713–E720. [CrossRef]
19. De Meyer, D.; Kottner, J.; Beele, H.; Schmitt, J.; Lange, T.; Van Hecke, A.; Verhaeghe, S.; Beeckman, D. Delphi procedure in core outcome set development: Rating scale and consensus criteria determined outcome selection. *J. Clin. Epidemiol.* **2019**, *111*, 23–31. [CrossRef]
20. StataCorp. *Stata Statistical Software: Release 16*; StataCorp LLC: College Station, TX, USA, 2019.
21. Diamond, I.R.; Grant, R.C.; Feldman, B.M.; Pencharz, P.B.; Ling, S.C.; Moore, A.M.; Wales, P.W. Defining consensus: A systematic review recommends methodologic criteria for reporting of Delphi studies. *J. Clin. Epidemiol.* **2014**, *67*, 401–409. [CrossRef]

22. Keeney, S.; Hasson, F.; McKenna, H. Consulting the oracle: Ten lessons from using the Delphi technique in nursing research. *J. Adv. Nurs.* **2006**, *53*, 205–212. [CrossRef]
23. Meijering, J.V.; Kampen, J.K.; Tobi, H. Quantifying the development of agreement among experts in Delphi studies. *Technol. Forecast. Soc. Chang.* **2013**, *80*, 1607–1614. [CrossRef]
24. Sohal, K.; Mason, D.; Birkinshaw, J.; West, J.; McEachan, R.; Elshehaly, M.; Cooper, D.; Shore, R.; McCooe, M.; Lawton, T.; et al. Connected Bradford: A Whole System Data Linkage Accelerator. *Wellcome Open Res.* **2022**, *7*, 26. [CrossRef]
25. The Bromley by Bow ActEarly Community Research Team. What Makes the Best Start in Life for Children in Tower Hamlets? [Internet]. London; 2021. Available online: https://actearly.org.uk/wp-content/uploads/2022/03/ActEarly-BBB-The-Best-Start-In-Life-Final-Report-for-publication.pdf (accessed on 22 May 2022).
26. Hug, L.; Alexander, M.; You, D.; Alkema, L. National, regional, and global levels and trends in neonatal mortality between 1990 and 2017, with scenario-based projections to 2030: A systematic analysis. *Lancet Glob. Health* **2019**, *7*, e710–e720. [CrossRef]
27. Naghavi, M.; Abajobir, A.A.; Abbafati, C.; Abbas, K.M.; Abd-Allah, F.; Abera, S.F.; Aboyans, V.; Adetokunboh, O.; Ärnlöv, J.; Afshin, A.; et al. Global, regional, and national age-sex specifc mortality for 264 causes of death, 1980–2016: A systematic analysis for the Global Burden of Disease Study 2016. *Lancet* **2017**, *390*, 1151–1210. [CrossRef]
28. Cao, X.; Hou, Y.; Zhang, X.; Xu, C.; Jia, P.; Sun, X.; Sun, L.; Gao, Y.; Yang, H.; Cui, Z.; et al. A Comparative, Correlate Analysis and Projection of Global and Regional Life Expectancy, Healthy Life Expectancy, and their GAP: 1995–2025. *J. Glob. Health* **2020**, *10*, 020407.
29. Petruccelli, K.; Davis, J.; Berman, T. Adverse childhood experiences and associated health outcomes: A systematic review and meta-analysis. *Child Abus. Negl.* **2019**, *97*, 104127. [CrossRef]
30. Boullier, M.; Blair, M. Adverse childhood experiences. *Paediatr. Child Health* **2018**, *28*, 132–137. [CrossRef]
31. Public Health England. PHE Strategy 2020-25 Executive summary [Internet]. London; 2019. Available online: https://assets.publishing.service.gov.uk/government/uploads/system/uploads/attachment_data/file/830105/PHE_Strategy_2020-25__Executive_Summary.pdf (accessed on 22 May 2022).
32. WHO Europe. Action Plan for the Prevention and Control of Noncommunicable Diseases in the WHO European Region [Internet]. Copenhagen; 2016. Available online: http://www.euro.who.int/en/who-we-are/governance (accessed on 22 May 2022).
33. Kennedy, A.C.; Prock, K.A. "I Still Feel Like I Am Not Normal": A Review of the Role of Stigma and Stigmatization Among Female Survivors of Child Sexual Abuse, Sexual Assault, and Intimate Partner Violence. *Trauma Violence Abus.* **2018**, *19*, 512–527. [CrossRef]
34. Meyrick, J.; Gray, D. Evidence-based patient/public voice: A patient and public involvement audit in the field of sexual health. *BMJ Sex. Reprod. Health* **2018**, *44*, 267–271. [CrossRef]
35. Powell, C. The Delphi technique: Myths and realities. *J. Adv. Nurs.* **2003**, *41*, 376–382. [CrossRef]

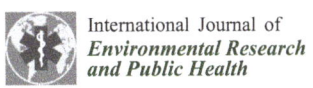

Systematic Review

Workplace Interventions to Reduce Occupational Stress for Older Workers: A Systematic Review

Daniel Subel [1,*], David Blane [2] and Jessica Sheringham [3]

[1] Institute of Epidemiology and Health Care, University College London, London WC1E 6BT, UK
[2] Faculty of Medicine, School of Public Health, Imperial College London, London SW7 2AZ, UK
[3] Department of Applied Health Research, University College London, London WC1E 6BT, UK
* Correspondence: daniel.subel.20@alumni.ucl.ac.uk

Abstract: The working life of individuals is now longer because of increases to state pension age in the United Kingdom. Older workers may be at particular risk in the workplace, compared with younger workers. Successful workplace interventions to reduce occupational stress amongst older workers are essential, but little is known about their effectiveness. The aim is to evaluate current evidence of the effectiveness of interventions for reducing stress in older workers in non-healthcare settings. Four database searches were conducted. The search terms included synonyms of "intervention", "workplace" and "occupational stress" to identify original studies published since 2011. Dual screening was conducted on the sample to identify studies which met the inclusion criteria. The RoB 2.0 tool for RCTs was used to assess the risk of bias. From 3708 papers retrieved, ten eligible papers were identified. Seven of the papers' interventions were deemed effective in reducing workplace stress. The sample size for most studies was small, and the effectiveness of interventions were more likely to be reported when studies used self-report measures, rather than biological measures. This review indicates that workplace interventions might be effective for reducing stress in older workers. However, there remains an absence of high-quality evidence in this field.

Keywords: intervention; workplace; occupational stress; older workers

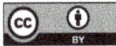

1. Introduction

By 2040, it is predicted that one in every two people of working age will be aged 65 or over [1]. The global ageing population has resulted in government concerns regarding the future of the workplace [2]. The increase in life expectancy and the lack of equitable social resources available has been a catalyst for most European governments to increase the state pension age [3].

Prolonging the working life of individuals cannot be done without due diligence and needs to be medically supervised, as suggested by MISPA (Mitigating Increases in the State Pension Age) [4]. Before governments can continue increasing state pension age, it needs to be assessed how this can be conducted, without damaging or harming the health of workers affected by these changes–particularly workers in physically demanding and highly stressful occupations.

Older workers face greater or different hazards to their health than younger workers. Bravo et al.'s [5] review found that in 50% of the papers they reviewed, older workers were at a much greater risk of fatal workplace injuries, when compared to their younger counterparts. Older workers are more likely to have pre-existing long-term health conditions, which can affect their capacity to work or the kinds of work they are able to sustain. There is also evidence that they experience greater sickness absence [6].

Stress—adverse reactions to excessive pressure—and burnout are recognised as a major risk to the health of all workers [7,8]. There is conflicting evidence whether older workers are at a greater risk of stress than younger workers [9]. It is clear, however, that older workers are likely to face different stressors to younger workers, not just through pressures within the workplace, but also through additional caring responsibilities outside of work [4]. Moreover, there is agreement that, despite legislation to prevent it, there is evidence that older workers are subject to age discrimination [10]. Therefore, interventions to improve workplace health in older workers may well need to be different to those of younger workers because it cannot be assumed that the problems they face, or the mechanisms by which interventions work, will be the same.

Based on currently available research, very little is known about this topic. Evidence of the effectiveness of workplace interventions for older workers is lacking. Poscia et al.'s [3] systematic review found a paucity of high-quality evidence on workplace health promotion for older workers. There was a suggestion that active workplace interventions help improve the health of older workers, but included studies used small, convenience samples not representative of the working population.

Pieper et al.'s [11] more recent review of reviews on workplace health promotion interventions found that psychological interventions, such as stress management, cognitive behavioural therapy and mindfulness-based interventions have the ability to significantly reduce stress. However, Pieper et al. found few reviews specifically focusing on older workers and they reported that there was insufficient evidence to conclude that psychological interventions were the most successful and effective to reduce occupational stress amongst older workers. Interventions were predominately targeted towards white-collar workers, teachers, and healthcare providers. Interventions for healthcare providers may be of limited generalisability to other settings, given the specific nature of healthcare settings and healthcare work and the hazards that may present in this environment. When assessing previous studies on this topic, the overwhelming majority focus upon younger people employed in advantaged occupations, using small cohort sizes. Furthermore, they use inconsistent and haphazard outcome measures to assess interventions' successes, which results in studies being unrepresentative, difficult to replicate and unable to demonstrate the impact on increased state pension age for older workers.

Before policy makers can enact changes to state pension age, they must have access to a sufficient level of high-quality research which has outlined the impact on individuals working longer, as well as interventions used to retain older workers. This information must also be accessible to employers, so they are made aware of the most successful interventions in the workplace to reduce occupational stress and maintain their workforce. This article intends to provide policy makers and employers a review of the current literature and research in this field. This study also has the potential to provide union representatives, and workers themselves, with evidence for them to vouch to their employers for adequate, appropriate, and successful interventions in their workplaces.

This systematic review sought to answer the question:

"What is the evidence of effectiveness of workplace interventions for reducing occupational stress in older workers outside of the healthcare sector?"

The objectives were to:

(1) Identify and appraise papers evaluating the effectiveness of workplace stress reduction interventions on older workers.
(2) Describe the types of interventions and measures of effectiveness used
(3) Summarise the evidence of effectiveness of interventions
(4) Identify existing knowledge gaps in the literature which require further research

2. Materials and Methods

2.1. Search Strategy

PRISMA guidelines for reporting systematic reviews were followed throughout the process of this review [12], see checklist in Supplementary Materials. Four database searches were conducted: OvidMedline, PsycInfo, Scopus and Web of Science. After an initial literature search, a PICO model was developed (see Table 1), which helped form the database search terms for the review [13]. Previously systematic reviews' search terms, including Pieper et al. [11] and Poscia et al. [3], helped to inform the search terms. The search term combinations were first applied in OvidMedline, which uses MeSH terms, and then modified and adapted for use in the other databases (see Table 2). In all the databases, the presence of key words was sought in "all fields", which would detect the terms in key words, titles, abstracts and full papers. Initially age terms were included in the search strategy, but this resulted in an improbably low number of results retrieved, so this term was dropped. The searches took place throughout the first week of August 2021, therefore only research published before 31 July 2021 were included in this review.

Table 1. The PICO model.

PICO Term	Detail
Population	Older workers, in the Organisation for Economic Co-Operation and Development (OECD) country, in non-health sector jobs.
Intervention	All interventions occurring in the workplace, including medication, educational and exercise interventions.
Control	Comparison with control conditions as described in each of the papers in the review
Outcome	Reduced workplace stress

Table 2. Search Terms.

Database	Programmes Search Terms	Setting Search Terms	Outcome Search Terms	Papers per Database
OvidMedline	Intervention.mp. OR Psychosocial Intervention/	Workplace/ OR Workplace.mp.	Burnout, Professional/OR Occupational Stress.mp. OR Stress, Psychological/OR Occupational Stress/OR Occupational Diseases	2444
Scopus	Intervention OR Programme OR Program	Workplace OR Office OR "Work Centre"	"Occupational Stress" OR "Professional Burnout" OR "Psychological Stress"	701
Web of Science	Intervention OR Programmes OR Program	Workplace * OR Office * OR "Work Centre"	"Occupational Stress" OR "Professional Burnout" OR "Workplace Stress" OR "Job Stress" OR "Psychological Stress"	964
PsycInfo	Exp Workplace Intervention/OR Intervention.mp. OR exp intervention	Exp Workplace Intervention/OR Workplace.mp.	Occupational Stress.mp. OR exp Occupational Stress/	469
Total Papers		3708 Papers		

* MeSH terms are indicated with a "/" after the search term. Programmes, setting and outcome search terms were combined with "AND" in each database.

2.2. Inclusion/Exclusion Criteria

Table 3 depicts the inclusion/exclusion criteria. Eligible papers had to report an intervention in a non-health sector workplace, specifically focusing on older workers. The papers had to have been conducted in an Organisation for Economic Co-operation and Development (OECD) country, to ensure findings have some relevance to the United Kingdom (UK) context [14]. Studies without a control group or baseline data, or without an aim of reducing workplace stress, were excluded. The authors did not set out to select papers which specified a specific control condition but sought papers which described what interventions were compared with. Qualitative papers, such as focus groups or interviews, were excluded from this review as quantitative papers were deemed to illustrate more objective results and are more likely to be conducted on a large number of participants.

Table 3. Inclusion/Exclusion Criteria.

Order	Criteria	Inclusion Criteria	Exclusion Criteria
1	Language		Paper not published in English
2	Date of Publication	Published between 1 January 2011–31 July 2021	
3	Access to Publication	Full Paper Access via UCL/Online	Paper not fully available online
4	Type of Paper		Papers without an Abstract
5	Publication Type	Original Studies Peer Reviewed Studies	Systematic Reviews Editorials Dissertations Not Fully Published Papers
6	Setting	Conducted in the UK or an OECD Country Reporting an intervention that was conducted in a workplace	Reporting interventions in health sector workplaces (e.g., a hospital)
7	Outcome Measured	Quantitative data on workplace stress or anxiety (burnout, perceived stress, measures of cortisol levels, etc.)	Change in outcome level not reported
8	Population Group	Reporting an intervention which provides data on its effects on older workers in the workforce	Data reported with no desegregation by workers age or no evidence that included workers would be considered as "older"
9	Study Design	Experimental Designs Randomised Controlled Trials Non-Randomised Trials Before and After Studies	Qualitative papers (i.e., interview, focus group or ethnographic studies reporting experience of impressions)
10	Study Aim	Where at least one of the objectives of the intervention or programme is to reduce workplace stress	

The definition of an older worker was developed by adapting multiple definitions from various sources. Firstly, if the paper classified the intervention or participants as older workers, regardless of the mean age, these interventions were deemed to be focused on older workers. Secondly, for OECD countries, the average age at which an individual reached normal pension age in 2016 was 63.7 years old for women and 64.3 years old for men [15]. If the mean age of participants in a paper were within 15 years of normal pension age, it was concluded that older workers were included in this intervention.

2.3. Study Selection and Screening

Papers from the four databases were exported to Microsoft Excel. Title and abstracts of all papers screened by DS (author and reviewer) and a secondary reviewer (AH). Any papers which were unclear or resulted in polarized views, were then resolved by discussion with a third reviewer and co-author (JS). After the title and abstract screening, the remaining papers underwent a full-text screening.

Each paper that met the inclusion criteria on screening was carefully assessed for its relevance to older workers. Papers that were specifically focused on older workers were placed in the primary dataset. Papers where data on the effectiveness of the intervention on older workers was included, but without a specific focus on older workers, comprised the secondary dataset.

2.4. Data Extraction and Critical Appraisal

Data were extracted from all eligible papers used a data extraction form by DS, with a sample checked by JS (see Appendix A: Data Extraction Form) to cover features including: study design and employment setting; the age of participants; nature of the intervention; reported effectiveness. Interventions were coded into three categories–psychological interventions, educational interventions, and physical interventions. Outcome measurements were grouped by whether self-report or biological samples were used to measure stress.

The RoB 2.0 tool (Risk of bias in randomised trials) [16] was used by DS and JS in each paper to form a judgement about the risk of bias across six different domains. The RoB 2.0 tool was chosen as it enabled the reviewers to form their own assessment of an article's quality, in regard to its risk of different types of biases. If a domain or the overall judgement was deemed to have a high risk of bias, this meant that the reviewers believed that there was an issue with the paper that substantially lowered their confidence in the results. Some concerns of bias indicated that a paper included an issue which could potentially lower the reviewer's confidence in the results. If the overall judgement was that the paper had a low risk of bias, this meant that the reviewers were confident that the study results were valid.

The included studies were described, and the characteristics and methods for ascertaining stress levels were summarised. Based upon what was written in each paper, the effectiveness of the interventions was summarised, using quantitative data to assess the success of each intervention.

3. Results

3.1. Characteristics of Included Studies

From 3708 papers identified in the database searches, ten papers met the inclusion criteria (Figure 1). Five papers had a specific focus on older workers (the primary dataset). A further five papers did not have a specific focus of the research on older workers (the secondary dataset). As the mean age of participants in both datasets were similar (see Table 4), they are considered as one dataset in the rest of the paper.

Five papers were conducted in the United States [17–21]; the other five originated from Europe (Germany [22], the Netherlands [23], Finland [24], Italy [25] and Norway [26]). The number of participants ranged from 14–779, with three studies have less than 40 participants. Only one study included over 500 participants [24] (see Table 4).

Three studies were conducted with university faculty staff [17,18,21], and three in manufacturing or technical environments [19,20,22]. Two studies were conducted amongst police officers [23,25]. The remaining two studies were conducted with office workers [24,26].

The age of participants was described in two ways (Table 4). Six studies described the age range of participants in the intervention; the upper limit for the age range was between 57 and 68; the lower limit for the age range was 18 to 50. Three papers only included participants over the age of 40, with Calogiuri et al.'s [26] paper using only participants older than 50 years old. In the seven papers that documented the mean age of participants, mean age was over 40.9 years. Five papers had a mean age of over 48 years [17,18,21,23,24].

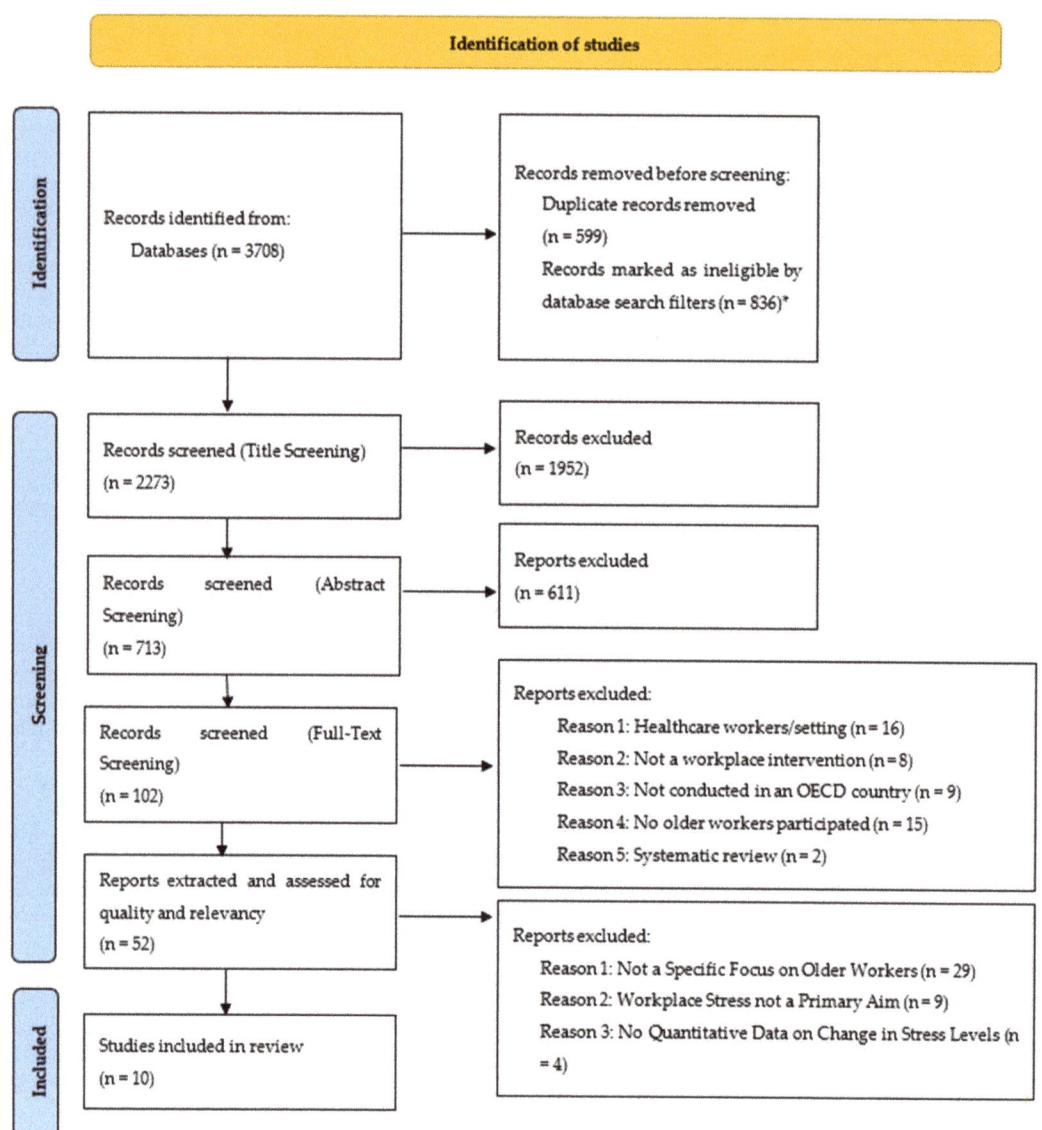

Figure 1. PRISMA Flow Chart (Adapted from Page et al. [12]) * Papers were automatically excluded using filters in the search databases where they were outside of our date range and language of publication.

Table 4. Description of Studies.

Study (First Author, Year)	Country	Study Design	Focus on Older Workers?	Participant's Occupation	Age of Participants	No. of Participants (and Dropouts)
			Primary Dataset			
Hughes, 2011 [17]	United States	Randomised Controlled Trial (RCT)	Yes	University Staff	51 (Mean)	423 (56 Dropouts)
Malarkey, 2013 [18]	United States	Randomised Controlled Trial	Yes	University Faculty Staff	50 (Mean)	186 (0 Dropouts)
Cook, 2015 [20]	United States	Randomised Controlled Trial	Yes	Tech Company Workers	59 (Median) * 50–68 (Range)	278 (0 Dropouts)
Fischetti, 2019 [25]	Italy	Randomised Controlled Trial	Yes	Police Officers	46.8 (Mean)	20 (0 Dropouts)
Calogiuri, 2016 [26]	Norway	Randomised Controlled Trial	Yes	Office Workers	49 (Median) * 41–47 (Range)	14 (3 Dropouts)
			Secondary Dataset			
Aikens, 2014 [19]	United States	Randomised Controlled Trial	No	Chemical Company Employees	41.5 (Median) * 18–65 (Range)	89 (23 Dropouts)
Largo-Wight, 2017 [21]	United States	Randomised Controlled Trial	No	University Office Staff	48.8 (Mean)	37 (0 Dropouts)
Limm, 2011 [22]	Germany	Randomised Controlled Trial	No	Lower and Middle Level Managers at a Manufacturing Plant	40.9 (Mean) 18–65 (Range)	174 (20 Dropouts)
Hoeve, 2021 [23]	Netherlands	Quasi-Experimental	No	Police Officers	49 (Mean) 30–63 (Range)	82 (19 Dropouts)
Ojala, 2019 [24]	Finland	Non-Randomised Trial	No	Public Sector Workers *	49.9 (Mean) 21–64 (Range)	779 (217 Dropouts)

* Median has been calculated by the researcher as the midpoint between the range. In Ojala's study, Public Sector. workers included construction and transport workers, office workers, food services and managerial specialists.

3.2. Risk of Bias

None of the papers had an overall high risk of bias (Table 5). Four papers were judged to have a low risk of bias. Some bias concerns were identified in six papers. In nine out of the ten papers there was a lack of detail on the randomisation of participants, which may have led to post-test reporting bias by participants exaggerating the effects of the intervention. Most papers showed a strong adherence to the intended intervention. Fischetti et al.'s [25] study showed a potential high risk of bias in the measurement of outcome. While the study used validated scales to assess stress, the score was high because of the study's pre-post evaluation design. It is possible that participants may be subject to bias in overestimating the effects of participation on their well-being.

Table 5. Results from the Risk of Bias Critical Appraisal.

Study (Author, Year)	Domain 1 (Randomisation Process)	Domain 2 (Deviations from intended Interventions)	Domain 3 (Missing Outcome Data)	Domain 4 (Measurement of Outcome)	Domain 5 (Selection of the Reported Results)	Domain 6 (Overall Bias)
Hughes, 2011 [17]	2	1	2	2	1	2
Malarkey, 2013 [18]	2	1	1	1	1	1
Aikens, 2014 [19]	2	2	1	1	1	1
Cook, 2015 [20]	2	1	2	2	1	2
Largo-Wight, 2017 [21]	2	1	1	2	2	2
Limm, 2011 [22]	2	1	1	2	1	1
Hoeve, 2021 [23]	1	1	1	1	1	1
Ojala, 2019 [24]	2	1	2	2	2	2
Fischetti, 2019 [25]	2	1	1	3	2	2
Calogiuri, 2016 [26]	2	1	2	2	2	2

Key for Table 5: 1 = Low Risk of Bias. 2 = Some Concerns. 3 = High Risk of Bias.

3.3. Study Methods

The most common form of intervention was psychological interventions ($n = 8$). Psychological interventions included mindfulness-based, cognitive behavioural therapy and stress management interventions. Three studies used physical interventions, which involved exercise, walking, weight training or circuit training programmes [20,25,26]. One paper included an educational intervention [17] focused on health education (Table 6).

Of the ten papers in this review, five papers [19,20,22,24,25] reported that the control group received no intervention during the research but were waitlisted to participate in the intervention at a later date. In Malarkey et al.'s [18] study, the participants in the control group received a lifestyle and educational intervention, compared with the mindfulness-based intervention that the experimental group received. Hughes et al.'s [17] study control group received a light level of health education compared with the experimental group, who received the health promotion intervention. Hoeve et al.'s [23] control group received a regular education intervention, without any mindfulness training. Two papers' control groups [21,26] had either an indoor standard work break or indoor exercise, compared to the experimental groups whose interventions were conducted outdoors. No conclusive pattern emerged between which control condition was in place and the outcome of the intervention. Table 6 illustrates that of the five interventions [19,20,22,24,25] in which the control group received no intervention, three of these papers reported an effective intervention in the experimental group.

Six papers conducted their interventions in the workplace offices, two papers were carried out via online means in the workplace, and a further two papers took place outside of the workplace, in green areas and nature.

All papers in this review used self-reported questionnaires to collect data on stress. Three of these papers also collected cortisol levels, either from saliva samples or blood tests [18,22,26]. Four of the papers used the Perceived Stress Scale Questionnaire to assess the level of psychological stress perceived in participants.

The shortest intervention took place over the course of two weeks [26]. Three of the papers' interventions took place for over six months, including follow up time [17,22,24]. The longest duration for intervention was Hughes et al.'s [17] 12-month study.

3.4. Study Findings

Changes in stress levels as a result of each intervention are reported in Table 6. In seven out of the ten studies [19,21–26], there was improvement in at least one measure of self-reported stress levels. However, none of the three studies that measured cortisol levels [18,22,26] found any significant differences between the intervention and the control group's cortisol levels.

Three interventions [17,18,20] showed no evidence of effectiveness on any measure. There were no consistent patterns in terms of the intervention type (psychological, physical educational), workplace setting or delivery method between effective and ineffective interventions.

Table 6. Description of Methods and Findings.

Study (Author, Year)	Intervention Type	Duration	Location	Outcome Measurement Method	Data Collection Type	Findings	Intervention Deemed Effective? [1]
				Low risk of bias			
Malarkey, 2013 [18]	Psychological	8 Weeks	Office	Perceived Stress Scale Questionnaire	Self-report	No significant differences were seen at follow-up	No
				Cortisol Levels	Blood test & Saliva sample	No significant changes were noted	
Aikens, 2014 [19]	Psychological	7 Weeks	Online	Perceived Stress Scale Questionnaire	Self-report	23.1% decline in perceived stress	Yes
Limm, 2011 [22]	Psychological	8 Months	Office	Stress Reactivity Scale (SRS)	Self-report	The reduction in SR in intervention group (from 54.5 to 50.2) was significantly higher than in the control group (from 54.5 to 52.7)	Mixed
				Salivary Cortisol Levels	Saliva samples	No effect observed	
				Depression, anxiety, and stress scale (DASS)	Self-report	General stress score decreased from a group mean of 1.05 to 0.58	
Hoeve, 2021 [23]	Psychological	6 Weeks	Office	Police Stress Questionnaire (PSQ-Op)	Self-report	Occupational Stress scores decreased from a group of 3.17 to 2.84	Yes
				Some bias concerns			
Hughes, 2011 [17]	Educational & Psychological	12 Months	Office	Perceived Stress Scale Questionnaire	Self-report	No quantitative data reported [2]	No
Cook, 2015 [20]	Physical & Psychological	3 Months	Online	Symptoms of Distress Likert scale questionnaire	Self-report	No difference between groups	No
				Coping with Stress questionnaire	Self-report	No differences between groups on coping with stress	
Largo-Wight, 2017 [21]	Psychological	4 Weeks	Outside	Perceived Stress Scale Questionnaire	Self-report	Mean PSSQ score decreased from 62.3 to 61.2 in intervention group, compared to 66.2 to 64.2 decrease from control group	Yes

Table 6. Cont.

Study (Author, Year)	Intervention Type	Duration	Location	Outcome Measurement Method	Data Collection Type	Findings	Intervention Deemed Effective? [1]
Ojala, 2019 [24]	Psychological	9 Months	Implied to be in Office	Bergen Burnout Inventory (BBI)	Self-report	Total BBI decreased from 36.9 to 33.9 in intervention group, at follow up	Yes
				Utrecht Work Engagement Scale (UWES)	Self-report	UWES increased from 4.3 to 4.5 in intervention group, at follow-up	
Fischetti, 2019 [25]	Physical & Education	8 Weeks	Office	Occupational Stress Indicator	Self-report	Scores for Job as a source of stress decreased from 30.7 to 25.2	Yes
				Short-Form 12 Questionnaire	Self-report	Increases in scores with significant changes from pre- to post-intervention (48.2 to 53.4)	
Calogiuri, 2016 [26]	Physical	2 Weeks	Outside	Physical Activity Affective Scale Questionnaire	Self-report	Higher ratings for PAAS, in relation to Positive Affect in the intervention group	Mixed
				Cortisol Awakening Response (CAR)	Blood Test	No significant differences between groups	

[1] For the Intervention Deemed Effective Column: Yes = the paper's authors classify the intervention as effectiveness and/or successful in the text of the paper. Mixed = the paper has unclear conclusions regarding the effective of the intervention report. No = the intervention was not deemed as being effective by the authors of the paper. [2] In Hughes et al.'s paper there are no quantitative data for stress levels in the main text. However, a supplementary paper with that data was said to be available via contact with the Journal or Author. After contacting both, no response was received.

4. Discussion

4.1. Main Findings

The evidence of the effectiveness of interventions to reduce stress in older workers was varied. Seven out of the ten papers reported some effectiveness in reducing self-reported stress in older workers as a result of interventions. Studies that measured cortisol levels did not report any reduction in stress. Most of the interventions were psychological in nature, but there was no difference in reported effectiveness between psychological, physical, or educational interventions. It should be noted that most of these interventions were only short-term, and therefore, longer-term impacts of these interventions are not clearly demonstrated.

4.2. Methodological Considerations

There were some important limitations in the studies included in the review. Firstly, the number of participants reported in each study was generally low, with three papers comprising studies of less than 40 participants and only one study with more than 500. Due to the low number of participants, it is difficult to generalise the results of these interventions to the broader population [27]. In most of the studies, participants had to volunteer to take part. In some studies, it was not clear how many employees that were eligible declined to take part so the acceptability of such interventions in the workplace cannot be concluded from this study.

Secondly, none of the ten papers observed the longer-term impacts of the interventions. Whilst papers stated or implied that the interventions were longer-term solutions to the problem of occupational stress amongst older workers, they provide no conclusive evidence of long-term benefit. The concern regarding the long-term effects associated with workplace interventions has also been discussed by others. Steenstra et al. [28] reported how the effect of interventions require a very long follow-up, which is extremely difficult to achieve and maintain. They concluded that the interventions' effect would most likely dilute over time and not result in any long-term benefits. Similarly, in this review, two out of the three papers which had interventions lasting more than 8 months were shown to have mixed or no effect on reducing workplace stress. This is suggestive evidence in support of Steenstra et al.'s conclusions that the impact of workplace interventions to reduce stress could have little to no long-term benefit if the intervention is not maintained in the workplace. It is also possible maintenance of a short-term intervention is not enough; workplaces may need different kinds of approaches to maintain reductions in stress levels in the longer term.

Thirdly, there was a range of self-report questionnaires used, which collected data on various aspects relating to stress, mental health, or other factors. When analysing the interventions, as different measurement outcomes are used, it can cause difficulties in understanding which intervention is the most effective.

There were some limitations also in the conduct of this review. Only papers published in English were included in the review. Studies which were written and published in other languages were removed at the first stage of screening. Whilst the majority of papers which were found in the database search stage of the review were written in English, those in other languages may have been beneficial to include in this review. Using free, online translation software to translate any non-English studies has become more common in academic reviews, and if this research was to be conducted again in the future, including non-English studies, and using translation software should be strongly considered. It was also beyond the scope of the review to include qualitative studies. Whilst these would not have definitely addressed questions of effectiveness, they could have provided useful insights into why intervention achieved their effects. The RoB 2.0 tool which was used for performing the critical appraisal does not prompt consideration of wider aspects of quality and relevance, for example, what the control conditions were. This could be seen as a potential limitation in several of the papers in the review.

A further challenge faced in this review was the ambiguity regarding the definition of an older workers. The initial search terms included specific terms and synonyms for "older worker". However, this resulted in a very small number of papers being retrieved. Therefore, this search term was removed and at abstract and full paper screening, the reviewers determined which papers focused on older workers and which did not. Eliminating "older workers" as a search term in the database search led to a potential risk that relevant literature, with a clear focus on older workers, may have been overlooked. However, "older worker" was hard to define partly because the classification of an older worker varies across countries. The ELSA (English Longitudinal Study of Ageing) and the JSTAR (Japanese Study of Ageing and Retirement) both describe workers over the age of 50 as "older workers", however, Kingston and Jagger [29] argue that cohort studies with the lower age limit of 50 to 65 years old, often have fewer very old people in the studies, therefore, are not fully representative of older workers. The nature of the risk of being an older worker varies in the context of workplace settings, occupations and job demands. For example, as seen in Fischetti et al.'s [25] and Hoeve et al.'s [23] research, police officers may be more at risk of injury at a younger age, due to the physical nature of their occupation. This may result in police officers aged 40 being deemed as older workers in their profession, although at their chronological age, in society and in other professional groups, they would be classified as younger. However, at this age, it is possible for some police officers that the nature of their work may change, to become more 'desk based'. In this case, the current workplace exposures may be more similar to office workers, but the prior exposures they faced from working in communities may have long lasting and distinct effects on their health that are not experienced by those who have spent their entire careers in office-based jobs. Due to the small number of studies identified, this review was not able to explore the differences in the nature of interventions across workplaces. This is needed in future because different causes of stress based upon a range of diverse types of employment may affect the sustainability and the effectiveness of interventions to reduce workplace stress.

4.3. Interpretation of Findings and Comparison to Previous Studies

Of the ten papers sourced for this review, only five reported a specific focus on older workers, demonstrating the lack of robust and available literature on this topic. This finding is consistent with older systematic reviews researching workplace interventions for older workers [3,11,28]. More than ten years ago, Crawford et al. [30] urged for more research to be conducted on health and safety management interventions for workers over the age of 50 in relation to the physical and psychological changes that occur when workers reach this age.

Interventions that used self-reported measures appeared more effective when compared to biological measures. However, it is important to note that self-reports and biological samples measure different things. Taking part in an intervention may improve subjective well-being in an individual, even if it has no biological effect. This does not imply that the intervention was unsuccessful or ineffective. Indeed, McDonald [31] suggests that gaining self-reported data from participants is the most logical way to learn more about an individual. Arguably, an individual's subjective well-being is what would keep them in the workplace.

Whilst it is understood that older workers might not always face more workplace stress compared to younger workers, they could be more at risk of specific stressors connected to responsibilities outside of work, age discrimination and physical health conditions that are more common in older age [32]. In the ten papers' interventions, there was not enough description regarding the extent to which specific stressors associated with older age were addressed. It is, however, significant that there were five studies that did not seek to focus on older workers, potentially overlooking distinct stressors. In these studies, it is also possible that the overall effectiveness could have been driven by higher effectiveness in younger populations but there was not sufficient data reported in these papers on effects by participant age to explore this. The context in which the interventions effect change may be important. Interventions in the workplace, which are promoted and supported by employers may encourage participants not only to take part in the intervention, but also to make changes to their lifestyle and behaviour, which, in turn, would ultimately improve their well-being and decrease their stress levels at work [33].

4.4. The Significance of the Review and Public Health Implications

Since Crawford et al.'s [30] review was undertaken, policy and demographic changes have lead to a higher proportion of older workers in many countries, increasing the importance of health and safety interventions for workers over the age of 50. The need for such research has not been addressed and the knowledge gaps that were present in the literature remain.

This review has demonstrated that there is still not sufficient research available for governments and policy makers to make an informed decision on the impact of increasing state pension age on the population. If they are determined to extend the working life of individuals, governments will need to ensure that there is no detriment to the health of older workers.

The lack of high-quality literature on this topic results in this review being unable to provide any definitive conclusions regarding the most effective and successful workplace intervention to deal with occupational stress. This systematic review can be updated to illustrate newly published literature about older workers' well-being in years to come. The significance of implementing a successful intervention to promote and maintain the health of older workers is vital for the longer-term wealth creation and sustaining of both the economy and health of the population [34].

This review has not shown an adequate amount of successful workplace interventions to support older workers' occupational stress to mitigate the public health implications of raising state pension age, as reported by MISPA [4]. More extensive and robust research is required to illustrate to both employers and policy makers that increasing state pension age will result in; increased morbidity and mortality rates for those in demanding occupations; overwhelming the already sparse healthcare services-both for occupational health and primary care; and, worsening the health for workers who are already ill. Careful considerations need to be made to ensure that older workers are not adversely harmed by increases to state pension age. It is fundamental that interventions, which have been proven successful for older workers, must be introduced into more workplaces to ensure a smoother transition for older workers who are now working longer.

5. Conclusions

As the population ages, and statutory pension age increase, the proportion of older workers will increase in the workplace. Older workers face distinct and sometimes greater risks to health and well-being compared with younger workers, which may place them at particular risk of stress. This review found some promising evidence that interventions in the workplace can improve self-reported stress in older workers in the short term. It also highlighted the paucity of studies with interventions specifically designed for older workers. Further studies are required to understand longer term impacts of workplace interventions on older workers and to elucidate what type of intervention is most likely to be effective in different workplace settings.

Supplementary Materials: The following supporting information can be downloaded at: https://www.mdpi.com/article/10.3390/ijerph19159202/s1, PRISMA 2020 Checklist.

Author Contributions: The idea of the study was developed by D.S. and J.S., with input from D.B. D.S. developed the study protocol and searched the four databases. The title and abstract screening process was conducted by D.S. J.S. supported the screening process as a third reviewer in events where a decision could not be agreed upon. The Critical Appraisal was undertaken by J.S. and D.S. D.S. drafted the manuscript. All three authors contributed to subsequent drafts and agreed upon the final manuscript for submission. All authors have read and agreed to the published version of the manuscript.

Funding: Jessica Sheringham is supported by the National Institute for Health and Care Research (NIHR) Applied Research Collaboration (ARC) North Thames. The views expressed in this publication are those of the authors and not necessarily those of the National Institute for Health and Care Research or the Department of Health and Social Care.

Institutional Review Board Statement: Not applicable.

Informed Consent Statement: Not applicable.

Data Availability Statement: Not applicable.

Acknowledgments: The authors wish to thank all who supported them throughout the project. Thank you to Hynek Pikhart and Martin Bobak at University College London (UCL) for their constructive feedback throughout the developmental stages. We also wish to give particular acknowledgement to both Anne Harte, who acted as the secondary reviewer during the screening and data extraction process and Jenny Lisle, who provided specialist input regarding the role of occupational health.

Conflicts of Interest: The authors declare no conflict of interest.

Appendix A

Table A1. Data Extraction Form from Primary Dataset.

	1	2	3	4	5
Study Number					
Data Set Decision	PRIMARY DATA SET	PRIMARY DATA SET	PRIMARY DATA SET	PRIMARY DATA SET	PRIMARY DATA SET
Study Information					
Database No.	WoS154	WoS321	O1587	O1320	O1544
Author(s)	Francesco Fischetti, Stefania Cataldi, Francesca Latino & Gianpiero Greco	Giovanna Calogiuri, Katinka Evensen, Andi Weydahl, Kim Andersson, Grete Patil, Camilla Ihlebaek and Ruth Raanaas	Royer F Cook, Rebekah K Hersch, Dana Schlossberg, Samantha L Leaf	William B. Malarkey, David Jarjoura, Maryanna Klatt	Susan L. Hughes, Rachel B. Seymour, Richard T. Campbell, James W. Shaw, Camille Fabiyi and Rosemary Sokas
Year	2019	2016	2015	2013	2011
Link to Article	https://rua.ua.es/dspace/bitstream/10045/96031/1/JHSE_14_Proc4_53.pdf	https://brage.inn.no/inn-xmlui/bitstream/handle/11250/2380639/Work_2015_Calogiuri.pdf?sequence=1&isAllowed=y	https://www.jmir.org/2015/3/e82	https://www.ncbi.nlm.nih.gov/pmc/articles/PMC3528077/	https://ajph.aphapublications.org/doi/full/10.2105/AJPH.2010.300082
Access Date	8 June 2022	8 June 2022	8 June 2022	8 June 2022	8 June 2022
Title of Article	"Effectiveness of multilateral training didactic method on physical and mental wellbeing in law enforcement"	Green exercise as a workplace intervention to reduce job stress. Results from a pilot study	A Web-Based Health Promotion Program for Older Workers: Randomized Controlled Trial	Workplace based mindfulness practice and inflammation: a randomized trial.	Comparison of two health-promotion programs for older workers.
Country	Italy	Norway	United States	United States	United States
Intervention					
Study Aim	to investigate the effects of an 8-week multilateral training program on physical and mental wellbeing in policemen	to explore possible effects of green-exercise interventions in the workplace on psychological and physiological indicators of stress.	to evaluate the impact of a multimedia Web-based health promotion program on central health attitudes and practices of older workers.	This study focused on working adults who could benefit from lifestyle intervention strategies. In comparing the mindfulness intervention to the lifestyle education program, we focused on three biologic measures of chronic stress and inflammation	to examine the effects of 2 worksite health-promotion interventions (compared with a health-education control) on older workers' healthy behaviors and health outcomes.
Type of Intervention	Multilateral training program on physical and mental well-being	Exercise-based Intervention	Web-based program to address a wide variety of health behavior topics, including physical activity, healthy eating, stress management, and tobacco cessation	Mindfulness Intervention	health-promotion intervention and health-education control
Duration of Intervention	8 Weeks	2 Weeks	3 months	8 weeks	12 months
Location of Intervention	Police Offices	outdoors in a green/nature area or in an indoor exercise-setting	Online intervention	University Offices	at university worksite
Study Design	Randomised Controlled Trial	Between Subjects Randomised Controlled Trial	Randomised Controlled Trial	randomized controlled trial	randomized controlled trial

Table A1. Cont.

Study Number	1	2	3	4	5
			Methods		
How were participants recruited?	recruited in the police offices of the Puglia region (Italy) between January and February 2019, healthy males belonging to the State Police voluntarily participated	healthy employees, sedentary or moderately active, in two workplaces in a small town in the north of Norway who responded to an invitation to participate in the study by e-mail	A recruitment flyer briefly describing the purpose of the study was emailed by company officials to all employees 50 years of age and older (approximately 2500 employees) located in multiple US offices of a global information technology company. The flyer stated that the study was being conducted by a research organization through a grant from the National Institutes of Health. The flyer also explained that participants would receive US $25 for completing the first questionnaire and US $25 for completing the second questionnaire, and that their name would be entered into a drawing in which 1 participant would receive US $500 during each questionnaire round. Interested employees who fit the inclusion criteria (age 50 and older) were instructed to contact the project staff directly by email or telephone.	PARTICIPANTS: were recruited from faculty and staff of The Ohio State University. Advertising promoted the trial as a life style intervention program and the types of interventions were not specified, with participants unaware of the intervention type until the first day of the actual intervention	Participants were recruited via announcements on staff listservs, targeted e-mails, staffed recruitment tables at events in highly trafficked buildings, and flyers posted throughout the university.
Occupation of Participants	Police Officers	Office Workers	employees of a large global information technology company	University Faculty Staff	Research participants were older support and academic staff at the University of Illinois at Chicago
Specific Focus on Older Workers?	No	No	Yes	Not specific - but mean age is high	Yes
Outcome Measurement	the sources of stress and coping strategies, and the physical and mental state of health perceived were measured by the Occupational Stress Indicator and the Short Form-12	Self-reported affective state was measured by the Physical Activity Affective Scale (PAAS), which place feeling states within four factors corresponding to the quadrants circumplex model of affect and arousal: 'Positive Affect', 'Tranquility', 'Negative Affect', and 'Fatigue' AND Two measures of cortisol as an indicator of stress were used: Cortisol Awakening Response (CAR) and serum concentration. Saliva samples were selfadministered by the subjects for the determination of the CAR the morning after each session.	Twelve items assessing the type of strategies one uses to cope with difficult situations and events. Questions are answered on a 4-point scale ranging from 1 (never) to 4 (almost always); higher score = better coping; Typical questions included "I often put things aside for a while to get perspective on them" and "I decide certain problems are not worth worrying about"	CRP, IL-6, Cortisol, BP and Perceived Stress Scale Questionnaires	We investigated change from baseline to 6 months and 12 months in 4 measures of stress. We used the Perceived Stress Scale to measure overall stress during the preceding month. We used a 4-item scale developed by Lorig et al. to assess health-related stress, and we used the Brief COPE to assess use of positive and negative coping behaviors

Table A1. Cont.

Study Number	1	2	3	4	5
Data Collection Style	Self report questionnaires	Self report questionnaires and Cortisol levels in serum were measured by professional nurses through blood test the morning after each session between 8:00 and 9:00 AM	self report survey	Via blood tests, saliva samples for cortisol and self reported questionnaires	self reported questionnaire
How were the Results analysed?	Pre and Post Intervention	Comparison to Control, and Pre and Post Intervention	Comparison to Control, and Pre and Post Intervention	Comparison to Control, and Pre and Post Intervention	Comparison to control and other intervention
Results					
No. of Participants	20	14	278	186	423
Dropout Rate	0 Dropouts	11: 3 dropouts/lost to f/u	Zero Dropouts	16 dropouts/lost to follow up	56 dropouts/lost to follow up
Age of Workers	Mean = 46.8 (SD 3.9)	Range = 41–57	Participants ranged in age from 50 to 68 years	Mean age = Education group—49, MBI-Id—51	Mean age = 51, participants were all aged 40 years and older
Any other condition of workers?	No	No	No	No—participants were excluded if they had a known condition which enhances inflammation and a psychiatric disorder other than depression	No
Change in Stress Levels	experimental group perceived less stress, showed a more realistic attitude towards the various working situations and a greater perception of physical and mental wellbeing than control group ($p < 0.05$).	Concerning the PAAS components, a significant effect of group was found for Positive Affect when corrected for baseline values, with higher ratings reported by the nature group No significant differences between groups were found for cortisol concentration in serum	There were no differences between the program and control groups on symptoms of distress or coping with stress. The estimated adjusted posttest different between program and control group is 0.01 for Coping with Stress	Cortisol at Baseline in Education group was 0.15, mean at follow up is 0.12; MBI-id group at baseline is 0.10 and followup mean is 0.11. The mindfulness intervention was effective as the MBI-Id group demonstrated greater self reported mindfulness than the education group at 2 months. This difference was sustained at 6 and 12 months: With measures of depression (CES-D), stress (Perceived Stress Scale), sleep quality (PSQI), no significant differences were found at 2-months. The global test across all five produced a p-value of 0.91. The PSS measure, however, asked the questions in reference to the past week rather than the past month as is the standard format, which permitted an evaluation of the intervention at completion.Using an extensive pre and post MBI-Id salivary cortisol sampling protocol we saw no decrease in cortisol levels	No significant differences were seen for COACH or RealAge participants on any of the 4 stress outcomes at either time point

Table A1. Cont.

Study Number	1	2	3	4	5
Intervention deemed effective/ successful	It has been found that police officers perceived fewer sources of pressure after intervention and specifically: working days are lived with less stress	Green-exercise at the workplace could be a profitable way to manage stress and induce restoration among employees.	Significant program effects were not shown on measures of stress	The trial was designed to test whether MBI-ld was superior to an education control in lowering cortisol, IL-6 and CRP immediately at the end of the interventions. We did not confirm this hypothesis. MBSR in smaller observational studies has been reported by some but not all investigators to lower cortisol levels when the intervention is compared to a wait list control group	The differences in the findings of our respective studies raises important questions about whether a dose—response relationship exists between comprehensiveness of services offered, and whether certain program components, such as incentives, are more effective and more critical than others.
Key Conclusions	public policies are needed to promote the practice of physical activities as continuing education, including leisure and sports activities, and to promote the psychological stability, work efficiency, changes in living habits, improvements in wellbeing and, therefore, improvements in quality of life.	it also provides some evidence that green-exercise interventions in the workplace can be a more valuable resource than 'traditional' indoor exercise in promoting health among employees, especially reducing psychological as well as physiological stress.	A Web-based health promotion program showed promise for making a significant contribution to the short-term dietary and exercise practices of older working adults. The findings suggest that a multimedia Web-based program could be a promising vehicle for delivering health promotion material to older working adults.	MBI-ld significantly enhanced mindfulness by 2 months and it was maintained for up to a year when compared to the education control. We did not see any significant changes in self-report measures for depressive symptoms, perceived stress, or sleep quality. Most but not all MBSR investigations have found improvements in these areas when the intervention is compared to a wait list control group. We have performed a randomized trial with a compressed MBSR intervention in which instruction and practice occurred in the workplace. This reduced the barriers commonly mentioned for non-participation in MBSR programs. Adherence to the program was greater than 90% for 8 weeks (evidenced by weekly attendance/practice sheets) even though the subjects were unaware that mindfulness meditation was one of the lifestyle interventions being offered. Additionally, mindfulness was achieved and sustained for at least one year. It is possible that a more intense intervention would have produced more significant effects. We conclude that MBI-ld should be more fully investigated as a low-cost self-directed complementary strategy for reducing inflammation.	If we can reach older adults while they are still working and engage them in sustained health-promotion activities, we may be able to delay morbidity onset, thereby reducing cost to employers as well as future Medicare expenditures

Table A1. *Cont.*

Study Number	1	2	3	4	5
			Discussion		
Author Identified Weaknesses	the small number of police officers recruited due to the difficulties encountered during the organizational phase in obtaining the necessary authorizations and having the subjects available. Moreover, the voluntary sample is not representative of the entire population of the law enforcement and therefore it is not possible to generalize the results. the results obtained could provide important indications for future studies aimed to know the effects of physical training with a multilateral approach on the occupational stress management	due to a small-sample size, the generalizability of the results is quite limited. Using a between-subjects design represented a further limitation. a within-subjects design was preferred as in previous studies it was shown that nature-based interventions can have long lasting effects on physiological parameters	the reliance on self-reports. because of the particular characteristics of the sample, caution should be exercised in generalizing these findings to workforces that are less educated and affluent	A limitation of our study was omission of wait list control group as the impact of the MBI-ld may have achieved significance in comparison, indicating the potential impact of such a workplace intervention.	the interventions were tested with staff at an inner-city university who may have had higher levels of education than do workers in other industries. Thus, the generalizability of the findings to workers in other settings requires further testing.

Table A2. Data Extraction Form from Secondary Dataset.

Study Number	6	7	8	9	10
Data Set Decision	SECONDARY DATASET	SECONDARY DATASET	SECONDARY DATASET	SECONDARY DATASET	SECONDARY DATASET
Database Number	WoS62	P144	O1594	O1575	O1130
Study Information					
Author(s)	Machteld Hoeve, Esther L. de Bruin, Floor van Rooij and Susan Bögels	Erin Largo-Wight, Peter S. Wlyudka, Julie W. Merten & Elizabeth A. Cuvelier	Birgitta Ojala, Clas-Håkan Nygård, Heini Huhtala, Philip Bohle and Seppo T. Nikkari	Heribert Limm, Harald Gündel, Mechthild Heinmüller, Birgitt Marten-Mittag, Urs M Nater, Johannes Siegrist, Peter Angerer	Kimberly A. Aikens, John Astin, Kenneth R. Pelletier, Kristin Levanovich, Catherine M. Baase, Yeo Yung Park, and Catherine M. Bodnar
Year	2021	2017	2019	2011	2014
Link to Article	https://link.springer.com/content/pdf/10.1007/s12671-021-01631-7.pdf	https://www.tandfonline.com/doi/pdf/10.1080/15555240.2017.1335211?needAccess=true	https://www.mdpi.com/1660-4601/16/1/80	https://oem.bmj.com/content/68/2/126?casa_token=4CAKgnx0h2wAAAAA%3Acw336eYaWoATNiEplkpbAJuA7PAdtiStdoNW0lXmrrJAAudRtJfdD0TEBaY6Rw8eeCpwbmjVvTs	http://affinityhealthhub.co.uk/d/attachments/mindfulness-goes-to-work-impact-of-an-online-intervention-1498490157.pdf
Access Date	8-June-2022	8-June-2022	8-June-2022	8-June-2022	8-June-2022
Title of Article	Effects of a Mindfulness-Based Intervention for Police Officers	Effectiveness and feasibility of a 10-minute employee stress intervention: Outdoor Booster Break	A Cognitive Behavioural Intervention Programme to Improve Psychological Well-Being	Stress management interventions in the workplace improve stress reactivity: a randomised controlled trial.	Mindfulness goes to work: impact of an online workplace intervention.
Country	Netherlands	United States	Finland	Germany	Michigan, United States
Intervention					
Study Aim	to increase knowledge on the effects of a mindfulness-based intervention in police officers and potential mechanisms of change by relating changes in facets of mindful awareness to changes in stress	to explore the feasibility and efficacy of a brief work break outside (Outdoor Booster Break) among office employees.	to evaluate a cognitive behavioural intervention as an early rehabilitation strategy to improve employees' well-being	to test the long-term effect of this SMI on acute perceived reactions to stress at work (stress reactivity) after 1 year, as the primary endpoint	to determine whether a mindfulness program, created for the workplace, was both practical and efficacious in decreasing employee stress while enhancing resiliency and well-being.
Type of Intervention	Mindfulness-based Intervention	Outdoor Booster Break environmental intervention	Cognitive Behavioural Intervention Programme	stress management intervention	online mindfulness workplace intervention
Duration of Intervention	6 Weeks	4 weeks	9 months	8 months	7 week
Location of Intervention	Police offices	University office	Not Specified—facilitated by an interdisciplinary, goal-oriented multi professional team (a doctor, an occupational physiotherapist, an occupational psychologist, and a nurse)	at worksite	Online (at work)
Study Design	Quasi Experimental Study Design	Randomised Controlled Trial	Non Randomised Controlled Trial	randomised controlled trial	randomized controlled study

Table A2. Cont.

Study Number	6	7	8	9	10
			Methods		
How were participants recruited?	Participants were recruited by the Dutch trade union. Before the training, during a company away day, members of the trade union had the opportunity to participate in a mindfulness 2-hour workshop, led by SB and one of the mindfulness trainers, in order to inform them about the possibility of participating in a mindfulness training.	A census of university office staff in the southeast in springtime was invited to participate	Participants were volunteers who met the inclusion criteria for the study: Being employed in the public sector and working as permanent or long-term temporary staff with at least one year of service.	All lower and middle level managers (n $\frac{1}{4}$ 262), each responsible for a specific unit within production and for the management of 50 workers, on average, were eligible. All participants were invited to a 1.5 h medical and psychological examination by an experienced team consisting of a psychologist (HL) and a physician (MH). Written informed consent was obtained. All volunteers were required to complete a battery of questionnaires, participate in a basic physical examination with blood sampling and collect saliva samples the next working day. This initial health check included feedback to each participant a few days later.	Participants were drawn from a sample of 600 Dow employees, located in Midland, Michigan, who had completed a health risk assessment (comprehensive questionnaire and biometrics) in the preceding 6 months. All employees are invited for health risk assessment with employees in given departments being scheduled throughout the year. This recruitment allowed for study access to a good cross section of employees because the standard process of invitations would include all elements of the employee base. Study participant recruitment occurred from March to April 2012 and consisted of one e-mail notification, which described the free mindfulness-based stress management program. The e-mail notification explained that the purpose of the program was to help employees reduce and manage workplace stress.
Occupation of Participants	Police Officers	University office staff	Public sector workers	lower and middle level managers at an international manufacturing plant located in Southern Germany	General employees at a chemical company
Specific Focus on Older Workers?	No	No	No	No	No
Outcome Measurement	Symptoms of stress were measured by four instruments that measure different types of stress, including general feelings of stress and tension, physical stress, occupational stress during police work, and stress symptoms that are related to a traumatic event (i.e., PTSD symptoms).	Perceived stress was measured two times–at pretest and posttest for both groups with a self-report perceived stress instrument. The Perceived Stress Questionnaire (PSQ).	The measurement tools used in this study were the Bergen Burnout Inventory (BBI) and the Utrecht Work Engagement Scale (UWES). BBI 15 was used to measure burnout. It includes three sub-dimensions: Exhaustion (five items), cynicism (five items), and sense of inadequacy (five items). UWES 9 was used to define three dimensions of work engagement: Vigour (three items), dedication (three items), and absorption (three items)	Self-reported stress reactivity was measured with the 29-item Stress Reactivity Scale (SRS). Biological stress indices were measured using levels of salivary cortisol as an indicator of hypothalamic-pituitary-adrenal axis activity, and salivary a-amylase, reflecting basal activity of the sympathetic nervous system	The Perceived Stress Scale (PSS-14) was used to assess participants' levels of psychological stress. The PSS-14 is a well-validated stress measurement tool whose items are designed to tap into how unpredictable, uncontrollable, and overloaded individuals find their lives
Data Collection Style	Self report questionnaires	self-reported perceived stress 4-point Likert type scale from participants	self reported questionnaire	self reported questionnaire and saliva samples	self reported questionnaire
How were the Results analysed?	Pre and Post Intervention, plus Follow Up	Comparison to control group, and pre and post intervention	Comparison to Control, and Pre and Post Intervention	Comparison to Control, and Pre and Post Intervention	Comparison to Control, and Pre and Post Intervention

Table A2. Cont.

Study Number	6	7	8	9	10
			Results		
No. of Participants	82	37 (Treatment had Outdoor Break, Control had Indoor Break)	779	174	89
Dropout Rate	19 dropouts	No Dropout Mentioned	217 dropouts	20 dropouts/lost to follow up	23 dropouts/failed to follow up
Age of Workers	30–63 (mean = 49)	Average age of 48.8	mean age of subjects was 49.9 years (range 21–64 years)	Mean age = 40.9. Aged 18–65 years with more than 2 years left before retirement	18–65
Any other condition of workers?	No	No	No	No	No
Change in Stress Levels	Improvement in mindful awareness (mindfulness total scale) was marginally significantly associated with a reduction in general feelings of stress and tension. Further, an increase in attention was significantly associated with reductions in general stress and occupational stress.	Observed average posttest stress scores were lower for both the control group and the treatment group (Mean PSQ Stress, Control Pre = 66.25, Control Post 64.25, Treatment Group Pre 65.25, Treatment Group Post 61.25). Posttest stress was 4.22 points lower (95% CI: or the treatment group compared to controls	Total BBI 15 values for the intervention group were 36.9 (standard deviation (SD) 11.8) at baseline and 33.9 (SD 12.3) at follow-up. The change from baseline was −3.0 ($p < 0.001$). Values for the control group were 37.6 (SD 12.2) at baseline and 37.5 (SD 14.4) at follow-up. The change from baseline was 0.1 ($p = 0.912$). The difference in changes between groups was statistically significant ($p = 0.023$).	The reduction in perceived stress reactivity in the intervention group (from 54.5 to 50.2) was significantly higher than in the control group (from 54.5 to 52.7). For cortisol, no effect of the intervention was observed. Self-perceived stress reactivity assesses typical cognitive, emotional and physiological reactions to different stressful situations. High stress reactivity scores have been shown to significantly correlate with a variety of other psychological measures of distress such as depression or anxiety.	perceived stress declined by 23.1% from baseline values in the follow up 6 months. Participants also reported a decline in weekly high stress episodes by 33%, which is a significant downward trend ($p < 0.001$).
Intervention deemed effective/successful	Police officers significantly benefited from the mindfulness-based intervention	taking a work break in general resulted in a reduction of stress among the employees. All employees benefited from a reduction of generalized stress after 4 weeks of daily work breaks. But, as expected, the participants randomized into the Outdoor Booster Breaks resulted in significantly greater reduction in stress over the 4-week study than the participants who took a standard indoor work break.	The principal finding of this study is a statistically significant improvement in several measures of psychosocial well-being (BBI 15, UWES, stress, depression) for participants who completed the cognitive behavioural intervention programme.	Our approach proved to be feasible in the workplace setting, it was well accepted and it produced selected favourable behavioural and physiological effects	The present findings have significant potential implications for corporate health and human performance. The program studied was a mindfulness intervention, which was modified in length, content, and messaging to fit workplace needs and delivered through an on-line platform that included personal coaching. Overall, the ESs obtained in this study were in the moderate to large range and were either maintained, or further improved, over time. This indicates that a shortened, Web-based mindfulness program can replicate the results of traditionally delivered MBSR.

Table A2. Cont.

Study Number	6	7	8	9	10
Key Conclusions	Mindfulness-based intervention appears beneficial for police officers. Further, increases in both attention and acceptance skills such as acting with awareness and non-judging seem to be most important in explaining reductions of stress in police officers.	This study points to several implications for employers and worksite health promoters. First, environmental stress interventions such as Outdoor Booster Breaks are relatively simple to implement. Creating healthy workplaces is a health promotion effort that may be more practical and feasible than many other labor-intensive health promotion efforts. Creating a healthful work environment—with the purposeful use of nature contact—is a simple and practical step to improve employee health and productivity. Environmental improvements require little, if any, commitment and effort from the employee. In a way, improving the workplace environment to foster health among employees is one way to "set the employees up for success."	This study suggests that a cognitive behavioural intervention achieved significant improvements in several measures of mental health. The results imply that this kind of intervention is needed to give early support on mental health issues for the working-age population.	SMI based on work stress theory, is effective in reducing perceived stress reactivity and sympathetic activation in lower and middle management employees. Other mental health parameters and ERI show a tendency towards improvement. These beneficial effects are present 1 year later.	This on-line mindfulness intervention seems to be both practical and effective in decreasing employee stress, while improving resiliency, vigor, and work engagement, thereby enhancing overall employee well-being.

Table A2. *Cont.*

Study Number	6	7	8	9	10
			Discussion		
Author Identified Weaknesses	we examined the effectiveness of an adapted corporate mindfulness training. Although adaptations to the work situation of police officers were made, such as in the enquiries and discussion after the meditations and the examples being used in exercises, no cultural adaptations were made to the content of the training, which could have diminished the positive effects. Second, findings might not be generalizable to the entire population of police officers. Although our sample size is larger than most earlier studies on the effects of mindfulness-based intervention in police officers, the number of participants was small due to attrition at post-test and follow-up: senior workers are generally overrepresented in unions in the Netherlands. Therefore, it should be kept in mind that the results may apply only to more experienced police officers and less to relatively young or inexperienced officers.	the sample size and group sizes were small. the generalizability of the findings to male workers. Future researchers should assess the impact of Outdoor Booster Breaks with greater male representation. Also perceived stress was the only outcome measured.	One limitation is that the participants represent a relatively small population in Finland. The intervention and control groups were selected partly according to the participants' own interests. Question-based research may suffer from bias if the participants feel satisfied with the service and therefore respond positively when they answer the second time.	the effects were only moderate and health effects still have to be demonstrated in longer follow-up studies. This also points to the fact that improving working conditions must remain a primary goal of stress prevention even though this is sometimes hard to attain in practice	this study had results from a relatively small number of participants ($n = 79$), creating the need for a larger randomized control trial to confirm the results. In addition, 12-month follow-up was not completed to avoid overburdening busy employees. This study limitation precludes us from making a more definitive assessment regarding the long-term effectiveness of the mindfulness intervention

References

1. Roberts, I. Taking age out of the workplace: Putting older workers back in? *Work. Employ. Soc.* **2006**, *20*, 67–86. [CrossRef]
2. Keese, M. *Live Longer, Work Longer: A Synthesis Report*; OECD Publishing: Paris, France, 2006.
3. Poscia, A.; Moscato, U.; La Milia, D.; Milovanovic, S.; Stojanovic, J.; Borghini, A.; Collamati, A.; Ricciardi, W.; Magnavita, N. Workplace health promotion for older workers: A systematic review. *BMC Health Serv. Res.* **2016**, *16*, 415–428. [CrossRef] [PubMed]
4. Possible Public Health Implications of Raising the State Pension Age and how to Mitigate Them—Mitigating Increases in the State Pension Age (MISPA). Available online: https://www.ucl.ac.uk/epidemiology-health-care/sites/epidemiology-health-care/files/mispa_long_text_final_version.pdf (accessed on 13 July 2022).
5. Bravo, G.; Viviani, C.; Lavallière, M.; Arezes, P.; Martinez, M.; Dianat, I.; Bragança, S.; Castellucci, H. Do older workers suffer more workplace injuries? A systematic review. *Int. J. Occup. Saf. Ergnonomics* **2020**, *28*, 1–30. [CrossRef] [PubMed]
6. Sickness Absence in the UK Labour Market—Office for National Statistics. Available online: https://www.ons.gov.uk/employmentandlabourmarket/peopleinwork/labourproductivity/articles/sicknessabsenceinthelabourmarket/2020/ (accessed on 3 June 2022).
7. Work-Related Stress and How to Manage It: Overview—Health and Safety Executive. Available online: https://www.hse.gov.uk/stress/overview.htm (accessed on 3 June 2022).
8. Health at Work—An Independent Review of Sickness Absence by Dame Carol Black and David Frost CBE. Available online: https://assets.publishing.service.gov.uk/government/uploads/system/uploads/attachment_data/file/181060/health-at-work.pdf (accessed on 3 June 2022).
9. Jones, M.; Latreille, P.; Sloane, P.; Staneva, A. Work-related health risks in Europe: Are older workers more vulnerable? *Soc. Sci. Med.* **2013**, *88*, 18–29. [CrossRef]
10. Blackham, A. *Extending Working Life for Older Workers: Age Discrimination Law, Policy and Practice*; Hart Publishing: Oxford, UK, 2016.
11. Pieper, C.; Schröer, S.; Eilerts, A. Evidence of Workplace Interventions—A Systematic Review of Systematic Reviews. *Int. J. Environ. Res. Public Health* **2019**, *16*, 3353. [CrossRef]
12. Page, M.; McKenzie, J.; Bossuyt, P.; Boutron, I.; Hoffmann, T.; Mulrow, C.; Shamseer, L.; Tetzlaff, J.; Akl, E.; Brennan, S.; et al. The PRISMA 2020 statement: An updated guideline for reporting systematic reviews. *BMJ* **2021**, *372*, 1–9.
13. Sayers, A. Tips and tricks in performing a systematic review. *Br. J. Gen. Pract.* **2008**, *58*, 136. [CrossRef]
14. List of OECD Member Countries—Ratification of the Convention on the OECD—OECD. Available online: https://www.oecd.org/about/document/ratification-oecd-convention.htm (accessed on 3 June 2022).
15. Current Retirement Ages—OECD. Available online: https://www.oecd-ilibrary.org/social-issues-migration-health/pensions-at-a-glance-2017/current-retirement-ages_pension_glance-2017-9-en;jsessionid=Dka7fyISbXMfYrchrezDCdWH.ip-10-240-5-16 (accessed on 3 June 2022).
16. Higgins, J.; Sterne, J.; Savović, J.; Page, M.; Hróbjartsson, A.; Boutron, I.; Reeves, B.; Eldridge, S. A revised tool for assessing risk of bias in randomized trials. *Cochrane Database Syst. Rev.* **2016**, *10* (Suppl. S1), 29–31.
17. Hughes, S.; Seymour, R.; Campbell, R.; Shaw, J.; Fabiyi, C.; Sokas, R. Comparison of Two Health-Promotion Programes for Older Workers. *Am. J. Public Health* **2011**, *101*, 883–890. [CrossRef]
18. Malarkey, W.; Jarjoura, D.; Klatt, M. Workplace based mindfulness practice and inflammation: A randomized trial. *Brain Behav. Immun.* **2013**, *27*, 145–154. [CrossRef]
19. Aikens, K.; Astin, J.; Pelletier, K.; Levanovich, K.; Baase, C.; Park, Y.; Bodnar, C. Mindfulness Goes to Work: Impact of an Online Workplace Intervention. *J. Occup. Environ. Med.* **2014**, *56*, 721–731. [CrossRef]
20. Cook, R.; Hersch, R.; Schlossberg, D.; Leaf, S. A Web-Based Health Promotion Program for Older Workers: Randomized Controlled Trial. *J. Med. Internet Res.* **2015**, *17*, e3399. [CrossRef]
21. Largo-Wight, E.; Wlyudka, P.; Merten, J.; Cuvelier, E. Effectiveness and feasibility of a 10-minute employee stress intervention: Outdoor Booster Break. *J. Workplace Behav. Health* **2017**, *32*, 159–171. [CrossRef]
22. Limm, H.; Gundel, H.; Heinmuller, M.; Marten-Mittag, B.; Nater, U.; Siegrist, J.; Angerer, P. Stress management interventions in the workplace improve stress reactivity: A randomised controlled trial. *Occup. Environ. Med.* **2011**, *68*, 126–133. [CrossRef]
23. Hoeve, M.; de Bruin, E.; van Rooij, F.; Bögels, S. Effects of a Mindfulness-Based Intervention for Police Officers. *Mindfulness* **2021**, *12*, 1672–1684. [CrossRef]
24. Ojala, B.; Nygård, C.; Huhtala, H.; Bohle, P.; Nikkari, S. A Cognitive Behavioural Intervention Programme to Improve Psychological Well-Being. *Int. J. Environ. Res. Public Health* **2019**, *16*, 80. [CrossRef]
25. Fischetti, F.; Cataldi, S.; Latino, F.; Greco, G. Effectiveness of multilateral training didactic method on physical and mental wellbeing in law enforcement. In Proceedings of the Spring Conferences of Sports Science. Costa Blanca Sports Science Events, Alicante, Spain, 14–15 June 2019.
26. Calogiuri, G.; Evensen, K.; Weydahl, A.; Andersson, K.; Patil, G.; Ihlebæk, C.; Raanaas, R. Green exercise as a workplace intervention to reduce job stress. Results from a pilot study. *Work* **2016**, *53*, 99–111. [CrossRef]
27. Polit, D.; Beck, C. Generalization in quantitative and qualitative research: Myths and strategies. *Int. J. Nurs. Stud.* **2010**, *47*, 1451–1458. [CrossRef]
28. Steenstra, I.; Cullen, K.; Irvin, E.; Van Eerd, D.; Alavinia, M.; Beaton, D.; Geary, J.; Gignac, M.; Gross, D.; Mahood, Q.; et al. A systematic review of interventions to promote work participation in older workers. *J. Saf. Res.* **2017**, *60*, 93–102. [CrossRef]

29. Kingston, A.; Jagger, C. Review of methodologies of cohort studies of older people. *Age Ageing* **2017**, *47*, 215–219. [CrossRef]
30. Crawford, J.; Graveling, R.; Cowie, H.; Dixon, K. The health safety and health promotion needs of older workers. *Occup. Med.* **2010**, *60*, 184–192. [CrossRef]
31. McDonald, J. Measuring Personality Constructs: The Advantages and Disadvantages of Self Reports, Informant Reports and Behavioural Assessments. *Enquire* **2008**, *1*, 75–94.
32. Griffiths, A. Designing and Managing Healthy Work for Older Workers. *Occup. Med.* **2000**, *50*, 473–477. [CrossRef]
33. Tetrick, L.; Winslow, C. Workplace Stress Manager Interventions and Health Promotion. *Annu. Rev. Organ. Psychol. Organ. Behav.* **2015**, *2*, 583–603. [CrossRef]
34. McDaid, D.; Park, A. Investing in mental health and well-being: Findings from the DataPrev project. *Health Promot. Int.* **2011**, *26*, 108–139. [CrossRef]

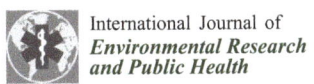

Review

Inequity in Access and Delivery of Virtual Care Interventions: A Scoping Review

Sabuj Kanti Mistry [1,2,*], Miranda Shaw [3], Freya Raffan [3], George Johnson [4], Katelyn Perren [4], Saito Shoko [5], Ben Harris-Roxas [6] and Fiona Haigh [5]

1. Centre for Primary Health Care and Equity, University of New South Wales, Sydney 2052, Australia
2. Department of Public Health, Daffodil International University, Dhaka 1207, Bangladesh
3. RPA Virtual Hospital, Sydney 2050, Australia; miranda.shaw@health.nsw.gov.au (M.S.); freya.raffan@health.nsw.gov.au (F.R.)
4. Sydney Institute for Women, Children and their Families, Sydney Local Health District, Sydney 2050, Australia; george.johnson@health.nsw.gov.au (G.J.); katelyn.perren@health.nsw.gov.au (K.P.)
5. Health Equity Research Development Unit (HERDU), Centre for Primary Health Care & Equity, The University of New South Wales, Sydney Local Health District, Sydney 2050, Australia; s.saito@unsw.edu.au (S.S.); f.haigh@unsw.edu.au (F.H.)
6. School of Population Health, University of New South Wales, Sydney 2052, Australia; b.harris-roxas@unsw.edu.au
* Correspondence: smitra411@gmail.com; Tel.: +61-406863358

Abstract: The objectives of this review were to map and summarize the existing evidence from a global perspective about inequity in access and delivery of virtual care interventions and to identify strategies that may be adopted by virtual care services to address these inequities. We searched *MEDLINE*, *EMBASE*, and *CINAHL* using both medical subject headings (MeSH) and free-text keywords for empirical studies exploring inequity in ambulatory services offered virtually. Forty-one studies were included, most of them cross-sectional in design. Included studies were extracted using a customized extraction tool, and descriptive analysis was performed. The review identified widespread differences in accessing and using virtual care interventions among cultural and ethnic minorities, older people, socioeconomically disadvantaged groups, people with limited digital and/or health literacy, and those with limited access to digital devices and good connectivity. Potential solutions addressing these barriers identified in the review included having digitally literate caregivers present during virtual care appointments, conducting virtual care appointments in culturally sensitive manner, and having a focus on enhancing patients' digital literacy. We identified evidence-based practices for virtual care interventions to ensure equity in access and delivery for their virtual care patients.

Keywords: inequality; health equity; health services; virtual care; COVID-19; scoping review

Citation: Mistry, S.K.; Shaw, M.; Raffan, F.; Johnson, G.; Perren, K.; Shoko, S.; Harris-Roxas, B.; Haigh, F. Inequity in Access and Delivery of Virtual Care Interventions: A Scoping Review. *Int. J. Environ. Res. Public Health* **2022**, *19*, 9411. https://doi.org/10.3390/ijerph19159411

Academic Editors: Jessica Sheringham and Sarah Sowden

Received: 19 May 2022
Accepted: 27 July 2022
Published: 1 August 2022

Publisher's Note: MDPI stays neutral with regard to jurisdictional claims in published maps and institutional affiliations.

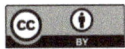

Copyright: © 2022 by the authors. Licensee MDPI, Basel, Switzerland. This article is an open access article distributed under the terms and conditions of the Creative Commons Attribution (CC BY) license (https://creativecommons.org/licenses/by/4.0/).

1. Introduction

Health inequities are referred to as those differences in health that are systemic, avoidable, unfair, and unjust [1]. A health equity approach recognises that not everyone has the same level of health or level of resources to address their health problems, and it may therefore be important apply different approaches in order to achieve similar health outcomes [2,3]. Health inequities are associated with a range of factors including age, gender, ethnicity, geographic location, and socioeconomic status [1,4]. A recent report has documented nine drivers of health inequity in relation to healthcare services: housing, income and wealth, health system and services, education, employment, social environment, transport, public safety, and physical environment [5]. Outcomes are determined by the dynamic interaction between service users and the health systems [6]. The World Health Organization (WHO) also identified gender, education, income, employment status, and ethnicity as the major factors associated with health inequity [7]. Health inequities are an established global phenomenon [8,9] and is a particular concern in a multicultural country with a history of settler colonialism, such as Australia [10,11]. Evidence demonstrates that the determinants of health inequity often lead to adverse health outcomes in the form of morbidities and mortality among vulnerable and marginalised populations [4,12,13].

Virtual care can be defined as "any interaction between patients and/or members of their care team occurring remotely, using technology with the aim of facilitating or maximising the quality and effectiveness of patient care" [14]. It has been identified as an approach that may partially address health inequities through improving access and availability of health services [15,16]. However, there are also concerns that virtual care services could exacerbate existing health inequities if services are not accessible, available, and acceptable to vulnerable population [17,18]. Virtual care interventions received particular attention during the COVID-19 pandemic, as many health services rapidly transitioned to providing virtual care services as an emergency method of reaching their clients [19]. The restriction of in-person health services and the rapid implementation of virtual care has been driven by necessity but also presents a significant opportunity to develop and strengthen the provision of virtual care [20–22]. However, this expansion in virtual care services using healthcare technologies also created the potential for the widespread digital divide to act as a potent barrier in successful implementation of virtual care interventions and a cause of health inequities. The digital divide is defined as disproportionate access and utilization of health technology and internet among certain population groups, characterised by their geographical, social, and geopolitical criteria or other features [23]. There are suggestions of a "digital paradox" where the "population groups that could potentially benefit most from digital innovations are the ones that would experience the highest barriers to access" [24].

Recently, several studies were conducted on the expansion of virtual care interventions, particularly in relation to the COVID-19 pandemic [25–27]. Many of these studies considered virtual care as a way of minimising the risk of COVID-19 transmission [26,28], to triage during emergency responses [21] and monitoring patients within their homes [21]. One such intervention is the RPA Virtual Hospital (rpavirtual), launched in February 2020 as a new model of care that combines integrated hospital and community care with digital solutions. It was the first service to introduce virtual care for COVID-19-stable patients in isolation in New South Wales, Australia, and has been demonstrated to be widely accepted by patients [29]. However, the potential equity issues related to rpavirtual and other similar virtual care interventions have not yet been adequately explored and described. Therefore, this scoping review aims to map and summarize the knowledge about equity issues in the access and delivery of virtual care interventions and to identify strategies to address potential inequities that may be adopted by virtual care services.

2. Materials and Methods

This scoping review is reported following the guidelines of PRISMA-ScR (Preferred Reporting Items for Systematic Reviews and Meta-analysis extension for Scoping Reviews) [30]. The review protocol is registered at the website of Centre for Primary Health Care and Equity, UNSW Sydney (https://cphce.unsw.edu.au/research/rapid-literature-review-identify-equity-issues-access-and-delivery-virtual-care, accessed on 1 March 2022), and PRISMA-ScR is provided in Supplementary Table S1.

2.1. Data Sources

We searched for peer-reviewed articles in electronic databases: *Medline*, *EMBASE*, and *CINAHL*. Both medical subject headings (MeSH) and free-text keywords were used to search relevant articles in these databases that were published in the English language between January 2010 and January 2021. The detailed search strategy is presented in Table 1.

Table 1. Search strategy.

Sl.	Search Terms
1	"telemedicine" [MeSH Terms] OR "telemedicine" [Text Word]
2	"tele medicine" [Text Word]
3	"telehealth" [Text Word]
4	"tele health" [Text Word]
5	"tele-health" [Text Word]
6	"e-health" [Text Word]
7	"teletherapy" [Text Word]
8	"virtual care" [Text Word]
9	"virtual health" [Text Word]
10	1 or 2 or 3 or 4 or 5 or 6 or 7 or 8 or 9
11	"disparit*" [Text Word]
12	"health equity" [MeSH Terms] OR "health equity" [Text Word]
13	"equit*" [Text Word]
14	"inequit*" [Text Word]
15	"inequalit*" [Text Word]
16	"healthcare disparities" [MeSH Terms] OR "health care disparities" [Text Word]
17	"health status disparities" [MeSH Terms] OR "health status disparities" [Text Word]
18	10 or 11 or 12 or 13 or 14 or 15 or 16 or 17
19	10 and 18

2.2. Study Selection

The articles yielded in the initial database searches were assessed by two independent reviewers in relation to the inclusion and exclusion criteria developed for this study (Box 1). All of the steps of study selection procedure were performed in Covidence (https://www.covidence.org, accessed on 1 March 2022). In the first stage, the title and abstract of the articles were assessed by two reviewers. The articles that passed this initial screening stage entered full text screening. The full texts of these articles were obtained, and more in-depth assessment was carried out against the inclusion and exclusion criteria. The reason for the exclusion for each of the articles was also noted at this stage. Any difference in assessment between the reviewers was resolved by discussion.

Box 1. Inclusion and exclusion criteria.

Inclusion criteria
- Published in English
- Published between January 2010 and January 2021
- Studies exploring equity in ambulatory services offered virtually
- Carried out in OECD countries
- Empirical studies

Exclusion criteria
- Published in language other than English
- Published before January 2010
- Studies not exploring equity in ambulatory services offered virtually
- Studies exploring robotic/tele-surgery
- Studies carried outside OECD countries
- Commentary/review/opinion pieces

2.3. Data Extraction

The data were extracted from the included studies in a Microsoft Excel template developed by the authors. Information including country, study setting, study design, study participants, characteristics of the intervention/study, type of virtual care modalities, type of inequity issues identified/addressed, main findings, summary of the results, and relevance to virtual care interventions were extracted.

2.4. Data Mapping

As the objective of scoping reviews is to map and summarize the available evidence, we performed descriptive analysis, which involved frequency counting and basic thematic coding [31].

3. Results

3.1. Search Results

Database searches yielded a total of 3021 articles, from which 1990 underwent screening after removal of the duplicates. The assessment of the title and abstract of the articles resulted in the exclusion of 1901 articles, and 89 articles underwent full-text screening. Finally, 41 articles satisfied the selection criteria and were included in the review (Figure 1). The detailed characteristics of the included studies are presented in Supplementary Table S2.

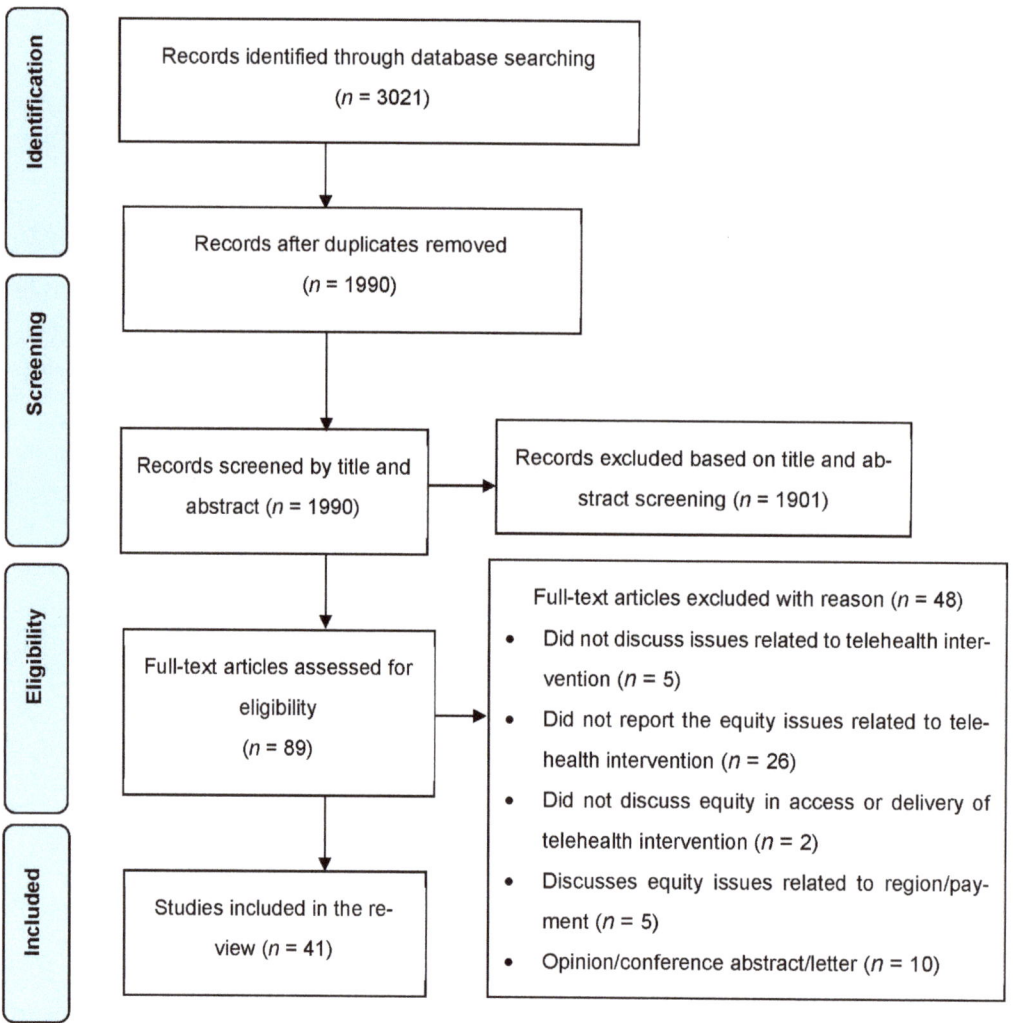

Figure 1. PRISMA diagram of study selection.

3.2. Study Settings

Of the forty-one included studies, thirty-one were conducted in the USA, three were carried out in Australia [32–34], two in Canada [35,36], one in Italy [37], one in China [38], one in Germany [39], one in Norway [40], and one in Scotland [41]. The studies were carried out either in a community or in a clinical setting, such as a hospital or primary care.

3.3. Study Designs

A range of study designs were used in the included studies. Twenty-three of the included studies followed a cross sectional design [5,32,34,36–55], five studies carried out retrospective analysis of the collected data [56–60], six studies followed cohort design [61–66], two were randomised controlled trials [67,68], and two followed a mixed-method design [33,69]. One study followed a combination of retrospective analysis and cross-sectional study design, [70] while the study design was not clear in two studies [35,71].

3.4. Type of Participants

The participants in most of the studies were adults, often with chronic conditions such as diabetes [45], cardiovascular disease [39], and mental health problems [61]. Most of the studies considered both native English speakers and those speaking languages other than English. Only a few studies considered all participants speaking a language other than English, such as Spanish [56] or Chinese [34]. Several studies examined outcomes of specific cultural and ethnic minorities. However, since most of the included studies were conducted in the USA, the population groups were mostly Black, Hispanic, and African American [46,48,50,54,55,60,66–68].

3.5. Virtual Care Modalities

The included studies considered several modalities of virtual care interventions ranging from video conferencing [37,41,42,44,46,48,49,51,57,59–64,66,67,71], teleconferencing [34,35,46,48,49,51,53,54,56–58,60,62,63,66,71], messaging [42,45,50], emails [42], health apps [5,39,40,50], patient portals [58,61,68,70], personal health records [59,61], and eHealth service use via the Internet [32,40,47,69].

The majority of the studies described the use of virtual visits (either video or audio) in comparison to face-to-face visit or video visit in comparison to audio/tele visit. Several video conferencing platforms, such as Zoom (https://zoom.us/, accessed on 1 March 2022) or Microsoft Teams (https://www.microsoft.com/en-au/microsoft-teams/group-chat-software/, accessed on 1 March 2022), were used to perform video visits in the reported studies. Some of the studies reported on non-synchronous communication tools such as text messaging, health apps, patient portals, or eHealth service use. Text messaging, health apps, or patient portals were generally used to book appointments with service providers, access health information, track health outcomes, or communicate with health service providers. On the other hand, eHealth services were offered to promote online learning, counselling, and information sharing, and these aims were accomplished through browsing search engines, health apps, social media, and video services.

3.6. Types of Inequity Issues Identified/Addressed

3.6.1. Cultural and Ethnic Inequities

Twenty-one studies [33,42,44–46,48,50,54,55,57,59–68,70] explored cultural and ethnic inequities in access to virtual care services and outcomes. The majority of these found that cultural and ethnic minorities, including those of African American, Black, Hispanic or Latinos, Asian American, Aboriginal and Torres Strait Islander, or Filipino descent, were less likely to access virtual care services compared to the White participants. For example, in their study, Schifeling and colleagues [60] found that non-White patients were less likely to have a video visit than White patients. Likewise, Walker et al. [68] found that African American patients used the patient portal less than White patients (40.4% difference, $p = 0.004$). However, four studies [42,44,50,65] reported a different result where the likelihood of using virtual care services was higher among the cultural and ethnic minorities compared to White participants.

3.6.2. Sociodemographic and Socio-Economic Inequities

Older people were identified as experiencing significant barriers to accessing and using virtual care services in most of the studies [5,32,36,38,39,41,43,45–50,55,60,61,63,65,68,70,71]. For example, Leng et al. [41] found that the patients under 60 years were over two times more likely to use video consulting (odds ratio (OR) 2.2, 95% CI 2.1–6.6). Nelson et al. [45] also pointed out that the probability of responding to texts tended to increase from about age 25 years until roughly age 50 years and then appeared to decrease with increasing age. Eberly et al. [64] further noted that younger participants were more likely to be engaged with video call appointments compared to telephone call. The only exception was reported by Pierce et al. [46], where age of 65 years and above was associated with higher odds of virtual care use (OR 1.21, 95% CI 1.05–1.40). It is also notable to mention that all nine studies [33,39,46,53,57,61,63–65] that explored the role of gender in accessing virtual care services found that females were less likely to use virtual care services compared to males. Two studies [63,65] also found that unmarried participants were less likely to access virtual care services. Meanwhile, Wegerman et al. [66] found that participants who were single or previously married (separated, divorced, widowed) had higher odds of completing a telephone appointment, while married participants were more likely to complete a video appointment.

Thirteen studies explored the use of virtual care in relation to the socioeconomic status of the participants, and all of these found that lower socioeconomic status was associated with lower use of virtual care services [5,32,33,38–40,47,48,50,51,61,63,67]. Alam et al. [32] reported that access to virtual care services was lower among participants from disadvantaged socioeconomic backgrounds. Likewise, other studies [5,33,38,40,48,50,51,61,63] also reported that low socioeconomic status was associated with decreased access to virtual care services. Not surprisingly, some of the included studies that explored the role of education in accessing virtual care services [5,32,33,38–40,47,48,50,67] also found that participants with lower education status were less likely to access the virtual care services.

3.6.3. Inequity Issues Related to Digital/eHealth Literacy

Seven studies [32,38,39,41,45,56,69] reported a lack of digital/eHealth literacy among the participants as a significant barrier to accessing virtual care services. Ernsting and colleagues [39] found that mHealth app users had higher levels of eHealth literacy compared to non-app users. A study [69] also reported that eHealth literacy increase was associated with a 3% increase in the number of searches for health information on the internet (beta = 0.03, 95% CI 0.00–0.06). Meanwhile, Leng et al. [41] found that higher computer proficiency correlated with an increased willingness to engage in video consultations.

3.6.4. Technological Inequities

Several studies [32,37,48,50] also found that improved access to digital devices and internet can increase the use of virtual care services. Arighi et al. [37] reported that issues such as a lack of devices (computers, phones, or tablets) with internet connection and poor internet connections were the main causes of failed virtual care. Alam et al. [32] pointed out that access to broadband internet services was associated with increased use of virtual care services.

4. Discussion

This review was conducted to explore inequity issues in relation to access to and delivery of virtual care interventions and to consider the international evidence of actions to address inequity issues that may be adopted by or provide learnings for rpavirtual and other similar virtual care interventions. The main drivers of inequity in access to virtual care identified in the literature review were relatively older age, unemployment, less income, lower education level, belonging to cultural or ethnic minorities, lack of access to digital devices or good internet connection, and lack of digital/eHealth literacy.

In recent times, due to the COVID-19 pandemic, virtual care interventions have been widely used due to restricted in-person health service delivery [25,26]. It has also been documented that the patient experience and their acceptance of virtual care during this pandemic has been generally good [72,73]. At the same time, it is also worth noting that the expansion of this digital innovation without due consideration of strategies to address inequity of access has the potential to increase health inequities due to poverty, digital health literacy, and lack of access to digital technology among some of the population [74].

Reviews carried out during the COVID-19 pandemic [75,76] also stressed the importance of virtual care interventions as an alternative to in-person health service delivery during a period of restrictions on face-to-face health service delivery. Doraiswami et al. (2020) [75] reported that virtual care could play a pivotal role in the health sector in future, but its feasibility and implementation in a resource-poor setting is challenging. In this regard, it is critical to mention that future virtual care interventions will be influenced by broader health and clinical governance agendas and directions in investment across systems.

While some recent reviews [77–79] have highlighted the effectiveness of virtual care as a way of delivering health care in a cost-effective way, with improved patient communication, outcomes, and satisfaction, the equity dimension of the virtual care interventions is not fully addressed in these reviews. The present review has helped to bridge the knowledge gap around inequity issues associated with virtual care and identified areas for further research.

The present review highlighted that access to virtual care services is particularly limited among patients from ethnic minorities, which suggests there is a need to carefully tailor services to ensure equitable access. Multilingual and culturally sensitive virtual care services can be of high value in this regard. For example, a culturally sensitive approach documented by Shaw et al. (2013) [34] could be to address cultural diversity in the developing of a virtual care intervention. This qualitative study was conducted among Chinese and Arabic patients and their carers to explore their willingness to take part in a telephone-based supportive-care intervention. The majority of the study participants supported the provision of a culturally sensitive intervention in their own language via an online platform. However, the participants identified that confidentiality of the clinical information was a concern and preferred an initial in-person appointment with patients to increase participation. It was also suggested that there should be the provision of an "on-call" support process initiated by patients to provide patients with access to assistance in times of high need between scheduled calls.

Access to virtual care services is linked to the level of digital literacy of the patients. For example, Ernsting et al. [39] and Guendelman et al. [69] strongly emphasised the importance of improving digital literacy of patients in order to address inequity of access to virtual care services. Older people and individuals with limited digital health literacy are less likely to access virtual care services and require targeted support. The present review indicates that availability of younger caregivers or caregivers with higher digital literacy can result in increased access to virtual care services [37].

Consideration of different levels of digital and health literacy across patients should be a part of routine planning for virtual care services. For example, an educational component can be incorporated in interventions to increase virtual care literacy among vulnerable patients. In addition, delivery methods can be updated, for example, by adapting portals to be comfortably used by less digitally literate patients or appropriately tailoring information or platforms to vulnerable patients.

Virtual care service delivery planning should consider the variances in service uptake between different socioeconomic classes. Access to digital resources influences a person's capacity to access and utilise virtual care. Research has also documented that the digital divide in terms of access to digital devices and strong internet connectivity is significant among people with lower level of education and lesser income [80,81]. When engaging patients with virtual care services, consideration should be given as to whether patients have access to appropriate devices and a reliable internet connection. rpavirtual and other similar virtual care interventions should include in their referral process that patients require devices and internet connection to access services.

This review was subject to some limitations. There are several synonyms used to represent inequity issues in the literature. While we were broad in searching the literature, we may still have missed some articles utilising different terminology. However, we explored both the MeSH terms and keywords to address this. We also limited our searches to three major databases, and there could be additional relevant articles available in other databases. We searched for only the peer-reviewed articles and therefore might have missed some grey publications.

We restricted our searches to English literature only, and therefore, we could miss relevant articles that are written in a language other than English. Furthermore, we only searched for studies published in last decade (January 2010–January 2021); therefore, we could miss some articles published before 2010 and after 2021.

5. Conclusions

This review highlights that while there is potential for virtual care to improve health service delivery, particularly during the COVID-19 pandemic, there can be widespread inequities in access to and delivery of virtual care interventions. These inequities are based on sociodemographic characteristics of the participants, such as age, gender, and ethnicity as well as other factors, such as access to appropriate digital technology, digital and health literacy, cultural acceptability, and trust and perceived quality of care. This review has identified several promising practices, such as the inclusion of young and educated caregivers, providing culturally sensitive interventions, and improving digital health literacy among patients. These strategies can be adopted by rpavirtual and other virtual care interventions to ensure equity in access and delivery of virtual care services. Future research should focus on how these promising practices can be implemented in clinical settings.

Supplementary Materials: The following supporting information can be downloaded at: https://www.mdpi.com/article/10.3390/ijerph19159411/s1, Table S1: Preferred Reporting Items for Systematic reviews and Meta-Analyses extension for Scoping Reviews (PRISMA-ScR) Checklist; Table S2: Characteristics of included studies.

Author Contributions: Conceptualization, S.K.M., M.S., B.H.-R., G.J. and F.H.; methodology, S.K.M., B.H.-R., G.J. and F.H.; formal analysis, S.K.M., F.R., G.J., K.P. and S.S.; writing—original draft preparation, S.K.M., K.P., S.S. and F.R.; writing—review and editing, M.S., G.J., B.H.-R. and F.H.; supervision, M.S., B.H.-R. and F.H.; project administration, S.K.M., M.S., B.H.-R., G.J., K.P. and F.H. All authors have read and agreed to the published version of the manuscript.

Funding: This research received funding from Sydney Local Health District.

Institutional Review Board Statement: Not applicable.

Informed Consent Statement: Not applicable.

Data Availability Statement: Not applicable.

Conflicts of Interest: The authors declare no conflict of interest.

References

1. Whitehead, M.; Dahlgren, G. *Policies and Strategies to Promote Social Equity in Health*; Institute for Future Studies: Stockholm, Sweden, 1991.
2. Braveman, P.; Gruskin, S. Defining equity in health. *J. Epidemiol. Community Health* **2003**, *57*, 254–258. [CrossRef]
3. Braveman, P. What are health disparities and health equity? We need to be clear. *Public Health Rep.* **2014**, *129* (Suppl. S2), 5–8. [CrossRef] [PubMed]

4. Baciu, A.; Negussie, Y.; Geller, A.; Weinstein, J.N.; National Academies of Sciences Engineering and Medicine. The root causes of health inequity. In *Communities in Action: Pathways to Health Equity*; National Academies Press: Washington, DC, USA, 2017.
5. Marrie, R.A.; Leung, S.; Tyry, T.; Cutter, G.R.; Fox, R.; Salter, A. Use of eHealth and mHealth technology by persons with multiple sclerosis. *Mult. Scler. Relat. Disord.* **2019**, *27*, 13–19. [CrossRef]
6. Levesque, J.-F.; Harris, M.F.; Russell, G. Patient-centred access to health care: Conceptualising access at the interface of health systems and populations. *Int. J. Equity Health* **2013**, *12*, 18. [CrossRef] [PubMed]
7. World Health Organization. Health Inequities and Their Causes. 2018. Available online: https://www.who.int/news-room/facts-in-pictures/detail/health-inequities-and-their-causes (accessed on 18 May 2022).
8. The Lancet. Taking urgent action on health inequities. *Lancet* **2020**, *395*, 659. [CrossRef]
9. Friel, S.; Marmot, M.G. Action on the social determinants of health and health inequities goes global. *Annu. Rev. Public Health* **2011**, *32*, 225–236. [CrossRef] [PubMed]
10. Zhao, Y.; You, J.; Wright, J.; Guthridge, S.L.; Lee, A.H. Health inequity in the northern territory, Australia. *Int. J. Equity Health* **2013**, *12*, 79. [CrossRef] [PubMed]
11. Flavel, J.; McKee, M.; Freeman, T.; Musolino, C.; van Eyk, H.; Tesfay, F.H.; Baum, F. The need for improved Australian data on social determinants of health inequities. *Med. J. Aust.* **2022**, *216*, 388–391. [CrossRef] [PubMed]
12. Garcia-Subirats, I.; Vargas, I.; Mogollón-Pérez, A.S.; De Paepe, P.; Da Silva, M.R.F.; Unger, J.P.; Borrell, C.; Vázquez, M.L. Inequities in access to health care in different health systems: A study in municipalities of central Colombia and north-eastern Brazil. *Int. J. Equity Health* **2014**, *13*, 10. [CrossRef] [PubMed]
13. Woodward, A.; Kawachi, I. Why reduce health inequalities? *J. Epidemiol. Community Health* **2000**, *54*, 923–929. [CrossRef]
14. Agency for Clinical Innovation. *Virtual Care in Practice*; Agency for Clinical Innovation: St. Leonards, NSW, Australia, 2021.
15. Khairat, S.; Haithcoat, T.; Liu, S.; Zaman, T.; Edson, B.; Gianforcaro, R.; Shyu, C.R. Advancing health equity and access using telemedicine: A geospatial assessment. *J. Am. Med. Inform. Assoc.* **2019**, *26*, 796–805. [CrossRef] [PubMed]
16. Barbosa, W.; Zhou, K.; Waddell, E.; Myers, T.; Dorsey, E.R. Improving Access to Care: Telemedicine Across Medical Domains. *Annu. Rev. Public Health* **2021**, *42*, 463–481. [CrossRef]
17. Katzow, M.W.; Steinway, C.; Jan, S. Telemedicine and health disparities during COVID-19. *Pediatrics* **2020**, *146*, e20201586. [CrossRef] [PubMed]
18. Velasquez, D.; Mehrotra, A. Ensuring the growth of telehealth during COVID-19 does not exacerbate disparities in care. *Health Aff. Blog* **2020**, *10*, 1–306. [CrossRef]
19. Harris-Roxas, B. The Impact and Effectiveness of Equity Focused Health Impact Assessment in Health Service Planning. Ph.D. Thesis, University of New South Wales, Sydney, Australia, 2014.
20. Chauhan, V.; Galwankar, S.; Arquilla, B.; Garg, M.; Di Somma, S.; El-Menyar, A.; Krishnan, V.; Gerber, J.; Holland, R.; Stawicki, S.P. Novel coronavirus (COVID-19): Leveraging telemedicine to optimize care while minimizing exposures and viral transmission. *J. Emergencies Trauma Shock.* **2020**, *13*, 20.
21. Hollander, J.E.; Carr, B.G. Virtually perfect? Telemedicine for COVID-19. *N. Engl. J. Med.* **2020**, *382*, 1679–1681. [CrossRef] [PubMed]
22. Denadai, R. COVID-19 pandemic as a driver for spreading virtual care globally: The future starts now. *Clinics* **2020**, *75*, e1967. [CrossRef] [PubMed]
23. López, L.; Green, A.R.; Tan-McGrory, A.; King, R.S.; Betancourt, J.R. Bridging the digital divide in health care: The role of health information technology in addressing racial and ethnic disparities. *Jt. Comm. J. Qual. Patient Saf.* **2011**, *37*, 437–445. [CrossRef]
24. Wong, B.L.H.; Maaß, L.; Vodden, A.; van Kessel, R.; Sorbello, S.; Buttigieg, S.; Odone, A.; Section, D.H.; European Public Health Association. The dawn of digital public health in Europe: Implications for public health policy and practice. *Lancet Reg. Health-Eur.* **2022**, *14*, 100316. [CrossRef] [PubMed]
25. Fisk, M.; Livingstone, A.; Pit, S.W. Telehealth in the context of COVID-19: Changing perspectives in Australia, the United Kingdom, and the United States. *J. Med. Internet Res.* **2020**, *22*, e19264. [CrossRef]
26. Monaghesh, E.; Hajizadeh, A. The role of telehealth during COVID-19 outbreak: A systematic review based on current evidence. *BMC Public Health* **2020**, *20*, 1193. [CrossRef] [PubMed]
27. Hutchings, O.R.; Dearing, C.; Jagers, D.; Shaw, M.J.; Raffan, F.; Jones, A.; Taggart, R.; Sinclair, T.; Anderson, T.; Ritchie, A.G. Virtual health care for community management of patients with COVID-19 in Australia: Observational cohort study. *J. Med. Internet Res.* **2021**, *23*, e21064. [CrossRef] [PubMed]
28. Legler, S.; Diehl, M.; Hilliard, B.; Olson, A.; Markowitz, R.; Tignanelli, C.; Melton, G.B.; Broccard, A.; Kirsch, J.; Usher, M. Evaluation of an intrahospital telemedicine program for patients admitted with COVID-19: Mixed methods study. *J. Med. Internet Res.* **2021**, *23*, e25987. [CrossRef] [PubMed]
29. Raffan, F.; Anderson, T.; Sinclair, T.; Shaw, M.; Amanatidis, S.; Thapa, R.; Nilsson, S.J.; Jagers, D.; Wilson, A.; Haigh, F. The Virtual Care Experience of Patients Diagnosed With COVID-19. *J. Patient Exp.* **2021**, *8*, 23743735211008310. [CrossRef] [PubMed]
30. Tricco, A.C.; Lillie, E.; Zarin, W.; O'Brien, K.K.; Colquhoun, H.; Levac, D.; Moher, D.; Peters, M.D.; Horsley, T.; Weeks, L.; et al. PRISMA extension for scoping reviews (PRISMA-ScR): Checklist and explanation. *Ann. Intern. Med.* **2018**, *169*, 467–473. [CrossRef] [PubMed]

31. Pollock, D.; Davies, E.L.; Peters, M.D.; Tricco, A.C.; Alexander, L.; McInerney, P.; Godfrey, C.M.; Khalil, H.; Munn, Z. Undertaking a scoping review: A practical guide for nursing and midwifery students, clinicians, researchers, and academics. *J. Adv. Nurs.* **2021**, *77*, 2102–2113. [CrossRef]
32. Alam, K.; Mahumud, R.A.; Alam, F.; Keramat, S.A.; Erdiaw-Kwasie, M.O.; Sarker, A.R. Determinants of access to eHealth services in regional Australia. *Int. J. Med. Inform.* **2019**, *131*, 103960. [CrossRef]
33. Foley, K.; Freeman, T.; Ward, P.; Lawler, A.; Osborne, R.; Fisher, M. Exploring access to, use of and benefits from population-oriented digital health services in Australia. *Health Promot. Int.* **2020**, *26*, 1105–1115. [CrossRef] [PubMed]
34. Shaw, J.; Butow, P.; Sze, M.; Young, J.; Goldstein, D. Reducing disparity in outcomes for immigrants with cancer: A qualitative assessment of the feasibility and acceptability of a culturally targeted telephone-based supportive care intervention. *Supportive Care Cancer* **2013**, *21*, 2297–2301. [CrossRef] [PubMed]
35. Arora, S.; Kurji, A.K.; Tennant, M.T. Dismantling sociocultural barriers to eye care with tele-ophthalmology: Lessons from an Alberta Cree community. *Clin. Investig. Med. Med. Clin. Exp.* **2013**, *36*, E57–E63. [CrossRef] [PubMed]
36. Mangin, D.; Parascandalo, J.; Khudoyarova, O.; Agarwal, G.; Bismah, V.; Orr, S. Multimorbidity, eHealth and implications for equity: A cross-sectional survey of patient perspectives on eHealth. *BMJ Open* **2019**, *9*, e023731. [CrossRef] [PubMed]
37. Arighi, A.; Fumagalli, G.G.; Carandini, T.; Pietroboni, A.M.; De Riz, M.A.; Galimberti, D.; Scarpini, E. Facing the digital divide into a dementia clinic during COVID-19 pandemic: Caregiver age matters. *Neurol. Sci.* **2021**, *42*, 1247–1251. [CrossRef] [PubMed]
38. Li, P.; Luo, Y.; Yu, X.; Wen, J.; Mason, E.; Li, W.; Jalali, M.S. Patients' Perceptions of Barriers and Facilitators to the Adoption of E-Hospitals: Cross-Sectional Study in Western China. *J. Med. Internet Res.* **2020**, *22*, e17221. [CrossRef] [PubMed]
39. Ernsting, C.; Stühmann, L.M.; Dombrowski, S.U.; Voigt-Antons, J.N.; Kuhlmey, A.; Gellert, P. Associations of Health App Use and Perceived Effectiveness in People with Cardiovascular Diseases and Diabetes: Population-Based Survey. *JMIR Mhealth Uhealth* **2019**, *7*, e12179. [CrossRef] [PubMed]
40. Hansen, A.H.; Bradway, M.; Broz, J.; Claudi, T.; Henriksen, Ø.; Wangberg, S.C.; Årsand, E. Inequalities in the Use of eHealth Between Socioeconomic Groups Among Patients with Type 1 and Type 2 Diabetes: Cross-Sectional Study. *J. Med. Internet Res.* **2019**, *21*, e13615. [CrossRef]
41. Leng, S.; MacDougall, M.; McKinstry, B. The acceptability to patients of video-consulting in general practice: Semi-structured interviews in three diverse general practices. *J. Innov. Health Inform.* **2016**, *23*, 141. [CrossRef]
42. Campos-Castillo, C.; Anthony, D. Racial and ethnic differences in self-reported telehealth use during the COVID-19 pandemic: A secondary analysis of a US survey of internet users from late March. *J. Am. Med. Inform. Assoc.* **2021**, *28*, 119–125. [CrossRef]
43. Gordon, N.P.; Hornbrook, M.C. Older adults' readiness to engage with eHealth patient education and self-care resources: A cross-sectional survey. *BMC Health Serv. Res.* **2018**, *18*, 220. [CrossRef]
44. Khoong, E.C.; Butler, B.A.; Mesina, O.; Su, G.; DeFries, T.B.; Nijagal, M.; Lyles, C.R. Patient interest in and barriers to telemedicine video visits in a multilingual urban safety-net system. *J. Am. Med. Inform. Assoc.* **2020**, *28*, 349–353. [CrossRef]
45. Nelson, L.A.; Mulvaney, S.A.; Gebretsadik, T.; Ho, Y.X.; Johnson, K.B.; Osborn, C.Y. Disparities in the use of a mHealth medication adherence promotion intervention for low-income adults with type 2 diabetes. *J. Am. Med. Inform. Assoc.* **2016**, *23*, 12–18. [CrossRef]
46. Pierce, R.P.; Stevermer, J.J. Disparities in use of telehealth at the onset of the COVID-19 public health emergency. *J. Telemed. Telecare* **2020**, 1–7. [CrossRef] [PubMed]
47. Potdar, R.; Thomas, A.; DiMeglio, M.; Mohiuddin, K.; Djibo, D.A.; Laudanski, K.; Dourado, C.M.; Leighton, J.C.; Ford, J.G. Access to internet, smartphone usage, and acceptability of mobile health technology among cancer patients. *Supportive Care Cancer* **2020**, *28*, 5455–5461. [CrossRef] [PubMed]
48. Rodriguez, J.A.; Betancourt, J.R.; Sequist, T.D.; Ganguli, I. Differences in the use of telephone and video telemedicine visits during the COVID-19 pandemic. *Am. J. Manag. Care* **2021**, *27*, 21–26. [CrossRef] [PubMed]
49. Severe, J.; Tang, R.; Horbatch, F.; Onishchenko, R.; Naini, V.; Blazek, M.C. Factors Influencing Patients' Initial Decisions Regarding Telepsychiatry Participation During the COVID-19 Pandemic: Telephone-Based Survey. *JMIR Form. Res.* **2020**, *4*, e25469. [CrossRef] [PubMed]
50. Spooner, K.K.; Salemi, J.L.; Salihu, H.M.; Zoorob, R.J. eHealth patient-provider communication in the United States: Interest, inequalities, and predictors. *J. Am. Med. Inform. Assoc.* **2017**, *24*, e18–e27. [CrossRef]
51. Tam, S.; Wu, V.F.; Williams, A.M.; Girgis, M.; Sheqwara, J.Z.; Siddiqui, F.; Chang, S.S. Disparities in the Uptake of Telemedicine During the COVID-19 Surge in a Multidisciplinary Head and Neck Cancer Population by Patient Demographic Characteristics and Socioeconomic Status. *JAMA Otolaryngol. Head Neck Surg.* **2020**, *147*, 209–211. [CrossRef]
52. Tong, T.; Myers, A.K.; Bissoonauth, A.A.; Pekmezaris, R.; Kozikowski, A. Identifying the barriers and perceptions of non-Hispanic black and Hispanic/Latino persons with uncontrolled type 2 diabetes for participation in a home Telemonitoring feasibility study: A quantitative analysis of those who declined participation, withdrew or were non-adherent. *Ethn. Health* **2020**, *25*, 485–494.
53. Van Veen, T.; Binz, S.; Muminovic, M.; Chaudhry, K.; Rose, K.; Calo, S.; Rammal, J.A.; France, J.; Miller, J.B. Potential of mobile health technology to reduce health disparities in underserved communities. *West. J. Emerg. Med.* **2019**, *20*, 799–803. [CrossRef]
54. Wang, Y.; Do, D.P.; Wilson, F.A. Immigrants' Use of eHealth Services in the United States, National Health Interview Survey, 2011–2015. *Public Health Rep.* **2018**, *133*, 677–684. [CrossRef]
55. Weber, E.; Miller, S.J.; Astha, V.; Janevic, T.; Benn, E. Characteristics of telehealth users in NYC for COVID-related care during the coronavirus pandemic. *J. Am. Med. Inform. Assoc.* **2020**, *27*, 1949–1954. [CrossRef]

56. Blundell, A.R.; Kroshinsky, D.; Hawryluk, E.B.; Das, S. Disparities in telemedicine access for Spanish-speaking patients during the COVID-19 crisis. *Pediatric Dermatol.* **2020**, *38*, 947–949. [CrossRef]
57. Gilson, S.F.; Umscheid, C.A.; Laiteerapong, N.; Ossey, G.; Nunes, K.J.; Shah, S.D. Growth of Ambulatory Virtual Visits and Differential Use by Patient Sociodemographics at One Urban Academic Medical Center During the COVID-19 Pandemic: Retrospective Analysis. *JMIR Med. Inform.* **2020**, *8*, e24544. [CrossRef] [PubMed]
58. Jiang, W.; Magit, A.E.; Carvalho, D. Equal Access to Telemedicine during COVID-19 Pandemic: A Pediatric Otolaryngology Perspective. *Laryngoscope* **2020**, *131*, 1175–1179. [CrossRef] [PubMed]
59. Kemp, M.T.; Williams, A.M.; Sharma, S.B.; Biesterveld, B.E.; Wakam, G.K.; Matusko, N.; Wilson, J.K.; Cohen, M.S.; Alam, H.B. Barriers associated with failed completion of an acute care general surgery telehealth clinic visit. *Surgery* **2020**, *168*, 851–858. [CrossRef] [PubMed]
60. Schifeling, C.H.; Shanbhag, P.; Johnson, A.; Atwater, R.C.; Koljack, C.; Parnes, B.L.; Vejar, M.M.; Farro, S.A.; Phimphasone-Brady, P.; Lum, H.D. Disparities in Video and Telephone Visits Among Older Adults During the COVID-19 Pandemic: Cross-Sectional Analysis. *JMIR Aging* **2020**, *3*, e23176. [CrossRef] [PubMed]
61. Abel, E.A.; Shimada, S.L.; Wang, K.; Ramsey, C.; Skanderson, M.; Erdos, J.; Godleski, L.; Houston, T.K.; Brandt, C.A. Dual Use of a Patient Portal and Clinical Video Telehealth by Veterans with Mental Health Diagnoses: Retrospective, Cross-Sectional Analysis. *J. Med. Internet Res.* **2018**, *20*, e11350. [CrossRef] [PubMed]
62. Chunara, R.; Zhao, Y.; Chen, J.; Lawrence, K.; Testa, P.A.; Nov, O.; Mann, D.M. Telemedicine and healthcare disparities: A cohort study in a large healthcare system in New York City during COVID-19. *J. Am. Med. Inform. Assoc.* **2021**, *28*, 33–41. [CrossRef] [PubMed]
63. Darrat, I.; Tam, S.; Boulis, M.; Williams, A.M. Socioeconomic Disparities in Patient Use of Telehealth During the Coronavirus Disease 2019 Surge. *JAMA Otolaryngol. Head Neck Surg.* **2021**, *147*, 287–295. [CrossRef]
64. Eberly, L.A.; Kallan, M.J.; Julien, H.M.; Haynes, N.; Khatana, S.A.M.; Nathan, A.S.; Snider, C.; Chokshi, N.P.; Eneanya, N.D.; Takvorian, S.U.; et al. Patient Characteristics Associated with Telemedicine Access for Primary and Specialty Ambulatory Care During the COVID-19 Pandemic. *JAMA Netw. Open* **2020**, *3*, e2031640. [CrossRef] [PubMed]
65. Jaffe, D.H.; Lee, L.; Huynh, S.; Haskell, T.P. Health Inequalities in the Use of Telehealth in the United States in the Lens of COVID-19. *Popul. Health Manag.* **2020**, *23*, 368–377. [CrossRef] [PubMed]
66. Wegermann, K.; Wilder, J.; Parish, A.; Niedzwiecki, D.; Gellad, Z.F.; Muir, A.J.; Patel, Y. Black, older, unmarried, and medicaid patients were less likely to complete hepatology video visits during COVID-19. *Hepatology* **2020**, *72* (Suppl. S1), 382A–383A.
67. Trief, P.M.; Izquierdo, R.; Eimicke, J.P.; Teresi, J.A.; Goland, R.; Palmas, W.; Shea, S.; Weinstock, R.S. Adherence to diabetes self care for white, African-American and Hispanic American telemedicine participants: 5 year results from the IDEATel project. *Ethn. Health* **2013**, *18*, 83–96. [CrossRef] [PubMed]
68. Walker, D.M.; Hefner, J.L.; Fareed, N.; Huerta, T.R.; McAlearney, A.S. Exploring the Digital Divide: Age and Race Disparities in Use of an Inpatient Portal. *Telemed. E-Health* **2020**, *26*, 603–613. [CrossRef]
69. Guendelman, S.; Broderick, A.; Mlo, H.; Gemmill, A.; Lindeman, D. Listening to Communities: Mixed-Method Study of the Engagement of Disadvantaged Mothers and Pregnant Women with Digital Health Technologies. *J. Med. Internet Res.* **2017**, *19*, e240. [CrossRef] [PubMed]
70. Gordon, N.P.; Hornbrook, M.C. Differences in Access to and Preferences for Using Patient Portals and Other eHealth Technologies Based on Race, Ethnicity, and Age: A Database and Survey Study of Seniors in a Large Health Plan. *J. Med. Internet Res.* **2016**, *18*, e50. [CrossRef]
71. Ferguson, J.M.; Jacobs, J.; Yefimova, M.; Greene, L.; Heyworth, L.; Zulman, D.M. Virtual Care Expansion in the Veterans Health Administration During the COVID-19 Pandemic: Clinical Services and Patient Characteristics Associated with Utilization. *J. Am. Med. Inform. Assoc. JAMIA* **2021**, *28*, 453–462. [CrossRef]
72. Shiferaw, K.B.; Mengiste, S.A.; Gullslett, M.K.; Zeleke, A.A.; Tilahun, B.; Tebeje, T.; Wondimu, R.; Desalegn, S.; Mehari, E.A. Healthcare providers' acceptance of telemedicine and preference of modalities during COVID-19 pandemics in a low-resource setting: An extended UTAUT model. *PLoS ONE* **2021**, *16*, e0250220. [CrossRef] [PubMed]
73. Isautier, J.M.; Copp, T.; Ayre, J.; Cvejic, E.; Meyerowitz-Katz, G.; Batcup, C.; Bonner, C.; Dodd, R.H.; Nickel, B.; Pickles, K.; et al. Lessons from the COVID-19 pandemic: People's experiences and satisfaction with telehealth during the COVID-19 pandemic in Australia. *MedRxiv* **2020**. [CrossRef]
74. Crawford, A.; Serhal, E. Digital health equity and COVID-19: The innovation curve cannot reinforce the social gradient of health. *J. Med. Internet Res.* **2020**, *22*, e19361. [CrossRef]
75. Doraiswamy, S.; Abraham, A.; Mamtani, R.; Cheema, S. Use of Telehealth During the COVID-19 Pandemic: Scoping Review. *J. Med. Internet Res.* **2020**, *22*, e24087. [CrossRef]
76. DelliFraine, J.L.; Dansky, K.H. Home-based telehealth: A review and meta-analysis. *J. Telemed. Telecare* **2008**, *14*, 62–66. [CrossRef] [PubMed]
77. Freed, J.; Lowe, C.; Flodgren, G.; Binks, R.; Doughty, K.; Kolsi, J. Telemedicine: Is it really worth it? A perspective from evidence and experience. *J. Innov. Health Inform.* **2018**, *25*, 14–18. [CrossRef] [PubMed]
78. Wang, X.; Zhang, Z.; Zhao, J.; Shi, Y. Impact of telemedicine on healthcare service system considering patients' choice. *Discret. Dyn. Nat. Soc.* **2019**, *2019*, 7642176. [CrossRef]

79. Kruse, C.S.; Krowski, N.; Rodriguez, B.; Tran, L.; Vela, J.; Brooks, M. Telehealth and patient satisfaction: A systematic review and narrative analysis. *BMJ Open* **2017**, *7*, e016242. [CrossRef] [PubMed]
80. Thomas, J.; Barraket, J.; Wilson, C.; Holcombe-James, I.; Kennedy, J.; Rennie, E.; Ewing, S.; MacDonald, T. *Measuring Australia's Digital Divide: The Australian Digital Inclusion Index 2020*; RMIT and Swinburne University of Technology: Melbourne, Australia, 2020.
81. Clare, C.A. Telehealth and the digital divide as a social determinant of health during the COVID-19 pandemic. *Netw. Modeling Anal. Health Inform. Bioinform.* **2021**, *10*, 26. [CrossRef] [PubMed]

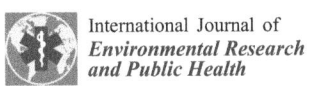

Article

Chronic Kidney Disease and Nephrology Care in People Living with HIV in Central/Eastern Europe and Neighbouring Countries—Cross-Sectional Analysis from the ECEE Network

Bartłomiej Matłosz [1,*], Agata Skrzat-Klapaczyńska [2], Sergii Antoniak [3], Tatevik Balayan [4], Josip Begovac [5], Gordana Dragovic [6], Denis Gusev [7], Djordje Jevtovic [8], David Jilich [9], Kerstin Aimla [10], Botond Lakatos [11], Raimonda Matulionyte [12], Aleksandr Panteleev [13], Antonios Papadopoulos [14], Nino Rukhadze [15], Dalibor Sedláček [16], Milena Stevanovic [17], Anna Vassilenko [18], Antonija Verhaz [19], Nina Yancheva [20], Oleg Yurin [21], Andrzej Horban [2] and Justyna D. Kowalska [2]

1. HIV Outpatient Clinic, Hospital for Infectious Diseases, Medical University of Warsaw, 02-091 Warszawa, Poland
2. Department of Adults' Infectious Diseases, Hospital for Infectious Diseases, Medical University of Warsaw, 02-091 Warszawa, Poland
3. Viral Hepatitis and AIDS Department, Gromashevsky Institute of Epidemiology and Infectious Diseases, 01001 Kyiv, Ukraine
4. National Center for Disease Control and Prevention, Yerevan 0002, Armenia
5. School of Medicine, University Hospital for Infectious Diseases, University of Zagreb, 10000 Zagreb, Croatia
6. Department of Pharmacology, Clinical Pharmacology and Toxicology, School of Medicine, University of Belgrade, 11000 Belgrade, Serbia
7. Botkin's Infectious Disease Hospital, First Saint-Petersburg State Medical University Named after I.P. Pavlov, 197022 Saint-Petersburg, Russia
8. Infectious Disease Hospital, Belgrade University School of Medicine, 11000 Belgrade, Serbia
9. Department of Infectious Diseases, 1st Faculty of Medicine, Charles University in Prague and Faculty Hospital Bulovka Hospital, 18000 Prague, Czech Republic
10. West Tallinn Central Hospital, 10111 Tallinn, Estonia
11. National Institute of Hematology and Infectious Diseases, South-Pest Central Hospital, National Center of HIV, 1007 Budapest, Hungary
12. Faculty of Medicine, Vilnius University, Vilnius University Hospital Santaros Klinikos, 08410 Vilnius, Lithuania
13. City TB Dispensary, 101000 Moscow, Russia
14. University General Hospital Attikon, Medical School, National and Kapodistrian University of Athens, 15772 Athens, Greece
15. Infectious Diseases, AIDS and Clinical Immunology Center, 112482 Tbilisi, Georgia
16. Faculty of Medicine in Plzeň, University Hospital Plzeň, Charles University, 30599 Plzen, Czech Republic
17. University Clinic for Infectious Diseases and Febrile Conditions, 1000 Skopje, North Macedonia
18. Global Fund Grant Management Department, Republican Scientific and Practical Center for Medical Technologies, 220004 Minsk, Belarus
19. Department for Infectious Diseases, Faculty of Medicine, University of Banja Luka, 78 000 Banja Luka, Republika Srpska, Bosnia and Herzegovina
20. Department for AIDS, Specialized Hospital for Active Treatment of Infectious and Parasitic Disease, 1000 Sofia, Bulgaria
21. Central Research Institute of Epidemiology, Federal AIDS Centre, 101000 Moscow, Russia
* Correspondence: bamat@mp.pl; Tel.: +48-22-3358-101

Abstract: Chronic kidney disease (CKD) is a significant cause of morbidity and mortality among patients infected with human immunodeficiency virus (HIV). The Central and East Europe (CEE) region consists of countries with highly diversified HIV epidemics, health care systems and socioeconomic status. The aim of the present study was to describe variations in CKD burden and care between countries. The Euroguidelines in the CEE Network Group includes 19 countries and was initiated to improve the standard of care for HIV infection in the region. Information on kidney care in HIV-positive patients was collected through online surveys sent to all members of the Network Group. Almost all centres use regular screening for CKD in all HIV (+) patients. Basic diagnostic tests for kidney function are available in the majority of centres. The most commonly used method

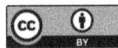

for eGFR calculation is the Cockcroft–Gault equation. Nephrology consultation is available in all centres. The median frequency of CKD was 5% and the main cause was comorbidity. Haemodialysis was the only modality of treatment for kidney failure available in all ECEE countries. Only 39% of centres declared that all treatment options are available for HIV+ patients. The most commonly indicated barrier in kidney care was patients' noncompliance. In the CEE region, people living with HIV have full access to screening for kidney disease but there are important limitations in treatment. The choice of dialysis modality and access to kidney transplantation are limited. The main burden of kidney disease is unrelated to HIV infection. Patient care can be significantly improved by addressing noncompliance.

Keywords: HIV; chronic kidney disease; Central and Eastern Europe

1. Introduction

Chronic kidney disease is a significant cause of morbidity and mortality among patients infected with the human immunodeficiency virus (HIV). The prevalence around the world in the HIV-infected population varies but, in most reports, it is estimated to be between 4.7% and 9.7% [1–5]. With effective antiretroviral therapy (ARV), life expectancy in individuals with HIV has increased. As a consequence, the spectrum of kidney diseases in people living with HIV has broadened, including not only HIV-related problems or drug toxicity but also renal damage from chronic noncommunicable diseases.

The Central and East Europe (CEE) region with a population of about 300 million consists of several countries with highly diversified HIV epidemics, health care systems and socio-economic status [6]. The data on kidney disease and health care in the region used to be scarce. In many reports regarding kidney disease prevalence and kidney care, the countries from the region are labelled as 'no data available' [5,7]. The availability of the data from the region is, however, improving and in the latest issue of the International Society of Nephrology Global Kidney Health Atlas, many of the blind spots were filled with data [8]. Still, the lack of national registries in the region remains a substantial obstacle to collecting reliable and comparable data. The ISN Global Kidney Health Atlas indicates 18 regional registries as the data source for Western Europe (out of 25 countries) and only 2 regional registries for the Central and Eastern Europe region (out of 19 countries). The resources available for kidney care seem to improve across the CEE region, although they still tend to lag behind other parts of Europe, especially in terms of low or very low rates of kidney transplantation [9].

As the data on renal disease in the population of people living with HIV are even more limited than in the general population, the present study aimed to investigate the state and limitations of care for chronic kidney disease and end-stage kidney disease in countries represented in the Euroguidelines in Central and Eastern Europe (ECEE) Network Group.

2. Materials and Methods

Euroguidelines in Central and Eastern Europe Network Group was initiated in February 2016 to compare and improve the standard of care for HIV infection in the region. Information on kidney care in HIV-positive patients was collected through online surveys sent to all members of the ECEE Network Group in November 2018. Respondents were ECEE members from 20 countries in the region (Albania, Armenia, Belarus, Bosnia and Herzegovina, Bulgaria, Croatia, Czech Republic, Estonia, Georgia, Greece, Hungary, Lithuania, Macedonia, Poland, Republic of Moldova, Romania, Russia, Serbia, Slovenia, Turkey and Ukraine).

The collected data were exported to the R statistical software. All analyses were performed using R software (version 3.6.2). The responses were based on real-world data, including centres' own databases. As all of the responders were practitioners actively involved in patient care, data regarding the availability of diagnostic tools and treatment relayed on their real experience. Some answers had to be analysed by country (e.g., coverage from public funding). In such cases, data received from the same country were used for validation purposes and then aggregated for by-country analysis.

Survey questions regarded institutional data, different aspects of nephrology care screening and diagnostic tests for kidney disease, availability of specialized nephrology care, burden and causes of kidney disease and guidelines employment. All survey questions can be found in Appendix A. The study did not include individual patient data and did not require ethical committee approval.

3. Results

The survey was sent to 43 members of the ECEE Network in 20 countries. We received 18 responses from 16 countries. According to the World Bank classification, among the responding countries, there were three lower–middle-income countries, five upper–middle-income countries and seven high–income countries. The vast majority of responding centres were described as treating PLWH as well as other infectious diseases (61%) and both hospital and outpatient-based (83%). The median population treated in a single centre was 1415 (IQR 600–2514) patients.

In most ECEE countries, the population of PLWH is relatively young with only four centres where patients > 65 years account for at least 10% of the population. In nine centres (50%), the proportion of elderly patients is less than 5%. We did not observe any significant correlation between age and the frequency of CKD. MSM was the most common route of HIV infection in 10 centres (55.5%). In six centres (33.3%), IVDU is a common route of infection (more than 25% of infected patients). In 11 centres (61.1%), the majority of patients receive ARV therapy within one year after HIV infection diagnosis.

All but one centre use regular screening for kidney disease in all HIV (+) patients irrespective of ARV therapy usually within 3–6 month intervals. Among basic diagnostic tests, creatinine and abdominal ultrasound are available in all centres. In a few centres, urinalysis and albumin-to-creatinine ratio are not available (11.1%, $n = 2$ and 27.8%, $n = 5$, respectively). NMR, biopsy, scintigraphy and cystatin are rarely available (less than 50% of centres). Only a few centres did not use eGFR (22%, $n = 4$) nor albumin (28%, $n = 5$) for chronic kidney disease screening (Figure 1). The most commonly used method for eGFR calculation is still the Cockcroft–Gault Equation, but the CKD-EPI Equation is used with a similar frequency (38.9%, $n = 7$ and 33.3%, $n = 6$, respectively). MDRD formula is used only in three centres (16.7%). In four centres (22.2%), the eGFR method is not known.

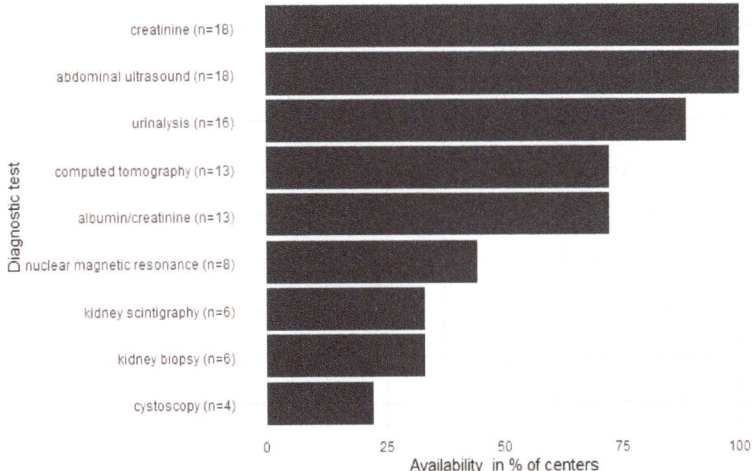

Figure 1. Availability of diagnostic tests.

Specialized nephrology consultation is available in all centres. In three centres, a nephrologist is available on-site on a regular basis. In nine centres, consultation is available on call, and in five centres, patients are referred for consultation to the external institution. Nevertheless, the waiting time for consultation in any of the centres is not longer than 1 month and in half of the cases, it is up to one week. In the majority of centres, nephrology care is provided without any fee, although in seven centres, patients have to partly contribute to costs.

The main causes of chronic kidney disease are not related to HIV infection. The majority of responders (55%) answered that the first most common cause of chronic kidney disease is comorbidity (i.e., hypertension and diabetes). As the second most common causes of CKD, antiretrovirals' and other drugs' nephrotoxicity were indicated most commonly (33% and 28% responses, respectively). The most common and second most common causes of chronic kidney disease are depicted in (Figure 2A,B).

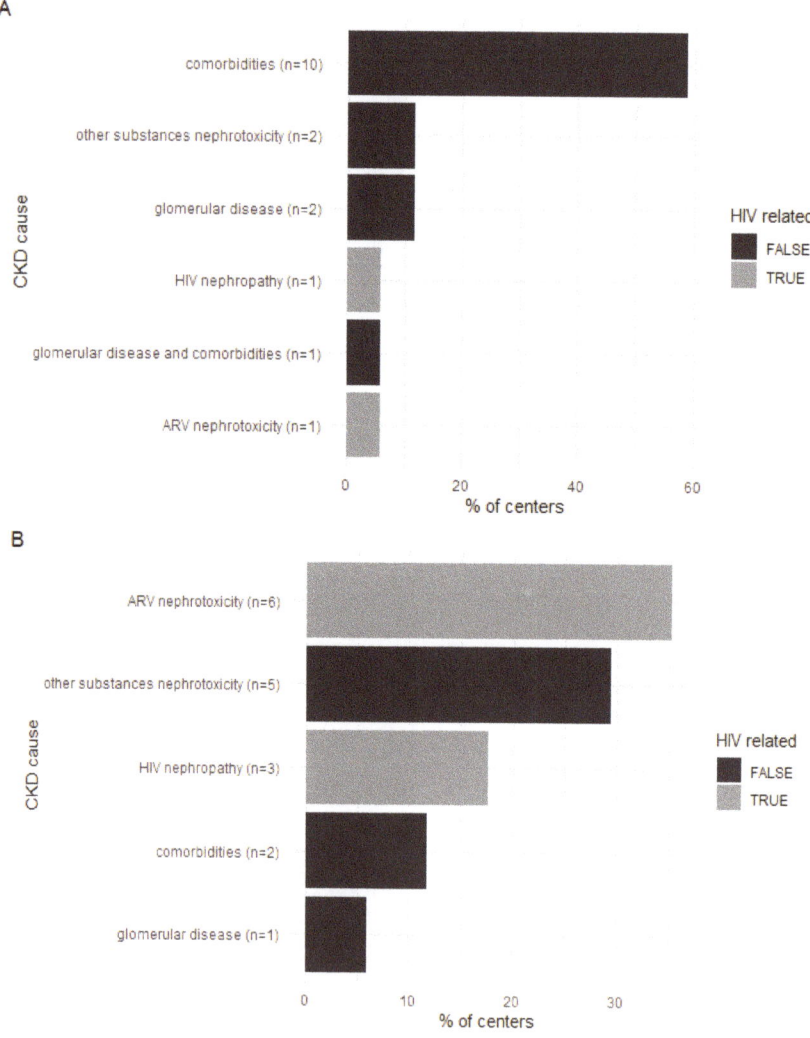

Figure 2. (**A**) The most common causes of CKD. (**B**) The second most common causes of CKD.

The median frequency of CKD was 5%, although there was significant variability between countries ranging from 0% to 20% of HIV-positive patients. With 37 reported cases out of over 58,000 individuals in care, end-stage renal disease is rare (0.06%) and only a few patients require RRT in most centres. Additionally, death resulting from end-stage renal disease is rare with no or single cases reported from almost all centres.

The only modality of treatment for ESRD completely covered from public funding (no matter of HIV status) in all ECEE countries is haemodialysis. Respondents from four countries declared that neither living nor deceased donor transplantation is founded on public funds. In five countries, the treatment of CKD complications and peritoneal dialysis is not covered. Only seven centres (38.9%) declared that all treatment options for ESRD (haemodialysis, peritoneal dialysis, and kidney transplantation) are available for HIV+ patients. In 11 centres (61.1%), the only treatment option was dialysis, and among them, in 6 centres (33.3%), only haemodialysis was possible.

In most centres, treatment of chronic kidney disease is the responsibility of a nephrologist or interdisciplinary team (72.2%). In five centres (27.8%), infectious disease specialists are primarily responsible for kidney care in people living with HIV. The most commonly indicated barrier in kidney care was patients' noncompliance (six centres). Other issues (i.e., health service availability, nephrologist availability, and distance from care point) were also common.

The most commonly used guidelines were EACS guidelines: eight centres (44.4%) use only EACS and seven centres (38.9%) both EACS and national ones. Guidelines adoption was usually described as moderate (61%) centres.

4. Discussion

The reported prevalence of CKD varied from 0 to 20% (median 5%). The highest rates (more than 10%) were observed in Hungary, Poland and Serbia. A very low prevalence of CKD (below 2%) was observed in Macedonia, Georgia, Estonia and Lithuania. In the general population, the prevalence of chronic kidney disease worldwide is 1.5–21% and in fact, it is highly variable in seemingly similar countries such as in Europe [7,10]. Significant differences were observed even within one country [11]. Aumann et al. showed that in different regions in Germany, the prevalence may be higher by a factor of 2. In the Pomerania region (SHIP-1 study) in Northeast Germany and the region of Augsburg in Southern Germany's Cooperative Health Research Study (KORA F4), the prevalence was 5.9% and 3.1% accordingly. The same is true for HIV-positive patients in Europe [2,12]. The population of people living with HIV across the ECEE countries network is widely variable. Our results show huge disparities in epidemics across quite a small geographical region. There are countries with a high prevalence of patients infected through intravenous drug use as well as countries with MSM population dominance. The prevalence of elderly patients in the HIV-infected population may vary from as high as 20% in some countries to almost no such patients, as reported in four countries where less than 1% of patients are aged 65 or more. This may result in different risk factors for chronic kidney disease in different countries. Although many authors attribute rising chronic kidney disease to the ageing HIV (+) population, we were not able to see any significant increase in the reported CKD prevalence in centres with a high proportion of elderly patients [13,14].

According to EACS guidelines, screening for renal disease (eGFR and urine protein) should be carried out in every HIV-positive patient at least once a year (with a wide range of every 3–12 months) [15]. In patients with risk factors for established CKD, the frequency of eGFR monitoring should be increased. Additionally, in patients with decreased eGFR or proteinuria, abdominal ultrasound should be performed. In this survey regarding kidney care clinical practice in people living with HIV, we observed general good availability of diagnostic tests and treatment in chronic kidney disease. Most of the kidney function tests were available in all centres and specialized nephrology care was provided without delay. It is worth mentioning that some centres still do not utilize urinary albumin/protein for screening for kidney disease which is required by EACS guidelines [15]. Poorer availability of some specialized diagnostic tests such as nuclear magnetic resonance imaging or kidney scintigraphy should not be a problem as almost all centres reported the possibility of patients' referral to a nephrologist for specialized care.

The definition of chronic kidney disease is based on the widely accepted KDIGO classification of CKD [16]. For GFR estimation, EACS guidelines recommend the use of the CKD-EPI formula, although it indicates that the abbreviated Modification of Diet in Renal Disease (MDRD) or the Cockcroft–Gault (CG) equation may be used as an alternative. KDIGO guidelines state that eGFR should be calculated with the CKD-EPI formula and an alternative creatinine-based GFR-estimating equation is acceptable only if it has been shown to improve the accuracy of GFR estimates compared to the 2009 CKD-EPI creatinine equation [16]. Almost all centres employ regular universal screening for kidney injury at 3–6 month intervals, which is even more frequent than required by EACS guidelines. The vast majority of the centres (67%) still use, for the estimation of GFR, equations other than the primarily recommended CKD-EPI equation. This fact may potentially have clinical significance as the CKD-EPI creatinine formula was validated in the HIV (+) population in many studies and seems to outperform other formulas by means of accuracy [17,18].

HIV may cause kidney injury in several ways. The classic kidney disease of HIV infection, HIV-associated nephropathy (HIVAN), causes rapid kidney function deterioration and, if not treated, usually leads to end-stage renal disease. The incidence of HIV-associated nephropathy decreased with the use of highly active antiretroviral therapy [19]. Additionally, a number of immune complex kidney diseases have been reported in patients with HIV infection, including membranous nephropathy, membranoproliferative and mesangial proliferative glomerulonephritis, and "lupus-like" proliferative glomerulonephritis [20,21]. However, the ageing cohort of HIV-positive patients may be at increased risk for kidney disease unrelated to direct HIV injury. Coinfections and comorbid or treatment-related diabetes and hypertension may play an important role [22]. The increasing role of traditional risk factors for CKD seems to be supported by the results of our survey. More than half of the centres indicated that comorbidity was the most common cause of CKD. Other commonly reported causes were nephrotoxicity of drugs and illegal substances. Only one centre reported HIV nephropathy as the main cause of chronic kidney disease. As the second most common causes of chronic kidney disease, ARV nephrotoxicity and other drugs' or illegal substances' nephrotoxicity were reported in the majority of centres.

Even in centres with a high prevalence of chronic kidney disease, end-stage renal disease was not a common problem. Only single cases of end-stage renal disease were reported. Only one country reported a significant number of patients requiring renal replacement therapy but not treated. The possible reasons include not only resource shortage but also patients' noncompliance indicated by many participating centres as an important obstacle in providing care. Noncompliance was also described in previous studies as a serious problem with more than 50% of patients not attending the scheduled consultations [23]. No country reported differences in kidney care for HIV and the general population. Some centres indicated that kidney transplantation is founded on the public health insurance system but there is no possibility for HIV (+) individuals for transplantation. This may indicate that access to care, in reality, is not truly equal. Another possible explanation is that in many ECEE countries, kidney transplant programs have a very limited capacity [24]. Thus, the availability of transplantation may be limited in general in those countries despite public funding.

In general, access to nephrology care for people living with HIV is seemingly good. All centres employ regular renal function screening and in the vast majority of centres, nephrology consultation is possible without a delay. Nevertheless, our findings showed the lack of treatment options for ESRD in HIV-positive patients in a substantial proportion of Central and Eastern Europe Countries. In the ECEE region, one country in four has no public funding for kidney transplantation (which is also true for HIV-negative individuals). The only renal replacement therapy reimbursed in all ECEE countries is haemodialysis. The fact that treatment of CKD complications is also not covered by public health insurance in many countries may negatively influence the patients' prognosis. Additionally, in many centres, chronic kidney disease treatment is solely the responsibility of the infectious disease specialists which is not optimal and is against current guidelines.

All centres indicate that there are barriers to kidney care access for HIV patients. The most commonly indicated obstacle was patients' noncompliance, although all the other answers (distance from care, nephrologist availability, and healthcare system access) were also commonly indicated.

There are some important limitations to be discussed. This was an online survey-based study where we preselected respondents based on our best knowledge of expertise and up-to-date acquaintance with epidemiological and clinical data in their centres. Secondly, the source of information on coinfection prevalence varied from personal communication to detailed epidemiological surveillance; thus, the weight of the data presented may vary significantly across countries.

5. Conclusions

In the ECEE region, people living with HIV have full access to screening for kidney disease. The screening might be improved by the employment of albuminuria screening in all centres. There are some important limitations in access to renal replacement therapy both regarding the choice of dialysis modality and kidney transplantation. It must be stated that those limitations are also true for the HIV (−) population. The main burden of kidney disease in the ECEE region is not directly related to HIV infection and treatment but comorbidity and patient care can be improved by addressing noncompliance.

Author Contributions: Conceptualization and methodology—J.D.K. and B.M.; formal analysis—B.M. and J.D.K.; data collection and curation—S.A., T.B., J.B., G.D., D.G., D.J. (Djordje Jevtovic), D.J. (David Jilich), K.A., B.L., R.M., A.P. (Aleksandr Panteleev), A.P. (Antonios Papadopoulos), N.R., D.S., M.S., A.V. (Anna Vassilenko), A.V. (Antonija Verhaz), N.Y., O.Y., J.D.K. and A.S.-K.; writing—B.M. and A.S.-K.; supervision—A.H.; project administration—A.S.-K.; funding acquisition—A.H. All authors have read and agreed to the published version of the manuscript.

Funding: The study has been funded by a research grant issued by the Research Development Foundation in Hospital for Infectious Diseases.

Institutional Review Board Statement: Not applicable.

Informed Consent Statement: Not applicable.

Data Availability Statement: Not applicable.

Conflicts of Interest: The authors declare no conflict of interest. The funders had no role in the design of the study; in the collection, analyses, or interpretation of data; in the writing of the manuscript; or in the decision to publish the results.

Appendix A

Survey questionnaire.
Access to nephrology care for HIV infected patients in CEE countries.
INSTITUTIONAL DATA

1. Contact info:

   First Name   _____
   Last Name   _____
   Country   _____
   City   _____
   Centre name (affiliation) _____
   E-mail   _____

2. Your center is:
    a. Mainly outpatient based [ ]
    b. Mainly hospital based [ ]
    c. Both hospital and outpatient based [ ]
3. Your center is:
    a. only for HIV infected patients [ ]
    b. for HIV infected and other infectious disease patients [ ]
    c. multidisciplinary center [ ]
    d. Other (please specify) _____ [ ]
4. How many HIV positive patients are in active care at your center (at least one visit in last year)?
    _____
5. What proportion of your patients is aged ≥65?
    _____%
6. What proportion of patients at your centre was infected through:
    a. MSM _____%
    b. IVDU _____%
7. In what proportion of your patients ARV treatment is introduced within one year after HIV infection is diagnosed?
    _____%

    NEPHROLOGY TESTING
8. What kidney tests are available for HIV positive patients at your institution:
    a. Serum creatinine [ ]
    b. Serum cystatin [ ]
    c. Urinalysis (dipstick test) [ ]
    d. Protein/creatinine or albumin/creatinine ratio in urine [ ]
    e. Abdominal ultrasound [ ]
    f. CT scan [ ]
    g. NMR scan [ ]
    h. Renal scintigraphy [ ]
    i. Kidney biopsy [ ]
9. At your institution screening tests (i.e., creatinine, eGFR) for chronic kidney disease (CKD) in HIV patients are:
    a. routinely performed in all HIV positive patients irrespective of ARV therapy [ ]
    b. routinely performed in patients on ARV therapy [ ]
    c. routinely performed only in selected groups or situations (please specify) [ ] _____
    d. not performed routinely [ ]
10. What screening test for CKD do you use in HIV-infected patients
    a. Serum creatinine [ ]
    b. eGFR [ ]
    c. Urine albumin or protein [ ]
    d. Other (please specify) _____ [ ]
11. How often do you perform screening tests for kidney injury in HIV+ patients?
    a. Every _____ months
    b. I do not perform screening [ ]

12. What method of eGFR calculation is routinely used at your centre:
    a. Cockcroft-Gault formula [ ]
    b. MDRD equation [ ]
    c. CKD EPI equation (creatinine) [ ]
    d. CKD EPI equation (creatinine + cystatin) [ ]
    e. It is provided by the laboratory, I do not know what method [ ]
    f. I do not use eGFR [ ]

NEPHROLOGY CARE

13. Is nephrologist consultation available for HIV infected patients?
    a. Yes, in my clinic daily or weekly [ ]
    b. Yes, in my clinic monthly [ ]
    c. Yes, in my clinic on call when demanded [ ]
    d. Yes, referral to the other center [ ]
    e. No, nephrology consultation is not available in my clinic for HIV+ patients [ ]

14. What is the waiting time for nephrology consultation?
    _____ days/weeks/months/years

15. Is specialized nephrology care in your country:
    a. publicly founded by government free at the point of delivery [ ]
    b. Publicly funded by government some fees at the point of delivery [ ]
    c. Mix of public and private funding systems [ ]
    d. Solely private and paid by the patient (out-of-pocket) [ ]

16. Is specialized nephrology care for general population and HIV+ patients the same or some restrictions apply:
    a. Yes, it is the same [ ]
    b. No, it is different (please describe _____) [ ]

CHRONIC KIDNEY DISEASE

17. What are the most common cases of chronic kidney disease in your patients:
    a. HIV nephropathy,
    b. glomerular disease,
    c. ARV nephrotoxicity,
    d. other drugs or illegal substances nephrotoxicity,
    e. comorbidities (i.e., diabetes mellitus, hypertension),
    f. unknown,
    g. other (please specify) _____
        - most common _____
        - second most common _____

18. At your center proportion of HIV+ patients with chronic kidney disease (eGFR < 60 mL/min) is _____%

19. What is the number of patients at your centre with end-stage renal disease (requiring renal replacement therapy—RRT):
    a. On dialysis _____
    b. After kidney transplantation _____
    c. Requiring RRT but not treated _____

20. How many patients died from kidney disease at your centre within last year?
    _____

21. Healthcare providers primarily responsible for chronic kidney disease care in HIV-positive patients:
    a. Nephrologists [ ]
    b. Infectious disease specialists [ ]
    c. Primary care physicians [ ]
    d. Multidisciplinary teams [ ]
    e. Other [ ]
22. What options are routinely available for patients requiring renal replacement therapy:
    a. hemodialysis [ ]
    b. peritoneal dialysis [ ]
    c. kidney transplantation [ ]
    d. none of them [ ]
23. Is renal replacement therapy (i.e., dialysis, transplantation) care for general population and HIV+ patients the same or some restrictions apply:
    a. Yes, it is the same [ ]
    b. No, it is different (please describe _____) [ ]
24. Which of the following services are covered from public founding:
    a. Dialysis
        i. Hemodialysis [ ]
        ii. Peritoneal dialysis [ ]
    b. Kidney transplantation
        i. living donor [ ]
        ii. deceased donor [ ]
    c. Management of CKD complications (i.e., anemia, bone disease) [ ]
25. Are there specific barriers to optimal kidney disease care for HIV positive patients in your country?
    a. Geography (distance from care)
    b. Nephrologist availability
    c. Patient non-compliance
    d. Healthcare system access
    e. Other (please specify) _____

GUIDELINES

26. Do you have national guidelines on HIV care?
    a. Yes [ ]
    b. No [ ]
27. When were your national/local guidelines updated?
    year _____
28. Does your national guidelines cover kidney disease management in HIV population?
    a. Yes [ ]
    b. No [ ]
29. What guidelines regarding kidney disease do you use at your centre?
    a. National guidelines [ ]
    b. EACS guidelines [ ]
    c. Other (please specify) _____ [ ]
    d. We do not use guidelines regarding kidney disease in HIV-positive patients [ ]

30. Adoption of guidelines regarding kidney disease in HIV-infected patients at your centre is:
    a. Not optimal
    b. Moderate
    c. Optimal
31. What are the obstacles that may prevent implementing guidelines regarding kidney disease in HIV-infected patients?

    _____

    If you have any other comments you can place it here:

    _____

References

1. Mocroft, A.; Kirk, O.; Gatell, J.; Reiss, P.; Gargalianos, P.; Zilmer, K.; Beniowski, M.; Viard, J.-P.; Staszewski, S.; Lundgren, J.D. Chronic renal failure among HIV-1-infected patients. *AIDS* **2007**, *21*, 1119–1127. [CrossRef] [PubMed]
2. Sorli, M.L.; Guelar, A.; Montero, M.; Gonzalez, A.; Rodriguez, E.; Knobel, H. Chronic kidney disease prevalence and risk factors among HIV-infected patients. *J. Acquir. Immune. Defic. Syndr.* **2008**, *48*, 506–508. [CrossRef] [PubMed]
3. Matlosz, B.; Pietraszkiewicz, E.; Firlag-Burkacka, E.; Grycner, E.; Horban, A.; Kowalska, J.D. Risk factors for kidney disease among HIV-1 positive persons in the methadone program. *Clin. Exp. Nephrol.* **2019**, *23*, 342–348. [CrossRef]
4. Calza, L.; Sachs, M.; Colangeli, V.; Borderi, M.; Granozzi, B.; Malosso, P.; Comai, G.; Corradetti, V.; La Manna, G.; Viale, P. Prevalence of chronic kidney disease among HIV-1-infected patients receiving a combination antiretroviral therapy. *Clin. Exp. Nephrol.* **2019**, *23*, 1272–1279. [CrossRef]
5. Ekrikpo, U.E.; Kengne, A.P.; Bello, A.K.; Effa, E.E.; Noubiap, J.J.; Salako, B.L.; Rayner, B.L.; Remuzzi, G.; Okpechi, I.G. Chronic kidney disease in the global adult HIV-infected population: A systematic review and meta-analysis. *PLoS ONE* **2018**, *13*, e0195443. [CrossRef]
6. Kowalska, J.D.; Oprea, C.; de Witt, S.; Pozniak, A.; Gokengin, D.; Youle, M.; Lundgren, J.D.; Horban, A. Euroguidelines in Central and Eastern Europe (ECEE) conference and the Warsaw Declaration—A comprehensive meeting report. *HIV Med.* **2017**, *18*, 370–375. [CrossRef]
7. Bruck, K.; Stel, V.S.; Gambaro, G.; Hallan, S.; Volzke, H.; Arnlov, J.; Kastarinen, M.; Guessous, I.; Vinhas, J.; Stengel, B.; et al. CKD Prevalence Varies across the European General Population. *J. Am. Soc. Nephrol.* **2016**, *27*, 2135–2147. [CrossRef] [PubMed]
8. International Society of Nephrology: ISN Global Kidney Health Atlas 2019. Available online: https://www.theisn.org/initiatives/global-kidney-health-atlas/ (accessed on 5 March 2022).
9. Spasovski, G.; Rroji, M.; Vazelov, E.; Basic Jukic, N.; Tesar, V.; Mugosa Ratkovic, M.; Covic, A.; Naumovic, R.; Resic, H.; Turan Kazancioglu, R. Nephrology in the Eastern and Central European region: Challenges and opportunities. *Kidney Int.* **2019**, *96*, 287–290. [CrossRef]
10. Mills, K.T.; Xu, Y.; Zhang, W.; Bundy, J.D.; Chen, C.-S.; Kelly, T.N.; Chen, J.; He, J. A systematic analysis of worldwide population-based data on the global burden of chronic kidney disease in 2010. *Kidney Int.* **2015**, *88*, 950–957. [CrossRef]
11. Aumann, N.; Baumeister, S.E.; Rettig, R.; Lieb, W.; Werner, A.; Doring, A.; Peters, A.; Koenig, W.; Hannemann, A.; Wallaschofski, H.; et al. Regional variation of chronic kidney disease in Germany: Results from two population-based surveys. *Kidney Blood Press. Res.* **2015**, *40*, 231–243. [CrossRef]
12. Gunter, J.; Callens, S.; de Wit, S.; Goffard, J.-C.; Moutschen, M.; Darcis, G.; Meuris, C.; van den Bulcke, C.; Fombellida, K.; Del Forge, M.; et al. Prevalence of non-infectious comorbidities in the HIV-positive population in Belgium: A multicenter, retrospective study. *Acta Clin. Belg.* **2018**, *73*, 50–53. [CrossRef] [PubMed]
13. Pelchen-Matthews, A.; Ryom, L.; Borges, A.H.; Edwards, S.; Duvivier, C.; Stephan, C.; Sambatakou, H.; Maciejewska, K.; Portu, J.J.; Weber, J.; et al. Aging and the evolution of comorbidities among HIV-positive individuals in a European cohort. *AIDS* **2018**, *32*, 2405–2416. [CrossRef] [PubMed]
14. Wong, C.; Gange, S.J.; Buchacz, K.; Moore, R.D.; Justice, A.C.; Horberg, M.A.; Gill, M.J.; Koethe, J.R.; Rebeiro, P.F.; Silverberg, M.J.; et al. First Occurrence of Diabetes, Chronic Kidney Disease, and Hypertension Among North American HIV-Infected Adults, 2000–2013. *Clin. Infect. Dis.* **2017**, *64*, 459–467. [CrossRef]
15. EACS Guidelines v.9.1. Available online: http://www.eacsociety.org/guidelines/eacs-guidelines/eacs-guidelines.html (accessed on 2 March 2020).
16. Kidney Disease: Improving Global Outcomes (KDIGO) CKD Work Group: KDIGO 2012 Clinical Practice Guideline for the Evaluation and Management of Chronic Kidney Disease. *Kidney Int. Suppl.* **2013**, *3*, 5–150.
17. Inker, L.A.; Wyatt, C.; Creamer, R.; Hellinger, J.; Hotta, M.; Leppo, M.; Levey, A.S.; Okparavero, A.; Graham, H.; Savage, K.; et al. Performance of creatinine and cystatin C GFR estimating equations in an HIV-positive population on antiretrovirals. *J. Acquir. Immune. Defic. Syndr.* **2012**, *61*, 302–309. [CrossRef] [PubMed]

18. Lucas, G.M.; Cozzi-Lepri, A.; Wyatt, C.M.; Post, F.A.; Bormann, A.M.; Crum-Cianflone, N.F.; Ross, M.J. Glomerular filtration rate estimated using creatinine, cystatin C or both markers and the risk of clinical events in HIV-infected individuals. *HIV Med.* **2014**, *15*, 116–123. [CrossRef] [PubMed]
19. Lescure, F.-X.; Flateau, C.; Pacanowski, J.; Brocheriou, I.; Rondeau, E.; Girard, P.-M.; Ronco, P.; Pialoux, G.; Plaisier, E. HIV-associated kidney glomerular diseases: Changes with time and HAART. *Nephrol. Dial. Transplant.* **2012**, *27*, 2349–2355. [CrossRef]
20. Wearne, N.; Swanepoel, C.R.; Boulle, A.; Duffield, M.S.; Rayner, B.L. The spectrum of renal histologies seen in HIV with outcomes, prognostic indicators and clinical correlations. *Nephrol. Dial. Transplant.* **2012**, *27*, 4109–4118. [CrossRef]
21. Haas, M.; Kaul, S.; Eustace, J.A. HIV-associated immune complex glomerulonephritis with "lupus-like" features: A clinicopathologic study of 14 cases. *Kidney Int.* **2005**, *67*, 1381–1390. [CrossRef]
22. Jotwani, V.; Li, Y.; Grunfeld, C.; Choi, A.I.; Shlipak, M.G. Risk factors for ESRD in HIV-infected individuals: Traditional and HIV-related factors. *Am. J. Kidney Dis.* **2012**, *59*, 628–635. [CrossRef]
23. Matlosz, B.; Firlag-Burkacka, E.; Horban, A.; Kowalska, J.D. Nephrology consultations incorporated into HIV care—Non-compliance is an important issue. *AIDS Care* **2017**, *29*, 226–230. [CrossRef] [PubMed]
24. Spasovski, G.; Busic, M.; Delmonico, F. Improvement in kidney transplantation in the Balkans after the Istanbul Declaration: Where do we stand today? *Clin. Kidney J.* **2016**, *9*, 172–175. [CrossRef] [PubMed]

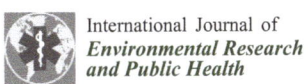

Article

Serious Injury in Metropolitan and Regional Victoria: Exploring Travel to Treatment and Utilisation of Post-Discharge Health Services by Injury Type

Jemma Keeves [1,2,*], Belinda Gabbe [2], Sarah Arnup [2], Christina Ekegren [3] and Ben Beck [2]

[1] Department of Physiotherapy, Epworth Hospital, Melbourne 3122, Australia
[2] Department of Epidemiology and Preventive Medicine, Monash University, Melbourne 3004, Australia
[3] Rehabilitation, Ageing and Independent Living Unit, Monash University, Melbourne 3004, Australia
* Correspondence: jemma.keeves@monash.edu

Abstract: This study aimed to describe regional variations in service use and distance travelled to post-discharge health services in the first three years following hospital discharge for people with transport-related orthopaedic, brain, and spinal cord injuries. Using linked data from the Victorian State Trauma Registry (VSTR) and Transport Accident Commission (TAC), we identified 1597 people who had sustained transport-related orthopaedic, brain, or spinal cord injuries between 2006 and 2016 that met the study inclusion criteria. The adjusted odds of GP service use for regional participants were 76% higher than for metropolitan participants in the orthopaedic and traumatic brain injury (TBI) groups. People with spinal cord injury (SCI) living in regional areas had 72% lower adjusted odds of accessing mental health, 76% lower adjusted odds of accessing OT services, and 82% lower adjusted odds of accessing physical therapies compared with people living in major cities. People with a TBI living in regional areas on average travelled significantly further to access all post-discharge health services compared with people with TBI in major cities. For visits to medical services, the median trip distance for regional participants was 76.61 km (95%CI: 16.01–132.21) for orthopaedic injuries, 104.05 km (95% CI: 51.55–182.78) for TBI, and 68.70 km (95%CI: 8.34–139.84) for SCI. Disparities in service use and distance travelled to health services exist between metropolitan Melbourne and regional Victoria following serious injury.

Keywords: serious injury; traumatic brain injury; orthopaedic injury; spinal cord injury; road trauma; access to healthcare; healthcare utilisation; geography

1. Introduction

Transport-related injuries are expected to become the third leading cause of disability worldwide by 2030 [1]. Despite advances in trauma care, people with orthopaedic injury, traumatic brain injury (TBI), and spinal cord injury (SCI) continue to experience long-term physical disability, psychological dysfunction, and interference from pain [2–4]. There is a need to understand whether long-term outcomes for people with serious transport-related injury can be improved through a coordinated and revised approach to post-discharge healthcare.

Urban and regional disparities in access to care exist, with people living in regional areas travelling further to access post-discharge healthcare after major trauma [5]. Both people with serious injury and health professionals have reported limited availability and difficulties accessing necessary care as barriers to health service delivery following injury, particularly for people living in regional areas [6–8]. It is unclear whether these barriers to post-discharge care are more significant for people in regional areas as a result of regionalised trauma system design, which centralises higher-level trauma centres in inner metropolitan areas.

Despite survivors of serious injury having long-term and complex healthcare needs, the level of specialised care provided beyond hospital discharge varies depending on the type of injury [4,5,9]. People with TBI and SCI are more likely to receive rehabilitation from specialised services due to the complexity of these injuries [10]. After an orthopaedic injury however, there is no clear pathway for rehabilitation once discharged from a major trauma centre [10]. Given the high prevalence of disability amongst trauma survivors, both with and without serious neurotrauma, consideration for the whole pathway of trauma care from acute management to specialised rehabilitation and community care is pertinent [10].

This novel study is the first to use geospatial analysis to clearly quantify the differences in travel to services and service use for people in different geographic areas by type of injury. The aim of this work was to understand how different injury populations use post-discharge health services across regional and metropolitan areas and explore the distances travelled to health services in the first three years following hospital discharge. Improving our understanding of post-discharge service utilisation is an important step in ensuring necessary services are accessible and available for people with transport-related serious injury.

2. Materials and Methods

2.1. Study Design

Our registry-based cohort study used linked data from the Victorian State Trauma Registry (VSTR) and Transport Accident Commission (TAC). Our study follows the Strengthening of Reporting of Observational Studies in Epidemiology checklist, see Appendix A [11].

Victoria is the second most populous state of Australia with a population of 6.46 million people, including over 2 million people residing outside the Greater Melbourne region [12]. Victoria has an inclusive trauma system consisting of two adults, and one paediatric, major trauma centres, which are located in metropolitan Melbourne.

The population-based VSTR collects data about all people with major trauma in Victoria, with major trauma defined as: (1) death due to injury; (2) an injury severity score (ISS; based on the abbreviated injury scale (AIS) 2005 version, 2008 update) >12; (3) admission to an intensive care unit >24 h; (4) or an injury requiring urgent surgery [13]. The registry has an opt-out rate <1% and includes data on prehospital care, pre-existing health conditions, injury characteristics and complications, and discharge information [13].

The TAC is Victoria's no-fault third-party insurer for people who have sustained a transport-related injury, covering medical treatment, rehabilitation, support services, and financial assistance. People are covered by the TAC if their injuries are sustained as a result of driving a car, motorcycle, bus, train, or tram. Cyclists injured in a collision with a moving or stationary motor vehicle (after 9 July 2014) are also covered by the TAC. Pedestrians are covered by the TAC when their injuries arise as a direct result of impact with a motor vehicle, motorcycle, train, or tram. Full details of eligible claimants and expenses covered by the TAC are outlined in the Transport Accident Act 1986 [14]. The TAC collect data pertaining to an individual claim, including detailed information regarding the post-discharge health services paid for by the TAC. These data include details of the date and type of service, service description, and where the service provider is located. The TAC provides these data to the VSTR, linked by claim number. A standardised and secure process is followed to ensure that no patient-level data are provided to the TAC by the VSTR.

2.2. Participants

Victorians who sustained major trauma from a transport-related event between 1 January 2006 and 31 December 2016 with a TAC compensation claim were identified within the VSTR. People were included if they sustained isolated orthopaedic injuries; a moderate to severe TBI or SCI; were aged 18 years or older at the time of injury; had three-years of TAC claims data; and resided in Victoria with a known residential address (Figure 1). The orthopaedic group consisted of people who had sustained an extremity injury with AIS score >1 and/or spine injury with AIS two or three and no other injury with AIS >1 [15]. Traumatic brain injury (TBI) cases were considered to be moderate or severe if they had a head injury with an AIS severity score >2 and the first recorded Glasgow coma scale (GCS) score <13, with or without other system injuries [15]. Mild traumatic brain injuries are not captured by the VSTR unless sustained with other system injures so were excluded from this study. Spinal cord injury was defined as an injury to the spine with an AIS severity score >3, with or without other injuries [15].

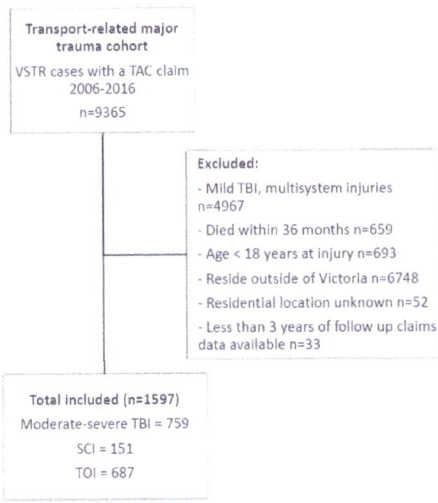

Figure 1. Flow diagram of inclusion criteria.

2.3. Variables

The three key outcomes of interest in this study were: service use, the number of trips per person and distance travelled to health services in the first three years following hospital discharge. Service use was defined as the percentage of participants who used a health service at some point within the study period. The number of trips per person refers to the number of times a health service was visited by service users. Distance travelled was the median trip distance per person from their residential location to the provider location, measured in kilometres.

Health services were categorised as: General Practitioner (GP), other medical professionals (e.g., neurologists, pathologists, psychiatrists, surgeons), mental health services (psychology, social work and case management), physical therapies (physiotherapy, exercise physiology, and hydrotherapy), and occupational therapy (OT). Speech pathology was excluded as this service was used almost exclusively by TBI participants.

2.4. Data Measurement

Demographic information, pre-existing health conditions, injury diagnosis and severity, and hospital length of stay and discharge status were extracted from the registry. Data relating to a TAC claim, client address, and service provider locations were provided by the TAC for all services funded between 1 January 2006 and 31 December 2019.

Each participant's residential address at the date of hospital discharge was mapped by their local government area (LGA) to the Accessibility/Remoteness Index of Australia 2016 (ARIA+) and categorised into major city, inner regional, or outer regional [16]. For analysis, the metropolitan group consisted of people living in 'Major Cities' and the regional group as people living in 'Inner Regional' or 'Outer Regional' areas (Figure 2). No participants were residing in 'Remote' or 'Very Remote' areas by the ARIA+ classification index. Socioeconomic status was categorised using The Index of Relative Socioeconomic Advantage and Disadvantage (IRSAD) according to LGA [17].

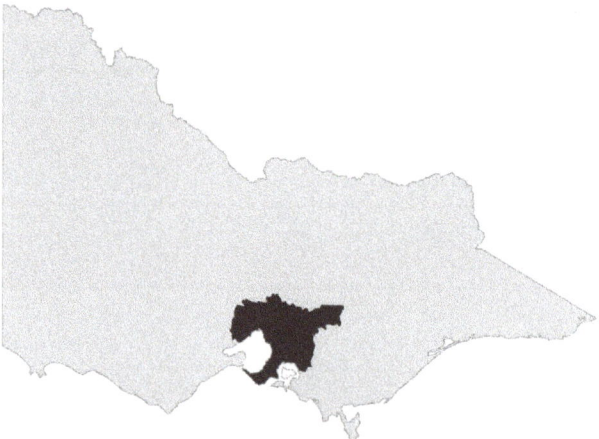

Figure 2. Boundaries for major cities (Greater Melbourne), dark grey, and regional. Victoria, light grey.

Geographic coordinates for each participant's address and service provider address were compiled through geocoding in RStudio version 3.5.1, and a random sample of 100 were manually checked using Google Maps [18]. Any incomplete provider address locations were entered manually using Google Maps to obtain coordinates. For a single provider it was possible for multiple locations to exist. We mapped the travel distances for all locations using Here Routing API (https://developer.here.com, accessed on 17 Febrary 2020) and used the shortest distance, assuming that people would visit the closest provider location to their homes.

2.5. Statistical Methods

Summary statistics were used to describe demographic information, injury characteristics, and service use outcomes. Medians and interquartile range were reported for skewed categorical variables and frequencies and percentages for continuous variables.

Regression models were used to provide estimates of the association between the outcomes of interest and region by injury type. Models were run for each outcome using region as an interaction term with injury type. All models were adjusted for the covariates of age group, sex, Charlson comorbidity index, ISS, and IRSAD based on factors known to impact healthcare utilization [19,20]. Multivariable logistic regression was used for service use (yes/no), and negative binomial regression was used for the number of trips per person, while a general estimating equation (GEE) was used to model distance travelled to services used. For the GEE, a Gaussian model and identity link was used, and an exchangeable correlation was assumed between trips to the same service within each individual. Adjusted odds ratios (OR) and incidence rate ratios (IRR), and the corresponding 95% confidence intervals were calculated for the logistic and negative binomial regression models, respectively. As distance travelled was positively skewed, the data were log transformed before modelling. Model fit was evaluated for concordance and discrimination using residual plots [21]. All analyses were completed in Stata Version 16.0 with the exception of the geospatial analyses which were conducted using RStudio version 3.5.1 [18].

3. Results

There were 9365 cases of transport-related major trauma identified from the VSTR; 17.1% (*n* = 1597) were eligible for this study (Figure 1). The characteristics of included participants for each injury group are presented in Table 1.

Table 1. Demographics and injury characteristics of participants.

	All Cases (1597)	TOI (687)	TBI (759)	SCI (151)
	n (%)	n (%)	n (%)	n (%)
Gender				
Male	1122 (70.3)	461 (67.1)	537 (70.8)	124 (82.1)
Female	475 (29.7)	226 (32.9)	222 (29.2)	27 (17.9)
Age group, years				
18–24	480 (30.1)	153 (22.1)	297 (39.1)	31 (20.5)
25–34	367 (23.0)	151 (22.0)	175 (23.1)	41 (27.2)
35–44	275 (17.2)	123 (17.9)	123 (16.2)	29 (19.2)
45–54	206 (12.9)	104 (15.1)	82 (10.8)	20 (13.2)
55–64	120 (7.5)	67 (9.8)	42 (5.5)	11 (7.3)
65–74	76 (4.8)	39 (5.7)	24 (3.1)	13 (8.6)
75+	73 (4.6)	51 (7.4)	16 (2.1)	6 (4.0)
Injury Severity Score, median (IQR)	20 (13–29)	13 (9–14)	29 (22–38)	29 (24–33)
CCI [22] weight (CCI) [1]				
0	857 (53.5)	521 (75.6)	235 (30.8)	101 (66.4)
1	582 (36.4)	126 (18.3)	424 (55.6)	33 (21.7)
>1	142 (8.9)	32 (4.6)	98 (12.9)	13 (8.6)
Acute hospital LOS (days), median (IQR)	13 (7–24)	8 (5–13)	18 (11–29)	24 (13–39)
Region (ARIA+ 2016)				
Major cities	1040 (65.1)	441 (65.2)	507 (66.8)	92 (60.9)
Inner regional	438 (27.4)	184 (26.8)	205 (27.0)	49 (32.5)
Outer regional	119 (7.5)	62 (9.0)	47 (6.2)	10 (6.6)
Socioeconomic status (IRSAD)				
1 (most disadvantaged)	268 (16.8)	128 (18.6)	118 (15.5)	22 (14.5)
2	168 (10.5)	72 (10.5)	81 (10.6)	15 (9.9)
3	309 (19.3)	128 (18.6)	150 (19.8)	31 (20.5)
4	432 (27.1)	189 (27.5)	202 (26.6)	41 (27.2)
5 (least disadvantaged)	420 (26.3)	170 (24.7)	208 (27.4)	42 (27.8)
Discharge destination				
Home	287 (18.0)	237 (34.5)	41 (5.4)	9 (6.0)
Other (e.g., inpatient rehabilitation)	1310 (82.0)	450 (65.4)	718 (94.6)	142 (94.0)
Road user [2]				
Motor vehicle driver or passenger	881 (55.2)	348 (50.6)	451 (59.5)	82 (53.9)
Motorcyclist	347 (21.7)	198 (28.8)	99 (13.0)	50 (32.9)
Pedestrian	244 (15.4)	85 (12.4)	154 (20.3)	6 (4.0)
Bicyclist	91 (5.7)	42 (6.1)	41 (5.4)	8 (5.3)

n = 19 missing [1]. n = 34 other or missing [2]. LOS = length of stay; IQR = interquartile range; CCI = Charlson comorbidity index, ARIA+ = Accessibility/Remoteness Index of Australia; IRSAD = Index of Relative Socio-economic Advantage and Disadvantage.

Across all injury groups, most participants were men and the median age was 33 years (IQR 23–48). Thirty-five percent of participants resided in regional areas. Most participants were injured in motor vehicle or motorcycle crashes. The SCI group had the longest length of acute hospital stay. In the first three years following hospital discharge, the 1597 participants visited health services 159,090 times for GP services, other medical appointments, mental health services, physical therapies, and OT (Table 2).

Figure 3 provides a summary of the key findings from the multivariable regression analysis for service use, number of trips, and distances travelled to services. More specific results from the models for each outcome and injury group are reported in each section below.

Table 2. All services used by participants in the first three years post-discharge by injury type.

	All Cases (n = 1597)		TBI (n = 759)		SCI (n = 151)		TOI (n = 687)	
	n	%	n	%	n	%	n	%
Physiotherapy	59,532	30.7	27,556	27.0	9667	31.7	22,309	36.5
Occupational Therapy	34,268	17.7	23,026	22.5	6557	21.5	4685	7.7
GP Consult	20,078	10.4	8791	8.6	2937	9.6	8350	13.7
Psychology	18,907	9.7	14,480	14.1	1285	4.2	3142	5.1
Nursing	13,289	6.9	2436	2.4	6032	19.8	4821	7.9
Medical (other)	10,972	5.7	6315	6.2	803	2.6	3854	6.3
Speech Therapy	8373	4.3	8143	7.9	165	0.5	65	0.1
Hydrotherapy	6917	3.6	1727	1.7	233	0.8	4957	8.1
Exercise Physiology	6832	3.5	1816	1.8	839	2.8	4177	6.8
Vocational counselling	4175	2.2	1720	1.7	359	1.2	2096	3.4
Social Work	1792	0.9	1203	1.2	313	1.0	276	0.5
Psychiatry	1584	0.8	1049	1.0	80	0.3	455	0.7
Podiatry	1193	0.6	348	0.3	551	1.8	294	0.5
Osteopathy	1017	0.5	306	0.3	112	0.4	599	1.0
Dental	990	0.5	864	0.8	55	0.2	71	0.1
Dietitian	800	0.4	511	0.5	186	0.6	103	0.2
Case Conferences	741	0.4	444	0.4	30	0.1	267	0.4
Chiropractor	680	0.4	380	0.4	66	0.2	234	0.4
Attendant carer	623	0.3	444	0.4	119	0.4	60	0.1
Paramedical (other)	557	0.3	443	0.4	36	0.1	78	0.1
Acupuncture	468	0.2	275	0.3	29	0.1	164	0.3
Optical	291	0.2	257	0.3	6	<0.1	28	<0.1
Total	194,079		102,534		30,460		61,085	

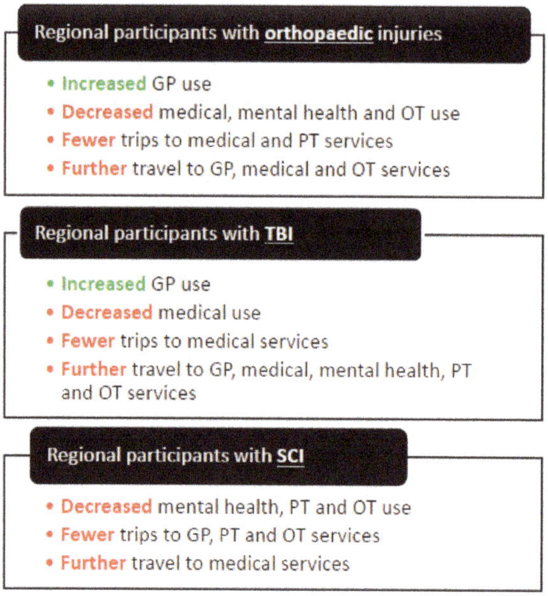

Regional participants with orthopaedic injuries
- Increased GP use
- Decreased medical, mental health and OT use
- Fewer trips to medical and PT services
- Further travel to GP, medical and OT services

Regional participants with TBI
- Increased GP use
- Decreased medical use
- Fewer trips to medical services
- Further travel to GP, medical, mental health, PT and OT services

Regional participants with SCI
- Decreased mental health, PT and OT use
- Fewer trips to GP, PT and OT services
- Further travel to medical services

Figure 3. Summary of key findings for regional participants compared with participants in major cities.

3.1. Service Use

The adjusted proportions of people using GP services were higher for regional participants in all injury groups (Figure 4). Across all other services, the adjusted proportions for service use were greater for people living in major cities compared with people living in regional areas, except for people with TBI accessing mental health services.

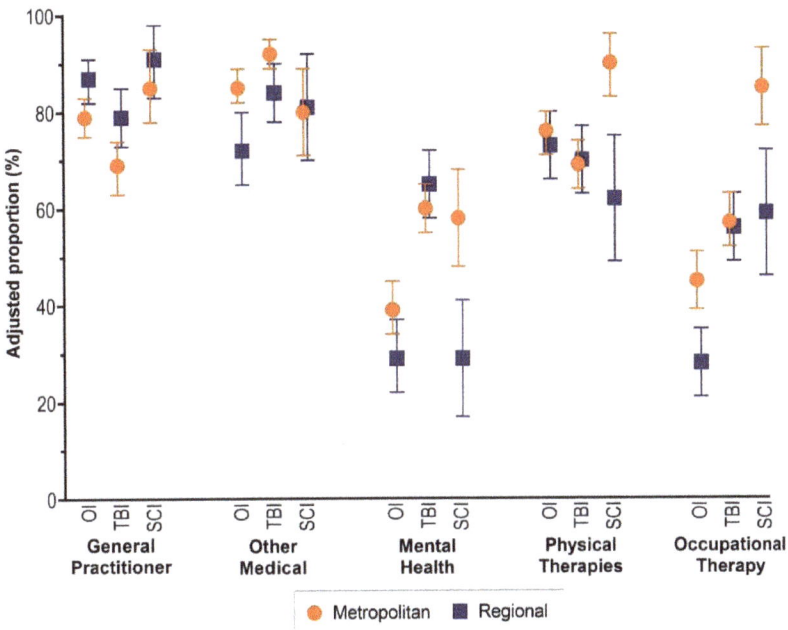

Figure 4. Adjusted proportion of service use by injury group and region.

In the orthopaedic and TBI groups, participants in regional areas, compared with major cities, had 76% higher adjusted odds of seeing a GP but 56% and 57% lower adjusted odds of attending other types of medical services, respectively (Table 3). In the orthopaedic group, participants in regional areas, compared with major cities, had 37% lower adjusted odds of attending mental health services and 45% lower adjusted odds of attending occupational therapy services. In the SCI group, participants in regional areas, compared with major cities, had 72% lower odds of accessing mental health, 82% lower adjusted odds of accessing physical therapies, and 76% lower adjusted odds of accessing OT services (Table 3).

Table 3. Regional variation in service use and number of trips per person in the first three years following hospital discharge determined by multivariable regression analysis.

	Participants Using Service (n, %)	Service Use, Adjusted OR (95%CI)	p *	Trips per Person, Median (IQR)	Adjusted IRR (95%CI)	p †
General Practitioner						
TOI						
Major cities	329 (74.6)	Reference		9 (4–22)	Reference	
Regional	206 (83.7)	1.76 (1.1–2.9)	0.02	9 (3–21)	0.81 (0.66–0.99)	0.04
TBI						
Major cities	370 (73.0)	Reference		9 (3–18)	Reference	
Regional	211 (83.7)	1.76 (1.1–2.8)	0.02	10 (4–22)	0.90 (0.75–1.1)	0.31

Table 3. Cont.

	Participants Using Service (n, %)	Service Use, Adjusted OR (95%CI)	p *	Trips per Person, Median (IQR)	Adjusted IRR (95%CI)	p †
SCI						
Major cities	80 (87.0)	Reference		18.5 (10.5–30)	Reference	
Regional	54 (91.5)	1.73 (0.5–5.4)	0.35	15 (6–23)	0.65 (0.5–0.9)	0.02
Medical Specialists						
TOI						
Major cities	360 (81.6)	Reference		5 (2–11)	Reference	
Regional	160 (65.0)	0.44 (0.28–0.70)	0.001	3 (2–8)	0.71 (0.6–0.9)	<0.001
TBI						
Major cities	477 (94.1)	Reference		8 (4–14)	Reference	
Regional	220 (87.3)	0.43 (0.24–0.78)	0.01	5 (3–9.5)	0.65 (0.6–0.8)	<0.001
SCI						
Major cities	76 (82.6)	Reference		4 (2–9.5)	Reference	
Regional	49 (83.1)	1.07 (0.42–2.70)	0.89	4 (2–8)	0.90 (0.6–1.2)	0.51
Mental Health						
TOI						
Major cities	158 (35.8)	Reference		11 (4–26)	Reference	
Regional	56 (22.8)	0.63 (0.41–0.96)	0.03	7 (4–23)	0.88 (0.6–1.3)	0.47
TBI						
Major cities	330 (65.1)	Reference		23.5 (8–54)	Reference	
Regional	169 (67.1)	1.23 (0.84–1.81)	0.29	16 (6–36)	0.78 (0.6–1.0)	0.05
SCI						
Major cities	57 (62.0)	Reference		14 (7–35)	Reference	
Regional	17 (28.8)	0.28 (0.1–0.6)	0.001	10 (4–17)	0.84 (0.5–1.5)	0.58
Physical Therapies						
TOI						
Major cities	322 (73.0)	Reference		42 (15–102)	Reference	
Regional	176 (71.5)	0.87 (0.57–1.33)	0.54	34 (14–74.5)	0.76 (0.6–0.9)	0.01
TBI						
Major cities	355 (70.0)	Reference		40 (14–85)	Reference	
Regional	181 (71.8)	1.08 (0.72–1.62)	0.71	34 (10–72)	0.81 (0.6–1.0)	0.07
SCI						
Major cities	84 (91.3)	Reference		87 (41–131.5)	Reference	
Regional	39 (66.1)	0.18 (0.07–0.45)	<0.001	46 (9–92)	0.63 (0.41–0.95)	0.03
Occupational Therapy						
TOI						
Major cities	165 (37.4)	Reference		9 (2–25)	Reference	
Regional	55 (22.4)	0.45 (0.29–0.69)	<0.001	4 (2–22)	0.76 (0.5–1.1)	0.17
TBI						
Major cities	317 (62.5)	Reference		30 (8–73)	Reference	
Regional	154 (61.1)	0.95 (0.65–1.39)	0.81	24.5 (5–57)	0.89 (0.7–1.2)	0.40
SCI						
Major cities	81 (88.0)	Reference		49 (14–93)	Reference	
Regional	39 (66.1)	0.24 (0.10–0.58)	0.001	11 (3–62)	0.55 (0.3–0.9)	0.01

* p value for the logistic regression analysis of service use. † p value for negative binomial regression analysis of number of trips, per person, for participants who used that service. p values in bold type are significant. IQR = interquartile range, OR = odds ratio, IRR = incidence rate ratio.

3.2. Number of Trips

For all injuries and service types, people in regional areas used fewer services than people residing in major cities after adjusting for covariates (Figure 5). Physical therapies were the most commonly used service across all injury groups. In the orthopaedic group, the mean number of trips for participants in regional areas, compared with major cities, was 29% lower for medical services and 24% lower for physical therapy services. In the TBI group, the mean number of trips for participants in regional areas, compared with major cities, was 35% lower for medical services. In the SCI group, the mean number of trips for participants in regional areas, compared with major cities, was 35% lower for GPs, 37% lower for physical therapy and 45% lower for OT services (Table 3).

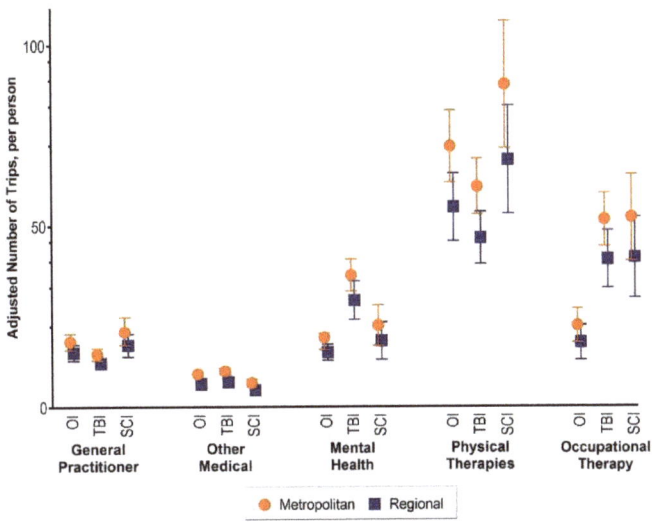

Figure 5. Adjusted number of trips to services in the first three years post-discharge by service type and injury group.

3.3. Distance Travelled

In the TBI group, participants in regional areas travelled significantly further to access all post-discharge health services compared with participants in major cities (Figure 6). In the SCI group, however, participants in regional areas travelled further only to attend medical services (RGM 2.66, 95%CI 1.63–4.36) (Figure 6). In the orthopaedic group, participants in regional areas travelled 1.4 times further to see a GP (95%CI 1.06–1.88), 2.26 times further to attend other medical services (95%CI 1.76–2.89), and 1.7 times further to OT services (95%CI 1.06–2.62) compared with participants in major cities.

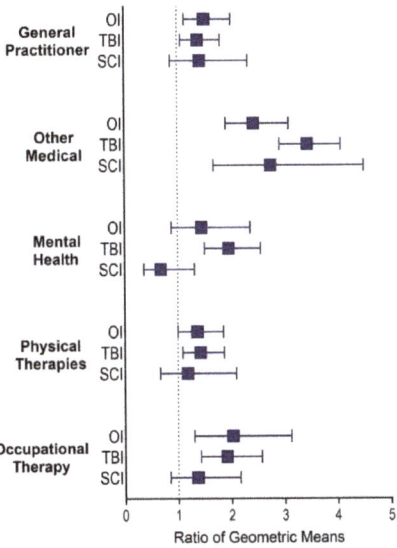

Figure 6. Ratio of geometric means for distance travelled by people in regional areas compared with major cities by injury group and service type.

For visits to medical services, the median trip distances for participants in regional areas with any injury type ranged from 68.70 km (95%CI: 8.34–139.84) to 104.05 km (95% CI: 51.55–182.78) (Figure 7). Comparatively, the median trip distances for participants in major cities with any injury type ranged from 9.44 km (95%CI 4.92–23.05) to 13.50 km (95% CI 6.65–25.59) (Figure 7).

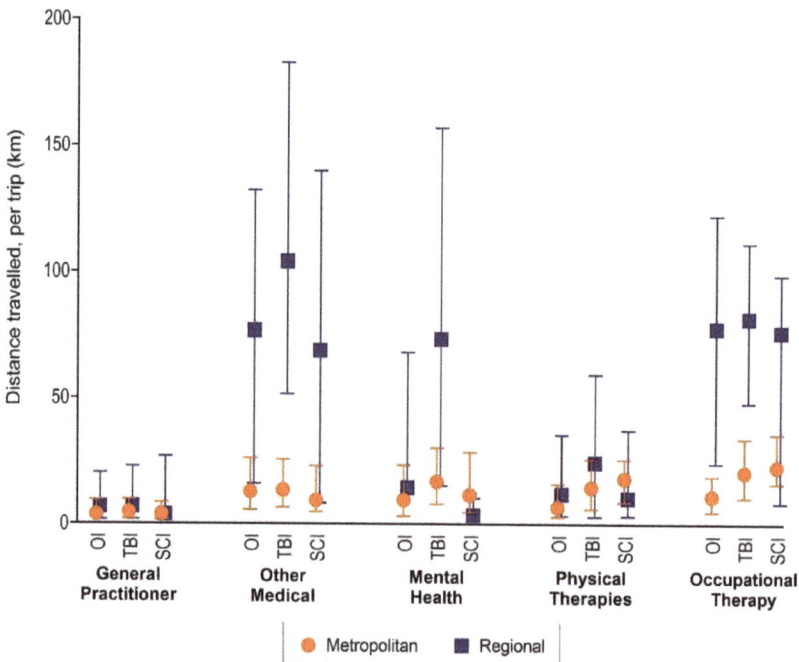

Figure 7. Median and IQR of raw distances travelled to healthcare by service type and injury group.

4. Discussion

In this study, we compared health service usage and distances travelled by people with transport-related orthopaedic, brain and spinal cord injuries across regional and metropolitan Victoria in the first three years following hospital discharge. For most services and injury types, people in regional areas used fewer services but travelled further to access them than people in metropolitan areas. People with orthopaedic injuries and TBI in regional areas had greater odds of seeing a GP compared with their metropolitan counterparts. This research provides an important contribution to our understanding of how geography impacts healthcare utilisation following major trauma.

We found that regional participants with orthopaedic injuries and TBI had greater odds of attending GP services than metropolitan participants, despite having to travel further. This may be explained by people in metropolitan areas living closer to trauma centres with better access to specialised rehabilitation providers, therefore being less reliant on their local GPs [23–25]. Following major trauma, GPs play a critical role in providing ongoing community support, monitoring for secondary complications of injury and psychosocial issues, and assisting in the patient's return to work [26]. For people living in metropolitan areas, it is possible that these issues may be monitored by a specialised rehabilitation team, including allied health and specialist physicians. Our findings highlight the importance of regional-based GPs having adequate knowledge of injury complications and a network of specialists that may be able to carry out shared virtual consultations to ensure timely and effective management closer to home [27].

Consistent with previous research, our findings suggest that people with serious injuries living in regional areas use fewer health services than their metropolitan counterparts [28–31]. Having to travel further to access healthcare for people in regional areas may limit accessibility [5,8,24]. Compounding the challenge of distance, transportation difficulties [6,8,29,32] and a limited availability of skilled providers [7,33] have been reported as barriers to accessing necessary services for people with orthopaedic injuries, TBI, and SCI, particularly for those in regional areas. A key consequence of reduced service use is that people with serious injuries living in regional areas often report higher levels of unmet care needs [25,30,34–36]. Ensuring the availability of local infrastructure or alternate service delivery methods is essential for people with serious injury due to the chronicity of the condition [8,34,37].

In this study, we found that for all injury types, people living in regional areas travelled further than people in metropolitan areas to access all services. However, after adjusting for covariates, our findings were more nuanced. People living in regional areas with TBI travelled significantly further to all health services than those in metropolitan areas, whereas for people with SCI, a significant difference was only found for travel to medical services, which was based on region. Due to the complexity and long-term issues associated with SCI, people with SCI may choose to live in areas where they can access necessary services [24]. In comparison, given the varying degree of severity of TBI, some people with TBI may place less importance on ease of service access and availability when deciding where they want to reside. These novel findings reinforce the importance of specialised telehealth services and outreach clinics for people in regional areas with TBI to reduce travel burden and ensure access to adequately skilled healthcare services.

In addition to considering alternate service delivery modes, at a systems level, this research contributes a new perspective for post-discharge care coordination for people with serious injury. Policy makers involved in the planning of healthcare pathways across the continuum of care should consider the extra distances travelled by people in regional areas and possible travel burden, which may impact post-discharge healthcare utilisation. Further research to understand patterns of health service utilisation for other groups at risk of health inequities, such as older adults, Aboriginal and Torres Strait Islander People, and culturally and linguistically diverse communities, particularly in regional areas, will further aid in improving healthcare planning.

Study Limitations

This population-based cohort study provides novel insights into geographic variations in healthcare use following transport-related orthopaedic, brain, and spinal cord injury. However, a limitation of this work was that due to multiple service provider locations being provided, we assumed that an individual attended the closest facility to their home and used the shortest trip distance. This study also only included services that were centre-based; therefore, for people with TBI and SCI, who are likely to have received services in the community or at home, the number of services used may be underrepresented. This also includes care from the Spinal Community Integration Service, a Victorian program that provides people with SCI assistance with returning home and participating in their communities in the first 12 months following discharge. Due to the nature of how these services are billed to the TAC, it was not possible to ascertain specific details of what services were provided on exact dates and at specific locations. However, as this was the same for both regional and metropolitan participants, this is unlikely to have impacted the regional variation within groups. It was also assumed that participants all travelled by car to attend services. Due to the reimbursement available for taxi travel and motorised travel expenses for TAC patients, it is most likely that participants would choose one of these options over human-powered or public transport.

5. Conclusions

Health service use following traumatic orthopaedic, brain, and spinal cord injury is complex and continues for years following the initial injury. This research has identified disparities in service use and distances travelled to health services across metropolitan and regional Victoria following serious injury. With people in regional areas using fewer services, except for GPs, and attending these services less often, there is a risk of unmet service needs for these individuals. An increased travel distance to services is one factor that may be contributing to the inequality in access to healthcare in regional areas compared with metropolitan areas. These findings reinforce the need for a review of how specialised rehabilitation services are delivered to people residing in regional areas following major trauma and whether access to post-discharge services is available to everyone long-term, regardless of where they reside. Further research exploring whether there is an association between service use, distance travelled, and health outcomes is necessary to ensure post-discharge care is optimised for people with serious injuries.

Author Contributions: Conceptualization, J.K., B.G., C.E. and B.B.; methodology, J.K., B.G., S.A. and B.B.; validation, J.K., B.G. and B.B.; formal analysis, J.K. and S.A.; resources, J.K.; data curation, J.K.; writing—original draft preparation, J.K.; writing—review and editing, J.K., B.G., S.A., C.E. and B.B.; visualization, J.K.; funding acquisition, J.K. All authors have read and agreed to the published version of the manuscript.

Funding: This research was funded in part by an Epworth Medical Foundation, Translational Research Grant. JK was supported by an Australian Government Research Training Program Scholarship. CE was supported by a National Health and Medical Research Council of Australia (NHMRC) Early Career Fellowship (1106633). BG was supported by an Australian Research Council Future Fellowship (FT170100048). BB was supported by an Australian Research Council Discovery Early Career Researcher Award Fellowship (DE180100825).

Institutional Review Board Statement: The study was conducted in accordance with the Declaration of Helsinki, and approved by the Monash University Human Research Ethics Committee (HREC) (Project ID 18433, 10 April 2019). The VSTR has ethics approval from the Department of Health and Human Services HREC (reference_11/14), Monash University and all trauma receiving hospitals.

Informed Consent Statement: Informed consent was obtained from all subjects involved in the study.

Data Availability Statement: Not applicable.

Acknowledgments: We thank the Victorian State Trauma Outcome Registry and Monitoring (VSTORM) group for providing VSTR data and Sue McLellan for their assistance with data preparation. We also express our appreciation to the TAC for the provision of data and their assistance in data preparation.

Conflicts of Interest: The authors declare no conflict of interest. The funders had no role in the design of the study; in the collection, analyses, or interpretation of data; in the writing of the manuscript; or in the decision to publish the results.

Appendix A

Table A1. Strengthening The Reporting of Observational Studies in Epidemiology (STROBE) statement checklist.

		Recommendation	Page
Title and abstract	1	(a) Indicate the study's design with a commonly used term in the title or the abstract	1
		(b) Provide in the abstract an informative and balanced summary of what was performed and what was found	1

Table A1. Cont.

		Recommendation	Page
Introduction			
Background/rationale	2	Explain the scientific background and rationale for the investigation being reported	1
Objectives	3	State specific objectives, including any prespecified hypotheses	2
Methods			
Study design	4	Present key elements of study design early in the paper	2
Setting	5	Describe the setting, locations, and relevant dates, including periods of recruitment, exposure, follow-up, and data collection	2–3
Participants	6	(a) Give the eligibility criteria and the sources and methods of selection of participants. Describe methods of follow-up	3–4
		(b) For matched studies, give matching criteria and number of exposed and unexposed	n/a
Variables	7	Clearly define all outcomes, exposures, predictors, potential confounders, and effect modifiers. Give diagnostic criteria, if applicable	4
Data sources/measurement	8	For each variable of interest, give sources of data and details of methods of assessment (measurement). Describe comparability of assessment methods if there is more than one group	2–3
Bias	9	Describe any efforts to address potential sources of bias	-
Study size	10	Explain how the study size was arrived at	Figure 1
Quantitative variables	11	Explain how quantitative variables were handled in the analyses. If applicable, describe which groupings were chosen and why	4
Statistical methods	12	(a) Describe all statistical methods, including those used to control for confounding	4
		(b) Describe any methods used to examine subgroups and interactions	4–5
		(c) Explain how missing data were addressed	n/a
		(d) If applicable, explain how loss to follow-up was addressed	n/a
		(e) Describe any sensitivity analyses	-
Results			
Participants	13	(a) Report numbers of individuals at each stage of study, e.g., numbers potentially eligible, examined for eligibility, confirmed eligible, included in the study, completing follow-up, and analysed	5
		(b) Give reasons for non-participation at each stage	n/a
		© Consider use of a flow diagram	Figure 1
Descriptive data	14	(a) Give characteristics of study participants (e.g., demographic, clinical, social) and information on exposures and potential confounders	Table 1
		(b) Indicate number of participants with missing data for each variable of interest	n/a
		(c) Summarise follow-up time (e.g., average and total amount)	5
Outcome data	15	Report numbers of outcome events or summary measures over time	5–8

References

1. World Health Organization. *World Health Organization Global Burden of Disease*; World Health Organization: Geneva, Switzerland, 2007.
2. Post, M.W.M.; van Leeuwen, C.M.C. Psychosocial issues in spinal cord injury: A review. *Spinal Cord* **2012**, *50*, 382–389. [CrossRef] [PubMed]
3. Dahm, J.; Ponsford, J. Comparison of long-term outcomes following traumatic injury: What is the unique experience for those with brain injury compared with orthopaedic injury? *Injury* **2015**, *46*, 142–149. [CrossRef] [PubMed]

4. Gabbe, B.J.; Simpson, P.M.; Cameron, P.A.; Ponsford, J.; Lyons, R.A.; Collie, A.; Harrison, J.E.; Ameratunga, S.; Nunn, A.; Braaf, S.; et al. Long-term health status and trajectories of seriously injured patients: A population-based longitudinal study. *PLoS Med.* **2017**, *14*, e1002322. [CrossRef] [PubMed]
5. Keeves, J.; Gabbe, B.J.; Ekegren, C.L.; Fry, R.; Beck, B. Regional variation in travel to health services following transport-related major trauma. *Injury* **2021**, *53*, 1707–1715. [CrossRef]
6. Gabbe, B.J.; Sleney, J.S.; Gosling, C.M.; Wilson, K.; Hart, M.J.; Sutherland, A.M.; Christie, N. Patient perspectives of care in a regionalised trauma system: Lessons from the Victorian State Trauma System. *Med. J. Aust.* **2013**, *198*, 149–152. [CrossRef]
7. Keeves, J.; Braaf, S.C.; Ekegren, C.L.; Beck, B.; Gabbe, B.J. Caring for people with serious injuries in urban and regional communities: A qualitative investigation of healthcare providers' perceptions. *Disabil. Rehabil.* **2020**, *43*, 3052–3060. [CrossRef]
8. Keeves, J.; Braaf, S.C.; Ekegren, C.L.; Beck, B.; Gabbe, B.J. Access to Healthcare Following Serious Injury: Perspectives of Allied Health Professionals in Urban and Regional Settings. *Int. J. Environ. Res. Public Health* **2021**, *18*, 1230. [CrossRef]
9. Ruseckaite, R.; Gabbe, B.; Vogel, A.P.; Collie, A. Health care utilisation following hospitalisation for transport-related injury. *Injury* **2012**, *43*, 1600–1605. [CrossRef]
10. *Victorian State Trauma Registry Annual Report 2019–2020*; Victorian State Trauma Outcomes Registry and Monitoring Group: Melbourne, Australia, 2021.
11. Von Elm, E.; Altman, D.G.; Egger, M.; Pocock, S.J.; Gøtzsche, P.C.; Vandenbroucke, J.P. The Strengthening the Reporting of Observational Studies in Epidemiology (STROBE) statement: Guidelines for reporting observational studies. *Bull. World Health Organ.* **2007**, *85*, 867–872. [CrossRef]
12. Australian Bureau of Statistics. Regional Population Growth, Australia, 2017–2018. Available online: www.abs.gov.au/ausstats/abs@.nsf/0/B7616AB91C66CDCFCA25827800183B7B?Opendocument (accessed on 9 July 2019).
13. Cameron, P.A.; Gabbe, B.J.; Cooper, D.J.; Walker, T.; Judson, R.; McNeil, J. A statewide system of trauma care in Victoria: Effect on patient survival. *Med. J. Aust.* **2008**, *189*, 546–550. [CrossRef]
14. Transport Accident Act 1986. Melbourne, Australia. 2020. Available online: https://www.legislation.vic.gov.au/in-force/acts/transport-accident-act-1986/151 (accessed on 1 September 2022).
15. Victorian State Trauma Registry Annual Report 2019–2020. Melbourne, Australia. Available online: https://www.monash.edu/__data/assets/pdf_file/0008/2706047/VSTR-Annual-Report-2019-20-WEB_FINAL.pdf (accessed on 1 September 2022).
16. Australian Bureau of Statistics. Australian Statistical Geography Standard (ASGS): Volume 5-Remoteness Structure, July 2011. Available online: http://www.ausstats.abs.gov.au/ausstats/subscriber.nsf/0/A277D01B6AF25F64CA257B03000D7EED/$File/1270055005_july%202011.pdf (accessed on 13 October 2020).
17. Pink, B. *Information Paper: An Introduction to Socio-Economic Indexes for Areas (SEIFA), 2006*; Australian Bureau of Statistics: Canberra, Australia, 2008.
18. Team, R.C. *R: A Language and Environment for Statistical Computing*; R Foundation for Statistical Computing: Vienna, Austria, 2020.
19. Ronca, E.; Scheel-Sailer, A.; Eriks-Hoogland, I.; Brach, M.; Debecker, I.; Gemperli, A. Factors influencing specialized health care utilization by individuals with spinal cord injury: A cross-sectional survey. *Spinal Cord* **2021**, *59*, 381–388. [CrossRef] [PubMed]
20. Gabbe, B.J.; Sutherland, A.M.; Williamson, O.D.; Cameron, P.A. Use of health care services 6 months following major trauma. *Aust. Health Rev.* **2007**, *31*, 628–632. [CrossRef] [PubMed]
21. Portney, L.G.; Watkins, M.P. *Foundations of Clinical Research: Applications to Practice*; Pearson/Prentice Hall: Upper Saddle River, NJ, USA, 2009; Volume 892.
22. Charlson, M.E.; Pompei, P.; Ales, K.L.; MacKenzie, C.R. A new method of classifying prognostic comorbidity in longitudinal studies: Development and validation. *J. Chronic Dis.* **1987**, *40*, 373–383. [CrossRef]
23. Touhami, D.; Brach, M.; Essig, S.; Ronca, E.; Debecker, I.; Eriks-Hoogland, I.; Scheel-Sailer, A.; Münzel, N.; Gemperli, A. First contact of care for persons with spinal cord injury: A general practitioner or a spinal cord injury specialist? *BMC Fam. Pract.* **2021**, *22*, 1–195. [CrossRef] [PubMed]
24. LaVela, S.L.; Smith, B.; Weaver, F.M.; Miskevics, S.A. Geographical proximity and health care utilization in veterans with SCI&D in the USA. *Soc. Sci. Med.* **2004**, *59*, 2387–2399. [CrossRef]
25. Kettlewell, J.; Timmons, S.; Bridger, K.; Kendrick, D.; Kellezi, B.; Holmes, J.; Patel, P.; Radford, K. A study of mapping usual care and unmet need for vocational rehabilitation and psychological support following major trauma in five health districts in the UK. *Clin. Rehabil.* **2021**, *35*, 750–764. [CrossRef]
26. Khan, F.; Baguley, I.J.; Cameron, I.D. 4: Rehabilitation after traumatic brain injury. *Med. J. Aust.* **2003**, *178*, 290–295. [CrossRef]
27. Jonnagaddala, J.; Godinho, M.A.; Liaw, S.-T. From telehealth to virtual primary care in Australia? a rapid scoping review. *Int. J. Med. Inform.* **2021**, *151*, 104470. [CrossRef]
28. Bell, N.; Kidanie, T.; Cai, B.; Krause, J.S. Geographic variation in outpatient health care service utilization after spinal cord injury. *Arch. Phys. Med. Rehabil.* **2017**, *98*, 341–346. [CrossRef]
29. Ronca, E.; Scheel-Sailer, A.; Koch, H.G.; Essig, S.; Brach, M.; Münzel, N.; Gemperli, A.; Group, S.S. Satisfaction with access and quality of healthcare services for people with spinal cord injury living in the community. *J. Spinal Cord Med.* **2020**, *43*, 111–121. [CrossRef]
30. Simpson, G.K.; Daher, M.; Hodgkinson, A.; Strettles, B. Comparing the Injury Profile, Service Use, Outcomes, and Comorbidities of People With Severe TBI Across Urban, Regional, and Remote Populations in New South Wales: A Multicentre Study. *J. Head Trauma Rehabil.* **2016**, *31*, E26–E38. [CrossRef] [PubMed]

31. Xia, T.; Iles, R.; Newnam, S.; Lubman, D.I.; Collie, A. Patterns of health service use following work-related injury and illness in Australian truck drivers: A latent class analysis. *Am. J. Ind. Med.* **2020**, *63*, 180–187. [CrossRef] [PubMed]
32. Legg, M.; Foster, M.; Jones, R.; Kendall, M.; Fleming, J.; Nielsen, M.; Kendall, E.; Borg, D.; Geraghty, T. The impact of obstacles to health and rehabilitation services on functioning and disability: A prospective survey on the 12-months after discharge from specialist rehabilitation for acquired brain injury. *Disabil. Rehabil.* **2022**, *44*, 5919–5929. [CrossRef] [PubMed]
33. Beatty, P.W.; Hagglund, K.J.; Neri, M.T.; Dhont, K.R.; Clark, M.J.; Hilton, S.A. Access to health care services among people with chronic or disabling conditions: Patterns and predictors. *Arch. Phys. Med. Rehabil.* **2003**, *84*, 1417–1425. [CrossRef]
34. Ronca, E.; Brunkert, T.; Koch, H.G.; Jordan, X.; Gemperli, A. Residential location of people with chronic spinal cord injury: The importance of local health care infrastructure. *BMC Health Serv. Res.* **2018**, *18*, 657. [CrossRef] [PubMed]
35. Mitsch, V.; Curtin, M.; Badge, H. The provision of brain injury rehabilitation services for people living in rural and remote New South Wales, Australia. *Brain Inj.* **2014**, *28*, 1504–1513. [CrossRef]
36. Archer, K.R.; Castillo, R.C.; MacKenzie, E.J.; Bosse, M.J.; Group, L.S. Perceived need and unmet need for vocational, mental health, and other support services after severe lower-extremity trauma. *Arch. Phys. Med. Rehabil.* **2010**, *91*, 774–780. [CrossRef] [PubMed]
37. Cox, R.J.; Amsters, D.I.; Pershouse, K.J. The need for a multidisciplinary outreach service for people with spinal cord injury living in the community. *Clin. Rehabil.* **2001**, *15*, 600–606. [CrossRef]

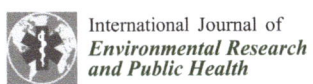

International Journal of
Environmental Research and Public Health

Review

A Scoping Review of Approaches to Improving Quality of Data Relating to Health Inequalities

Sowmiya Moorthie [1,*], Vicki Peacey [2], Sian Evans [3], Veronica Phillips [4], Andres Roman-Urrestarazu [1], Carol Brayne [1] and Louise Lafortune [1]

1. Cambridge Public Health, Interdisciplinary Research Centre, University of Cambridge, Cambridge CB2 0SZ, UK
2. Cambridgeshire County Council, Alconbury, Huntingdon PE28 4YE, UK
3. Local Knowledge Intelligence Service (LKIS) East, Office for Health Improvements and Disparities, UK
4. Medical Library, School of Clinical Medicine, University of Cambridge, Cambridge CB2 0SP, UK
* Correspondence: sam71@medschl.cam.ac.uk

Abstract: Identifying and monitoring of health inequalities requires good-quality data. The aim of this work is to systematically review the evidence base on approaches taken within the healthcare context to improve the quality of data for the identification and monitoring of health inequalities and describe the evidence base on the effectiveness of such approaches or recommendations. Peer-reviewed scientific journal publications, as well as grey literature, were included in this review if they described approaches and/or made recommendations to improve data quality relating to the identification and monitoring of health inequalities. A thematic analysis was undertaken of included papers to identify themes, and a narrative synthesis approach was used to summarise findings. Fifty-seven papers were included describing a variety of approaches. These approaches were grouped under four themes: policy and legislation, wider actions that enable implementation of policies, data collection instruments and systems, and methodological approaches. Our findings indicate that a variety of mechanisms can be used to improve the quality of data on health inequalities at different stages (prior to, during, and after data collection). These findings can inform us of actions that can be taken by those working in local health and care services on approaches to improving the quality of data on health inequalities.

Keywords: health inequalities; health disparities; data quality; public health

1. Introduction

Health inequalities are often defined as "differences in health across the population and between different groups" [1]. The study of health inequalities aims to better understand factors that contribute to unfair differences in the status of people's health to address them and achieve fairer and more inclusive health care. Inequalities in health can arise because of differences in the care that people receive and the opportunities they have to lead healthy lives, including differences in health status (e.g., life expectancy), quality and experience of care, and wider determinants of health [1].

Data analysis to improve understanding of health gaps is an important exercise that contributes to an aspiration for fair and inclusive health. Good data is vital for understanding inequality in health service provision and health outcomes, and necessary for informing and evaluating attempts to improve care or reduce inequality. In the United Kingdom, health inequalities are identified by analysing data across socio-economic factors, geography, and specific characteristics including those protected in law such as sex, ethnicity or disability, and socially excluded groups. However, the quality of data underpinning these analyses can be improved [2–4]. Good-quality data are data that are fit for the purpose; therefore, criteria on what constitutes "good" can vary. Dimensions such as completeness, accuracy, relevance, availability, and timeliness of data can be assessed to determine data quality [5].

Several policy reports released in the UK have highlighted the importance of improving the quality of data used for the identification and monitoring of health inequalities [6,7]. In particular, identifying and reducing inequalities linked to ethnicity are a key part of expectations in terms of improving NHS services [8]. Recommendations from these reports include ensuring consistent reporting and analysis of data on ethnicity, health, and health care and documenting and evaluating best practices [6]. The need for better data coverage across all age groups and allowing self-identification, particularly around ethnicity, has also been recommended [9].

Health inequalities have been increasing in England over the past 10 years and the COVID-19 pandemic has starkly highlighted inequalities that exist [10,11]. The pandemic has also demonstrated that collecting data at speed and using healthcare data in flexible and creative ways is possible [12]. This has renewed emphasis on the need for action to address inequalities at both national and system levels. This includes initiatives to improve data and make better use of data to address health inequalities [13,14]. A comprehensive understanding of the evidence base on how data quality can be improved and what has been shown to work is essential to inform the myriad of initiatives in the UK to address health inequalities.

The aim of this work was to identify and review the evidence base on approaches taken within the healthcare context to improve the quality of the data used for the identification and monitoring of health inequalities. The specific objectives were to describe the approaches that have been used or recommended to improve the quality (availability, completeness, accuracy, relevance, and timeliness) of data for identification of health inequalities, to describe the approaches that have been used or recommended to improve the quality of data for monitoring changes in health inequalities, and to describe the evidence base for the effectiveness of such approaches or recommendations.

2. Methods

2.1. Article Identification and Selection

A systematic literature search was conducted in the databases Medline (via Ovid), Embase (via Ovid), Global Health (via Ebscohost), Cinahl (via Ebschohost), and Web of Science (Core Collection) in September 2021 using search terms relating to data, data quality, and specific terms such as protected characteristics and tailoring them for each database (detailed search terms in Supplementary Materials). Search terms were deliberately broad to maximise the identification of relevant work, as more specific preliminary searches did not identify papers that were already known to be relevant. The searches were not date-limited initially. However, because legislation and guidance in the United Kingdom around recording data on health inequality characteristics has changed considerably in the last 10 years, we subsequently discarded reports published prior to January 2010. Papers that were published after 2010 but reported on data collected before 2010 were included. We undertook citation searching to identify other sources of information not identified in the database searches. In addition, a grey literature search was conducted using the advanced search function in Google. The search terms 'improving data quality health inequalities' were used; searches were restricted to .pdf file types. The first five pages of the search were examined for any documents that could be included. All results were limited to the English language.

2.2. Inclusion and Exclusion Criteria

Protocols for scoping reviews are not eligible for publication in PROSPERO; however, we have presented our findings as much as possible according to PRISMA guidelines [15] (Supplementary Materials). Peer-reviewed scientific journal publications, as well as grey literature, were included in this review if they described mechanisms to improve data quality relating to the identification and monitoring of health inequalities. Work that focused solely on improving the quality of data on health outcomes was not included, nor was work that simply evaluated data quality rather than presented attempts to improve data quality.

Two reviewers (SM and ARU) independently carried out primary screening of titles and abstracts to identify articles eligible for inclusion based on our eligibility criteria. A third reviewer (LL) reviewed all articles selected for inclusion and those marked as unsure and resolved any disagreements between the reviewers. The decision made by the third reviewer was final for inclusion or exclusion. Two reviewers (LL and SM) screened full-text articles for further assessment of eligibility for inclusion in this review. Discussion was undertaken to resolve any discrepancies. Figure 1 shows the search and selection outcomes for each stage of the review process.

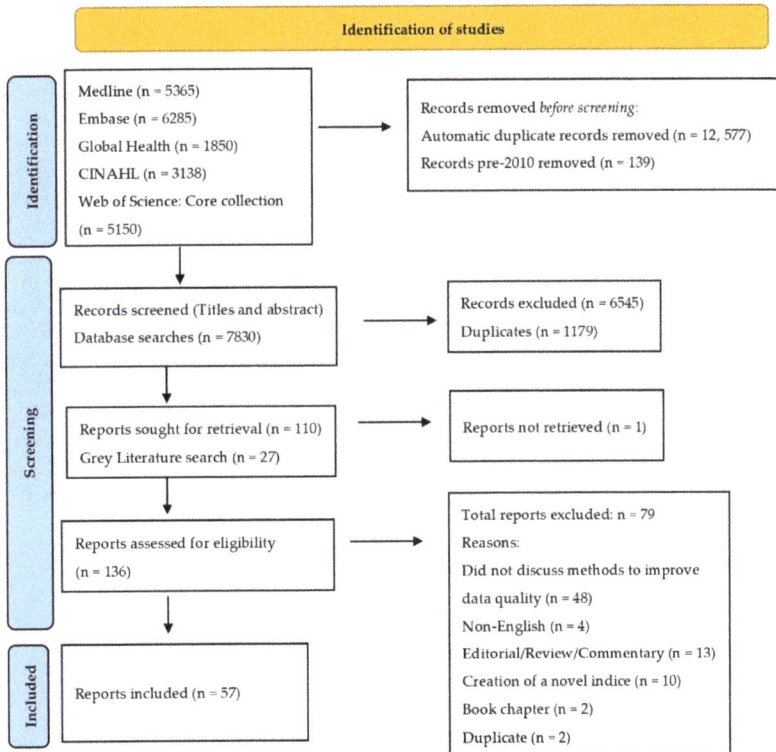

Figure 1. Flow diagram of included and excluded studies.

2.3. Data Extraction and Synthesis

Data extraction was carried out using an iterative process. One author (SM) read all papers eligible for inclusion, grouped them into broad categories based on the main type of data that was discussed (ethnicity, gender/sexual orientation, social determinants, general, or other), and extracted relevant text from sections of the papers that provided recommendations, methods, or approaches to improving data quality. Papers were categorised as "general" if they did not specify a particular inequality dimension or were across several dimensions. All the papers were subsequently read by at least one other author (VP, SE, or LL) to confirm and supplement the extraction before coding and to ensure quality and consistency. Any discrepancies in data extraction were resolved through discussion. A thematic analysis was then conducted by one reviewer (SM) to identify themes, which were then summarised narratively and validated by another reviewer (LL). There was heterogeneity in the included reports in terms of the subject matter and approaches used. This precluded us from using traditional quality-assurance measures for critiques of the papers.

3. Results

The initial database search revealed 21,788 records. Following automatic de-duplication and removal of articles published pre-2010, 7830 articles were identified for primary screening. A total of 110 articles met the eligibility criteria for retrieving full texts after primary screening. A further 27 reports were identified by the grey literature search. Seventy-nine studies were excluded following assessment of full texts. The main reason for exclusion was a lack of discussion on mechanisms to improve data quality. A total of 57 publications were included in the review. Table 1 provides a summary of the characteristics of these reports. Most were peer-reviewed publications ($n = 49$) with the remainder being grey literature ($n = 8$). Many were reporting on data related to the dimension of ethnicity ($n = 31$) or were more general across indicators related to health inequalities ($n = 15$). A smaller number were identified that were focused on dimensions of sexual orientation and gender ($n = 6$), or on specific areas such as infectious diseases, learning disabilities, or cardiovascular care. Most were from the US or UK. None of the studies identified were high on the traditional hierarchy of evidence, and in most cases the approaches that were used for improving data quality had several elements that could not be disaggregated.

Table 1. Included studies and characteristics.

Author, Year	Title	Type of Data Discussed	Distal Factors	Wider Actions to Enable Improvements in Data Collection	Data Collection Instruments, Systems, and Standardisation	Methodological Approaches to Improve Data Quality and Accuracy
Abouzeid, M et al. 2014 [16]	The potential for measuring ethnicity and health in a multicultural milieu—the case of type 2 diabetes in Australia	Ethnicity	✓	✓	✓	✓
Allen, VC et al. 2011 [17]	Issues in the Assessment of "Race" Among Latinos: Implications for Research and Policy	Ethnicity	✓	✓	✓	
Anderson, ML et al. 2018 [18]	Deaf Qualitative Health Research: Leveraging Technology to Conduct Linguistically and Sociopolitically Appropriate Methods of Inquiry	Disability		✓	✓	
Andrews, RM 2011 [19]	Race and Ethnicity Reporting in Statewide Hospital Data: Progress and Future Challenges in a Key Resource for Local and State Monitoring of Health Disparities	Ethnicity	✓	✓	✓	
Azar, KMJ et al. 2012 [20]	Accuracy of Data Entry of Patient Race/Ethnicity/Ancestry and Preferred Spoken Language in an Ambulatory Care Setting	Ethnicity		✓	✓	
Becker, T et al. 2021 [21]	Data Disaggregation with American Indian/Alaska Native Population Data	Ethnicity	✓	✓	✓	✓
Berry C et al. 2013 [22]	Moving to patient reported collection of race and ethnicity data Implementation and impact in ten hospitals	Ethnicity			✓	
Beltran VM et al. 2011 [23]	Collection of social determinants of health measures in U.S. national surveillance systems for HIV, viral hepatitis, STDs, and TB	Infectious disease	✓	✓	✓	✓
Bilheimer LT et al. 2010 [24]	Data and Measurement Issues in the Analysis of Health Disparities	General	✓	✓	✓	✓
Block RG et al. 2020 [25]	Recommendations for improving national clinical datasets for health equity research	General		✓	✓	✓
Blosnich JR et al. 2018 [26]	Using clinician text notes in electronic medical record data to validate transgender-related diagnosis codes	Gender				✓
Bozorgmehr, K et al. 2017 [16]	How Do Countries' Health Information Systems Perform in Assessing Asylum Seekers' Health Situation? Developing a Health Information Assessment Tool on Asylum Seekers (HIATUS) and Piloting It in Two European Countries	General			✓	
Cahill SR et al. 2016 [27]	Inclusion of Sexual Orientation and Gender Identity in Stage 3 Meaningful Use Guidelines: A Huge Step Forward for LGBT Health	Gender	✓			
Chakkalakal RJ et al. 2015 [28]	Standardized Data Collection Practices and the Racial/Ethnic Distribution of Hospitalized Patients	Ethnicity			✓	✓

Table 1. Cont.

Author, Year	Title	Type of Data Discussed	Distal Factors	Wider Actions to Enable Improvements in Data Collection	Data Collection Instruments, Systems, and Standardisation	Methodological Approaches to Improve Data Quality and Accuracy
Chen Y et al. 2018 [29]	Racial Differences in Data Quality and Completeness: Spinal Cord Injury Model Systems' Experiences	Ethnicity		✓	✓	
Clarke LC et al. 2016 [30]	Validity of Race, Ethnicity, and National Origin in Population-base Cancer Registries and Rapid Case Ascertainment Enhanced with a Spanish Surname List	Ethnicity				✓
Craddock L et al., 2016 [31]	Assessing race and ethnicity data quality across cancer registries and EMRs in two hospitals	Ethnicity	✓		✓	
Cruz, TM 2020 [32]	Perils of data-driven equity: Safety-net care and big data's elusive grasp on health inequality	General		✓		
Cruz, TM 2021 [33]	Shifting Analytics within US Biomedicine: From Patient Data to the Institutional Conditions of Health Care Inequalities	General	✓	✓	✓	
Davidson E et al., 2021 [34]	Raising ethnicity recording in NHS Lothian from 3% to 90% in 3 years: processes and analysis of data from Accidents and Emergencies	Ethnicity	✓	✓		✓
Derose, SF et al. 2013 [35]	Race and Ethnicity Data Quality and Imputation Using US Census Data in an Integrated Health System: The Kaiser Permanente Southern California Experience	Ethnicity	✓		✓	✓
Donald C and Ehrenfeld JM 2015 [36]	The Opportunity for Medical Systems to Reduce Health Disparities Among Lesbian, Gay, Bisexual, Transgender and Intersex Patients	Gender	✓	✓	✓	
Escarce, J et al. 2011 [37]	Collection Of Race and Ethnicity Data By Health Plans Has Grown Substantially, But Opportunities Remain To Expand Efforts	Ethnicity	✓	✓	✓	
Fortune, N et al. 2020 [38]	The Disability and Wellbeing Monitoring Framework: data, data gaps, and policy implications	Disability	✓	✓	✓	
Frank, J and Haw S 2011 [39]	Best Practice Guidelines for Monitoring Socioeconomic Inequalities in Health Status: Lessons from Scotland	Gender		✓	✓	✓
Fremont, A et al. 2016 [40]	When Race/Ethnicity Data Are Lacking: Using Advanced Indirect Estimation Methods to Measure Disparities	Ethnicity			✓	✓
Haas, AP et al. 2015 [41]	Collecting Sexual Orientation and Gender Identity Data in Suicide and Other Violent Deaths: A Step Towards Identifying and Addressing LGBT Mortality Disparities	Gender	✓		✓	
Hannigan, A et al. 2019 [42]	Ethnicity recording in health and social care data collections in Ireland: where and how is it measured and what is it used for?	Ethnicity	✓	✓		✓

Table 1. Cont.

Author, Year	Title	Type of Data Discussed	Distal Factors	Wider Actions to Enable Improvements in Data Collection	Data Collection Instruments, Systems, and Standardisation	Methodological Approaches to Improve Data Quality and Accuracy
Jorgensen S et al., 2010 [13]	Responses of Massachusetts hospitals to a state mandate to collect race, ethnicity and language data from patients: a qualitative study	Ethnicity	✓	✓	✓	
Khunti, K et al. 2021 [44]	The need for improved collection and coding of ethnicity in health research	Ethnicity			✓	
Knox et al. 2019 [45]	The challenge of using routinely collected data to compare hospital admission rates by ethnic group: a demonstration project in Scotland	Ethnicity	✓			✓
Liu, L et al. 2011 [46]	Challenges in Identifying Native Hawaiians and Pacific Islanders in Population-Based Cancer Registries in the U.S.	Ethnicity				✓
Mathur et al., 2013 [47]	Completeness and usability of ethnicity data in UK-based primary care and hospital databases	Ethnicity	✓			✓
Pinto, AD et al. 2016 [48]	Building a Foundation to Reduce Health Inequities: Routine Collection of Sociodemographic Data in Primary Care	General		✓	✓	
Polubriaginof, FCG et al. 2019 [49]	Challenges with quality of race and ethnicity data in observational databases	Ethnicity		✓	✓	
Ryan et al. 2012 [50]	Use of name recognition software, census data and multiple imputation to predict missing data on ethnicity: application to cancer registry records	Ethnicity				✓
Russell AM et al. 2017 [51]	Identifying people with a learning disability: an advanced search for general practice	Learning disability				✓
Saperstein, A. 2012 [52]	Capturing complexity in the United States: which aspects of race matter and when?	Ethnicity			✓	
Shah, SN et al. 2014 [53]	Measuring and Monitoring Progress Toward Health Equity: Local Challenges for Public Health	General	✓	✓	✓	✓
Siegel, B et al. 2012 [54]	A Quality Improvement Framework for Equity in Cardiovascular Care: Results of a National Collaborative	General		✓	✓	
Smith L et al., 2017 [55]	Comparison of ethnic group classification using naming analysis and routinely collected data: application to cancer incidence trends in children and young people	Ethnicity				✓
Smylie, J and Firestone M 2015 [56]	Back to the basics: Identifying and addressing underlying challenges in achieving high quality and relevant health statistics for indigenous populations in Canada	Ethnicity		✓		

Table 1. Cont.

Author, Year	Title	Type of Data Discussed	Distal Factors	Wider Actions to Enable Improvements in Data Collection	Data Collection Instruments, Systems, and Standardisation	Methodological Approaches to Improve Data Quality and Accuracy
Tan-McGrory, A et al. 2018 [57]	A patient and family data domain collection framework for identifying disparities in pediatrics: Results from the pediatric health equity collaborative	General		✓	✓	
Thorlby R et al. 2011 [58]	How Health Care Organizations Are Using Data on Patients' Race and Ethnicity to Improve Quality of Care	Ethnicity	✓	✓	✓	✓
Wang KR et al. 2020 [59]	Information Loss in Harmonizing Granular Race and Ethnicity Data: Descriptive Study of Standards	Ethnicity		✓	✓	
Webster P and Sampangi S, 2014 [60]	Did We Have an Impact? Changes in Racial and Ethnic Composition of Patient Populations Following Implementation of a Pilot Program	Ethnicity	✓	✓	✓	
Wei-Chen, L et al. 2016 [61]	Improving the Collection of Race, Ethnicity, and Language Data to Reduce Healthcare Disparities: A Case Study from an Academic Medical Center	General		✓	✓	
Wolff, M et al. 2017 [62]	Measuring Sexual Orientation: A Review and Critique of US Data Collection Efforts and Implications for Health Policy	Gender	✓	✓	✓	✓
Zhang XZ et al. 2019 [63]	Role of Health Information Technology in Addressing Health Disparities Patient, Clinician, and System Perspectives	General	✓	✓	✓	✓
Hutt P and Gilmour S 2010 [64]	Tackling inequalities in general practice	General	✓	✓	✓	
Scottish Government 2020 [65]	Improving data and evidence on ethnic inequalities in health: Initial advice and recommendations from the expert reference group on ethnicity and COVID-19	Ethnicity	✓	✓	✓	✓
NHS England, 2020 [66]	Advancing mental health equalities strategy	General	✓	✓	✓	
NHS, 2019 [67]	NHS Mental Health Implementation Plan 2019/20–2023/24	General	✓	✓	✓	
NHS Race and Health Observatory, 2021 [68]	Ethnic health inequalities and the NHS: Driving progress in a changing system	Ethnicity	✓	✓	✓	
Scobie S, Spencer J and Raleigh V, 2021 [4]	Ethnicity coding in English health service datasets	Ethnicity	✓	✓	✓	✓
NHS England, 2019 [69]	Improving identification of people with a learning disability: guidance for general practice	Learning disability		✓	✓	
National Services Scotland, 2017 [70]	Measuring use of health services by equality group	General		✓	✓	✓
Total citations		57	26	28	43	27

3.1. Distal Initiatives

The mechanisms and approaches that were upstream of data collection and analysis, but which impacted on these, were grouped under the theme "distal initiatives". A total of 26 reports stated that policy and legislative imperatives such as mandating data collection led to improvements and consistency in data quality (Table 1). This is through making it a priority and incentivising data collection and leading to the creation of data systems that facilitate such efforts [4,53,58]. Reports also evidenced how data collection had improved since the introduction of mandates and the prioritisation of ethnicity data collection [4,19,31,42,43,45,47,58,65]. In the UK, the Equality Act 2010 and incentivisation under the Quality and Outcomes Framework (QOF) had a significant impact on the completeness of ethnicity data [45,47]. Mathur et al. (2014) [47] describe how the proportion of patients with a valid self-reported ethnicity record changed over time (1995 to 2011) in English hospital data and GP data (via the Clinical Practice Research Datalink, which covered 6% of all GP practices in 2012). The proportion of people with a usable ethnicity recording in Hospital Episode Statistics (HES) inpatient data jumped from 50% to just under 70% in one year between 2000 and 2001. Between 2008 and 2011, the proportion with a usable record also changed from around 20% to around 50% in the HES A&E and outpatient data. The authors do not discuss what lay behind the improvement in HES data quality. Collection of sexual identity, gender, and behaviour, whilst lagging behind, have also been impacted by legislation that is incentivising data collection [33,62]. Furthermore, given the sensitive and private nature of information such as ethnicity, disability, gender, and sexual orientation, legal safeguards to ensure nondiscrimination on the basis of this information are also important factors that impact on data collection efforts [42,45].

3.2. Wider Actions to Enable Improvements in Data Quality

While mandating data collection leads to improvements in data quality, it needs to be supported by wider actions to enable organisations to put in place mechanisms to improve data quality at source [4,23,31,32]. Of the included reports, 38 provided evidence that achieving senior-level buy-in [4,34,42,45,65], the development of staff training programmes [19,20,22,24,25,27,29,31,32,35–37,49,54,58,61,62], guidance on how to use data [19,29,34,37], engagement activities with citizens, patients, and communities [17,25,29,49,56,58,65], and training on analysis of source data all contribute to efforts to improve data quality [19,20,24,25,27,29,31,32,35,36,54,58,61,62].

Senior-level buy-in is needed to prioritise data collection and put in place systems, such as IT infrastructure, to enable data collection, as well as utilisation of the data for service improvement. Davidson et al. (2021) report that obtaining executive-level buy-in was crucial for recording and improving ethnicity data collection in NHS Lothian [34]. Reports have shown that this can be achieved by demonstrating the value of data collection and analysis [19]. Using the data to demonstrate how outcomes or experiences vary for different groups, while also recognising the limitations of the data, created an awareness and interest in inequalities. This should result in an improvement spiral, driving a demand for better-quality data that in turn creates more interest in the intelligence based on that data [19,29]. Several papers reported the deliberations and recommendations of multidisciplinary groups created specifically to address issues in data quality in specific areas such as disability [38], paediatrics [57], deaf communities [18], and COVID-19 and ethnicity [65], or more broadly [68]. These examples demonstrate the value of multidisciplinary groups in informing efforts and developing effective solutions for improving data collection and analysis efforts.

Staff reluctance was cited in many reports as a key factor that may hinder attempts to improve data quality [4,19,20,29,71]. This was due to a lack of knowledge about the importance and use of the data, combined with staff reluctance to offend patients by asking for sensitive information. Training programmes were able to address this barrier and also assuage concerns relating to the use of systems to collect such data [20,22,24,25,27,29,31,35,49,54,58]. In addition, the development of guidance on using data was cited as a mechanism to improve data completeness and quality [4,34,43,68]. Training staff in communicating the rationale for data collection to the public and patients and on describing the parameters required was also a mechanism to improve data collection [34,60]. This was through building trust and openness between data collectors and providers [36,58]. One study suggested that ethnic matching could be one way of avoiding refusal during data collection [29].

In addition to staff reluctance, patients or the public may also be reluctant to provide data, or data collection instruments may not be appropriately developed for them. Several papers cited the importance of patient, public, or community involvement in initiatives to collect data or develop instruments such as surveys in data collection [27,58]. This involvement can help shape the questions that are asked and avoid marginalisation [17,36,38,56,63].

3.3. Data Collection Instruments, Systems and Standardisation

Many reports cited that data quality and granularity are impacted by the lack of standardised definitions. This creates pragmatic and logistical issues for data collection [19,21,71] through a lack of uniformity in data collection instruments such as surveys, as well as in IT systems that assign codes to different categories of data. Lack of standardised definitions and coding practices can cause major challenges when attempts are made to link data and in further analysis [63]. The introduction of standardised categories, or certain fields that are compulsory to complete as part of the design of IT systems, were mechanisms that were used to improve the recording and the quality of data [28,60–62]. Two papers recommended that consistency in coding and naming across different surveillance systems was also a way to enable consistency and more efficient linkage of sociodemographic data [23,25].

The importance of periodically revisiting these categories and ensuring their relevance was also shown to be an important activity [59]. Audit processes to monitor the completeness and accuracy of data and the methods used in data collection were discussed [20,70]. These processes allowed the assessment of data quality to put in place mechanisms for quality improvement [31]. One paper [16] reported on an instrument that could be used to compare and benchmark health information systems; however, it is unclear to what extent such tools are utilised or practical. Many grey literature reports in the UK recommended standardised protocols for collecting and recording ethnicity data as a mechanism to improve quality [4,65,67,70]. The importance of ensuring systems are in place to enable this was also discussed [31,38,63].

Improving the granularity and data fields available for individuals to self-assign their ethnicity or other characteristics was also shown to improve the completeness of data. For example, providing more options for self-reporting reduced the unknown ethnicity in certain studies [60]. This was achieved through providing more options (which are sometimes more relevant) to survey responders, resulting in less selection of the "unknown" category. Several reports used multidisciplinary groups to develop better understanding of the data that professionals from diverse disciplines thought should and can be collected [38,57,65,69].

3.4. Methodological Approaches to Improve Data Completeness and Accuracy

In addition to efforts to improve data at source, we also identified reports that described methods for improving data completeness and accuracy using statistical or other approaches ($n = 27$). This included data linkage, using proxy variables, or imputation through other methodologies [24].

Mathur et al. (2014) [47] found that when patients appeared in both the Clinical Practice Research Datalink (CPRD) and the Hospital Episode Statistics (HES) datasets with a usable ethnicity code in both datasets, the code was the same category in just 73% of cases. They found that when patients appeared in both datasets, completeness of usable ethnicity data in the CPRD increased from 78.7% to 97.1% once ethnicity data from HES was added. Knox et al. (2016) [45] looked at hospital admission rates by ethnicity in Scotland between 2009 and 2015, using the most recently recorded ethnicity to populate all admissions for that patient. This reduced the numbers of episodes with missing ethnicity from 24% to 15%, and the researchers completed the missing data for the remaining 15% by assigning those cases to ethnic groups in proportion to the distribution of known ethnicity by age and sex.

A number of imputation techniques can also be used to obtain more complete data; however, different methodologies have limitations and strengths [24,26]. Examples of the methods used include randomly assigning ethnicity, for example, on the basis of the distribution in the observed dataset or using a reference dataset [70], and using geographic location or probabilistic methods to infer ethnicity [35,50,51,58].

Several studies have investigated the use of algorithms to improve the completeness of ethnicity data by assigning ethnicity codes to individuals on the basis of their names, when self-identified data is missing [24,30,35,40,46,50,55,70]. The utility of this approach is recognised to differ considerably across countries because of significant variations in the composition of the population. Smith et al. (2017) [55] used the 'Onomap' software to categorise children and young people in the Yorkshire cancer registry as white, South Asian, or 'other' on the basis of their name, and also took ethnicity information from HES where this was recorded. Eleven per cent had missing HES ethnicity data and Onomap classified most of these patients. However, it is not clear whether these name-derived classifications were accurate, and these categories are very broad. The use of different methods to assign ethnicity did result in some different estimates of ethnic variation in cancer incidence, demonstrating the importance of accurate data.

Ryan et al. (2012) [50] also used Onomap and an additional name recognition software, Nam Pehchan [72], to predict the ethnicity of cases in a regional cancer registry who were missing this information following linkage with hospital inpatient data. They found that the software packages were accurate at predicting South Asian ethnicity but poor for other groups. They also looked at predicting ethnicity based on geographical area of residence but found this was also a poor predictor.

One paper also described the use of read codes to identify patients with learning difficulties (LD). NHS England issued guidance in October 2019 on improving the identification of people on the general practice LD register [69]. This required GPs to use a list of codes provided to check that all eligible patients were included on the practice LD register. The impact of this guidance on the numbers of patients on the register does not appear to have been evaluated. However, there was previous work evaluating the use of diagnostic read codes that found that this approach did identify small numbers of additional people who should have been on the register, and some further patients were found using specific descriptive codes [51]. The authors concluded that searching read codes to improve practice LD registers was quick and viable but not sufficient to capture most of the people eligible for inclusion, particularly those with milder learning difficulties. There does not appear to be evidence on how best to identify the remaining patients who could be included.

4. Discussion

Our scoping review identified a variety of mechanisms by which data quality in relation to health inequalities can be improved (Table 2). While the focus of many of the papers is on ethnicity data, many of the findings are also applicable to other dimensions of health inequalities because of the similarities in the issues that impact on data collection. There were relatively few papers that discussed improvements of data related to socio-economic status; however, this might be because such data are collected through other means, rather than self-reporting, and the practice for collating this data is better established. There were also relatively few papers that discussed improvement of data relating to gender and sexual orientation or disability. In addition, while some included papers discussed the issue of intersectionality, the impact in terms of data analysis or data collection were often not fully explored.

Table 2. Summary of best practices.

Theme	Point in the Data Pathway	Actions
Distal factors	Upstream of data collection and analysis	Mandating data collection Legal safeguards to ensure nondiscrimination Legislation incentivising data collection Prioritisation in policy
Wider actions to enable improvements in data collection	Preparing for data collection	Achieving senior-level buy-in in organisations involved in data collection Engagement activities with citizens, patients, and communities Staff training programmes on purpose and mechanisms for data collection Developing guidance on how data can be used Demonstration of the value of data collection and analysis for organisations
Data collection instruments, systems, and standardisation	Data collection	Using multidisciplinary groups to inform data collection instruments, systems, and standardisation Creating standardised definitions and coding practices across organisations Improving granularity of data fields Developing standardised processes for collecting and recording data Developing audit processes to monitor data quality aspects Creating IT systems to facilitate data collection Periodic revision of definitions and categories
Methodological approaches to improve data quality and accuracy	Data analysis	Linking with other data sources Use of proxy variables Imputation

We have classified the mechanisms that can be used to improve the quality of data on health inequalities as more distal or proximal to the source data. Distal factors that impact on data quality include legislation and policies that are in place to ensure and mandate collection of data to enable addressing health inequalities. While many countries recommend the monitoring of data related to equality and discrimination, the extent to which this is implemented and actioned for health varies. Much of this is due to the differing structures of health systems and legislation that are in place globally. These distal factors impact on the ability to collect data related to equality and discrimination. For example, in the UK, the duty of data collection falls with public bodies [42], whereas this is not necessarily the case in other countries. Nevertheless, several included reports evidenced the fact that legalisation and policy were key contributors to the success of high-quality data collection efforts. Mechanisms to enact these policies and enable data collection form the next series of mechanisms to improve data quality. Reports described a variety of mechanisms, such as senior-level buy-in, staff training programmes, patient and public involvement, needed to enable creation of data systems that take into consideration the purpose of data collection and are timely and relevant.

Data pertaining to health inequalities may be collected by different organisations involved in health and care provision. They may collect these data for different purposes, meaning that the granularity of information requirements may differ. In addition, definitions in relation to many protected characteristics such as gender and ethnicity vary and evolve over time. This is because these are composite social constructs, attempting to bring together a number of different elements. For example, ethnicity is a composite of cultural factors, language, and ancestry, amongst others. This is evidenced by reports from the UK [4] that do not make a strong distinction between race and ethnicity, though work from the US distinguishes between these concepts, particularly when considering people from a Hispanic/Latinx background. Furthermore, these concepts change over time, meaning minority groups can change in size and new groups may become more prevalent. Many reports cited that redefinition of how populations are categorised in relation to characteristics related to health inequalities is needed over time [24,29,36]. For example, it is now more common to collect data that allows us to identify a subcategory of White Eastern European, or distinguish between Black African groups. Similarly, few would have included 'nonbinary' as a possible answer option to a question on gender five years ago. Thus, engagement across citizens, providers, and those creating data systems is needed to ensure the data that are collected are acceptable, relevant, and fit for purpose, and yet retain the ability to compare across time to monitor change and assess the impact of policies and interventions that aim to prevent and reduce health inequalities.

The report of improvements to data collected by NHS Lothian is a good example of the multi-layered approach that is needed to improve data quality [34]. The Scottish government and the Commission for Racial Equality requested the Scottish health boards to improve the recording of patient ethnicity data, and all boards were required to produce an action plan with progress measures. Davidson et al. (2020) report an impressive increase in the proportion of patients with a recording of ethnicity from 3% to over 90% in just three years (between 2008 and 2012). The authors attribute this improvement to several factors, chief amongst these being the decision to make ethnicity a mandatory field in the hospital data systems. Other important factors were thought to include the training of individuals responsible for data collection, awareness raising with relevant clinical and management staff and sharing a clear purpose and vision, and executive buy-in from senior clinical and management colleagues to ensure staff were able to prioritise recording these data. Making it clear to staff how ethnicity information is used was also important to maintain their motivation to collect these data. In this case, the data were used to demonstrate that rates of A&E use by ethnic minority groups did not appear to be linked to rates of registration in primary care. The progress made by NHS Lothian is in contrast to many other NHS Boards in Scotland where, over the same period, recording remained poor or improved much more slowly, despite an identical governance and legal context [73].

The importance of staff training is also evidenced by some older studies. A review by Iqbal et al. (2009) showed that staff training was the main intervention for which there was evidence of data quality improvements for patient ethnicity, followed by adequate resources to allow data collection and use [74]. Training should be tailored to the local context and explain why it is important to gather standardised data on patient ethnicity, what the data will be used for, and how to ask the questions and record responses. The review also recommended collecting self-reported ethnicity as routine during GP registration.

Self-reported data are the gold standard for certain data such as gender and ethnicity that can inform studies of health inequality. However, the work included for this review has identified a wide range of reasons why individuals may be reluctant to share personal data relevant to these characteristics. A paper from NHS Scotland points out that different settings can have substantially different rates of refusal (for ethnicity data reporting), which suggests different organisational approaches to asking for and recording the information [70]. High rates of refusal (or high use of an 'other' category) can be compared against peer organisations and could likely be brought down by learning from successful approaches elsewhere. Improving public and patient understanding of why this information is being collected and how it will be used can also encourage efforts to improve data collection and, therefore, quality. Nevertheless, there will likely always be some people who decline to give information on their ethnicity, or other personal information not perceived to be directly relevant to their immediate care, and it is important to recognise their right to decline to provide this.

It can take time to put in place a best practice that leads to the collection of good-quality data in relation to health inequalities. In addition, as evidenced by many of the reports, this may still lead to incomplete data with inaccuracies. Thus, mechanisms that can improve the accuracy, quality, and completeness of available data are also important. We identified studies that reported the use of methodologies such as linkage, imputation, and the use of proxy variables. However, there are several limitations to these methods. Using naming software or linked data to improve the completeness of ethnicity data takes considerable time and analytical expertise and is not ideal for producing useful up-to-date routine reports for health services [50,55]. However, the studies that examined the use of naming software took place at a time when recording ethnicity for hospital inpatients was much poorer. It seems likely that their findings have less relevance today when hospital data are much less likely to be missing data on patient ethnicity, given that both studies were of cancer patients (who are likely to appear in HES data). Using naming software to estimate ethnicity may still have utility when data cannot be linked to hospital or other data, but clearly this approach to filling ethnicity-data gaps needs caution. It is likely to struggle more with mixed-ethnicity individuals (an increasing proportion of the UK population) and is unlikely to be able to produce the detail necessary to distinguish between subgroups.

Data linkage has been evaluated for its utility in reducing missing data. If the same individual is identifiable in two datasets, information from one dataset can be used to check or complete the information in the other. Data linkage can be powerful for 'filling in the gaps' and has been used by NHS Digital to increase coverage of ethnicity data during the COVID-19 pandemic [75]. However, using data linkage to improve ethnicity data on a routine basis, so that it can be useful for producing near-real-time intelligence to inform services and policy, is challenging given the requirements for analyst capacity and time [24]. Improving data through data linkage also requires having a resource to link to that contains accurate self-reported ethnicity data and has high coverage across the population. In England, this resource could potentially be census data, HES data, or GP data, or death certification data for people who have died. However, there are issues with each of these sources. Census data is very sensitive and not easy to access and is only updated every 10 years. GP data is known to have patchy coverage. Recent HES data has better completeness for the people included in the dataset, but coverage is an issue because of the requirement that patients have been hospital users. Using ethnicity data from death certificates is also likely to bring accuracy issues as, of course, ethnicity cannot be self-reported in these cases and, in fact, often mismatches the data in hospital records. Even within the group of patients who appear in the HES data, using HES as a source of accurate ethnicity data may be inadequate.

This scoping review has some strengths in that we used a systematic approach to identify as many reports as possible discussing different mechanisms to improve data quality. Yet, it is likely that there are reports that we missed, especially in the form of grey literature, because of the broad nature of the subject matter. The majority of the reports were from the UK or US. This might be a result of our search terms not being optimal. Other factors include the extent to which health inequalities monitoring has been implemented and is a priority as part of healthcare delivery [76,77]. Nevertheless, this work identified evidence for several distal and proximal approaches that can be taken within the healthcare context of the United Kingdom to improve the quality of the data used for the identification and monitoring of health inequalities. Some of these approaches may be transferable to other healthcare contexts. However, given differences in definitions and drivers of health inequalities and provision of health care around the globe, they may not apply to the same extent.

5. Conclusions

Accurate and timely data are essential in identifying inequalities in health and care, in understanding where inequalities occur and which groups are affected, and in assessing the impact of interventions. Despite this, many health-related datasets either do not routinely collect important dimensions of inequality or are limited by poor-quality data. Where data are available, they may not always be used to the best extent. Our review identified that a variety of effective mechanisms are available and can be utilised to improve data quality. These include those that are distal and impact on data collection, or those that are more proximal to the source data and can aid in data analysis. Given the renewed emphasis on the need for action to address health inequalities at both a national and a system level, it is important to understand how systems can easily implement the mechanism described in our review. This will likely require working with senior leaders, staff, and analysts to gain buy-in and identify effective ways to implement mechanisms to address issues with data quality. Further work is underway to understand how best to support health and care staff to act on the evidence identified in this review to improve the quality of data relating to health inequalities within their organisations and local systems.

Supplementary Materials: The following supporting information can be downloaded at https://www.mdpi.com/article/10.3390/ijerph192315874/s1: Search Terms and PRISMA-ScR checklist. Reference [15] is cited in the supplementary materials.

Author Contributions: S.M.: V.P. (Vicki Peacey), S.E. and L.L. conceived the study objective and design. V.P. (Veronica Philips) carried out the searches. A.R.-U. contributed to screening the titles. S.M. and L.L. carried out the scoping review with feedback from S.E., C.B. and V.P. (Vicki Peacey) All authors contributed to the original drafting, reviewing, and editing of the manuscript. All authors have read and agreed to the published version of the manuscript.

Funding: SM: LL, SE, ARU are supported in part by the NIHR Applied Research Collaboration East of England (ARC EoE). NIHR Applied Research Collaboration East of England, grant number G104017. The views expressed are those of the author(s) and not necessarily those of the NHS, the NIHR, or the Department of Health and Social Care or Cambridgeshire County Council.

Institutional Review Board Statement: Not applicable.

Informed Consent Statement: Not applicable.

Data Availability Statement: Data can be made available on request.

Conflicts of Interest: The authors declare no conflict of interest.

References

1. Public Health England. COVID-19 Place-Based Approach to Reducing Health Inequalities. PHE Publications Gateway Number: GOV-8343. 2020. Available online: https://www.gov.uk/government/publications/health-inequalities-place-based-approaches-to-reduce-inequalities (accessed on 20 January 2022).
2. NHS England. NHS Operational Planning and Contracting Guidance 2021/22. 2021. Available online: https://www.england.nhs.uk/operational-planning-and-contracting/ (accessed on 20 January 2022).
3. NHS England/ Equality and Health Inequalities Team. Monitoring Equality and Health Inequalities: A position Paper. 2015. Available online: https://www.england.nhs.uk/wp-content/uploads/2015/03/monitrg-ehi-pos-paper.pdf (accessed on 20 January 2022).
4. Scobie, S.; Spencer, J.; Raleigh, V. Ethnicity Coding in English Health Service Datasets. 2021. Available online: https://www.nhsrho.org/news/ethnicity-coding-in-english-health-service-datasets/ (accessed on 20 January 2022).
5. The Government Data Quality Hub. The Government Data Quality Framework. 2020. Available online: https://www.gov.uk/government/publications/the-government-data-quality-framework/the-government-data-quality-framework (accessed on 19 November 2022).
6. Public Health England. Local Action on Health Inequalities Understanding and Reducing Ethnic Inequalities in Health. 2018. Available online: publishing.service.gov.uk/government/uploads/system/uploads/attachment_data/file/730917/local_action_on_health_inequalities.pdf (accessed on 20 January 2022).
7. Public Health England. *COVID-19: Review of Disparities in Risks and Outcomes*; PHE Publications Gateway Number: GW-1447; Public Health England: London, UK, 2020.
8. NHS England. Third Phase of NHS Response to COVID-19. NHS. 2020. Available online: https://www.england.nhs.uk/coronavirus/publication/third-phase-response/ (accessed on 20 January 2022).
9. Office for National Statistics. Equalities Data Audit, Final Report. 2018. Available online: https://www.ons.gov.uk/methodology/methodologicalpublications/generalmethodology/onsworkingpaperseries/equalitiesdataauditfinalreport (accessed on 20 January 2022).
10. Marmot, M. *Fair Society, Healthy Lives: The Marmot Review*; Marmot Review: London, UK, 2010.
11. Marmot, M.; Allen, J.; Boyce, T.; Goldblatt, P.; Morrison, J. *Health Equity in England: The Marmot Review 10 Years On*; Institute of Health Equity: London, UK, 2020.
12. Office for Health Improvement and Disparities. Beyond the Data one Year on—Companion Narrative Data and Literature. 2021. Available online: https://www.london.gov.uk/what-we-do/health/health-inequalities/london-health-inequalities-strategy (accessed on 20 January 2022).

13. Centre for Equalities and Inclusion. Available online: https://www.ons.gov.uk/aboutus/whatwedo/programmesandprojects/onscentres/centreforequalitiesandinclusion (accessed on 24 January 2022).
14. NHS Race and Health Observatory. Available online: https://www.nhsconfed.org/networks-countries/nhs-race-and-health-observatory (accessed on 24 January 2022).
15. Tricco, A.C.; Lillie, E.; Zarin, W.; O'Brien, K.K.; Colquhoun, H.; Levac, D.; Moher, D.; Peters, M.D.J.; Horsley, T.; Weeks, L.; et al. PRISMA Extension for Scoping Reviews (PRISMA-ScR): Checklist and Explanation. *Ann. Intern. Med.* **2018**, *169*, 467–473. [CrossRef] [PubMed]
16. Bozorgmehr, K.; Goosen, S.; Mohsenpour, A.; Kuehne, A.; Razum, O.; Kunst, A.E. How Do Countries' Health Information Systems Perform in Assessing Asylum Seekers' Health Situation? Developing a Health Information Assessment Tool on Asylum Seekers (HIATUS) and Piloting It in Two European Countries. *Int. J. Environ. Res. Public Health* **2017**, *14*, 894. [CrossRef] [PubMed]
17. Allen, V.C.; Lachance, C.; Rios-Ellis, B.; Kaphingst, K.A. Issues in the Assessment of "Race" Among Latinos: Implications for Research and Policy. *Hisp. J. Behav. Sci.* **2011**, *33*, 411–424. [CrossRef] [PubMed]
18. Anderson, M.L.; Riker, T.; Gagne, K.; Hakulin, S.; Higgins, T.; Meehan, J.; Stout, E.; Pici-D'Ottavio, E.; Cappetta, K.; Craig, K.S.W. Deaf Qualitative Health Research: Leveraging Technology to Conduct Linguistically and Sociopolitically Appropriate Methods of Inquiry. *Qual. Health Res.* **2018**, *28*, 1813–1824. [CrossRef]
19. Andrews, R.M. Race and Ethnicity Reporting in Statewide Hospital Data: Progress and Future Challenges in a Key Resource for Local and State Monitoring of Health Disparities. *J. Public Health Manag. Pract.* **2011**, *17*, 167–173. [CrossRef]
20. Azar, K.M.J.; Moreno, M.R.; Wong, E.C.; Shin, J.J.; Soto, C.; Palaniappan, L.P. Accuracy of Data Entry of Patient Race/Ethnicity/Ancestry and Preferred Spoken Language in an Ambulatory Care Setting. *Health Serv. Res.* **2012**, *47*, 228–240. [CrossRef]
21. Becker, T.; Babey, S.H.; Dorsey, R.; Ponce, N.A. Data Disaggregation with American Indian/Alaska Native Population Data. *Popul. Res. Policy Rev.* **2021**, *40*, 103–125. [CrossRef]
22. Berry, C.; Kaplan, S.A.; Mijanovich, T.; Mayer, A. Moving to patient reported collection of race and ethnicity data: Implementation and impact in ten hospitals. *Int. J. Health Care Qual. Assur.* **2014**, *27*, 271–283. [CrossRef]
23. Beltran, V.M.; Harrison, K.M.; Hall, H.I.; Dean, H.D. Collection of social determinant of health measures in U.S. national surveillance systems for HIV, viral hepatitis, STDs, and TB. *Public Health Rep.* **2011**, *126* (Suppl. S3), 41–53. [CrossRef]
24. Bilheimer, L.T.; Klein, R.J. Data and Measurement Issues in the Analysis of Health Disparities. *Health Serv. Res.* **2010**, *45*, 1489–1507. [CrossRef]
25. Block, R.G.; Puro, J.; Cottrell, E.; Lunn, M.R.; Dunne, M.J.; Quinones, A.R.; Chung, B.W.; Pinnock, W.; Reid, G.M.; Heintzman, J. Recommendations for improving national clinical datasets for health equity research. *J. Am. Med. Inform. Assoc.* **2020**, *27*, 1802–1807. [CrossRef]
26. Blosnich, J.R.; Cashy, J.; Gordon, A.J.; Shipherd, J.C.; Kauth, M.R.; Brown, G.R.; Fine, M.J. Using clinician text notes in electronic medical record data to validate transgender-related diagnosis codes. *J. Am. Med. Inform. Assoc.* **2018**, *25*, 905–908. [CrossRef]
27. Cahill, S.R.; Baker, K.; Deutsch, M.B.; Keatley, J.; Makadon, H.J. Inclusion of Sexual Orientation and Gender Identity in Stage 3 Meaningful Use Guidelines: A Huge Step Forward for LGBT Health. *LGBT Health* **2016**, *3*, 100–102. [CrossRef]
28. Chakkalakal, R.J.; Green, J.C.; Krumholz, H.M.; Nallamothu, B.K. Standardized data collection practices and the racial/ethnic distribution of hospitalized patients. *Med. Care* **2015**, *53*, 666–672. [CrossRef]
29. Chen, Y.; Lin, H.Y.; Tseng, T.S.; Wen, H.; DeVivo, M.J. Racial Differences in Data Quality and Completeness: Spinal Cord Injury Model Systems' Experiences. *Top. Spinal Cord Inj. Rehabil.* **2018**, *24*, 110–120. [CrossRef]
30. Clarke, L.C.; Rull, R.P.; Ayanian, J.Z.; Boer, R.; Deapen, D.; West, D.W.; Kahn, K.L. Validity of Race, Ethnicity, and National Origin in Population-based Cancer Registries and Rapid Case Ascertainment Enhanced with a Spanish Surname List. *Med. Care* **2016**, *54*, e1–e8. [CrossRef]
31. Craddock Lee, S.J.; Grobe, J.E.; Tiro, J.A.; Lee, S.J.C. Assessing race and ethnicity data quality across cancer registries and EMRs in two hospitals. *J. Am. Med. Inform. Assoc.* **2016**, *23*, 627–634. [CrossRef]
32. Cruz, T.M. Perils of data-driven equity: Safety-net care and big data's elusive grasp on health inequality. *Big Data Soc.* **2020**, *7*. [CrossRef]
33. Cruz, T.M. Shifting Analytics within US Biomedicine: From Patient Data to the Institutional Conditions of Health Care Inequalities. *Sex. Res. Soc. Policy* **2022**, *19*, 287–293. [CrossRef]
34. Davidson, E.M.; Douglas, A.; Villarroel, N.; Dimmock, K.; Gorman, D.; Bhopal, R.S. Raising ethnicity recording in NHS Lothian from 3% to 90% in 3 years: Processes and analysis of data from Accidents and Emergencies. *J. Public Health* **2021**, *43*, e728–e738. [CrossRef]
35. Derose, S.F.; Contreras, R.; Coleman, K.J.; Koebnick, C.; Jacobsen, S.J. Race and Ethnicity Data Quality and Imputation Using US Census Data in an Integrated Health System: The Kaiser Permanente Southern California Experience. *Med. Care Res. Rev.* **2013**, *70*, 330–345. [CrossRef] [PubMed]
36. Donald, C.; Ehrenfeld, J.M. The Opportunity for Medical Systems to Reduce Health Disparities Among Lesbian, Gay, Bisexual, Transgender and Intersex Patients. *J. Med. Syst.* **2015**, *39*, 178. [CrossRef]
37. Escarce, J.J.; Carreón, R.; Veselovskiy, G.; Lawson, E.H. Collection of Race and Ethnicity Data by Health Plans Has Grown Substantially, But Opportunities Remain to Expand Efforts. *Health Aff.* **2011**, *30*, 1984–1991. [CrossRef] [PubMed]

38. Fortune, N.; Badland, H.; Clifton, S.; Emerson, E.; Rachele, J.; Stancliffe, R.J.; Zhou, Q.S.; Llewellyn, G. The Disability and Wellbeing Monitoring Framework: Data, data gaps, and policy implications. *Aust. N. Z. J. Public Health* **2020**, *44*, 227–232. [CrossRef] [PubMed]
39. Frank, J.; Haw, S. Best Practice Guidelines for Monitoring Socioeconomic Inequalities in Health Status: Lessons from Scotland. *Milbank Q.* **2011**, *89*, 658–693. [CrossRef]
40. Fremont, A.; Weissman, J.S.; Hoch, E.; Elliott, M.N. When Race/Ethnicity Data Are Lacking: Using Advanced Indirect Estimation Methods to Measure Disparities. *Rand Health Q.* **2016**, *6*, 16.
41. Haas, A.P.; Lane, A.; Working Grp, P. Collecting Sexual Orientation and Gender Identity Data in Suicide and Other Violent Deaths: A Step Towards Identifying and Addressing LGBT Mortality Disparities. *LGBT Health* **2015**, *2*, 84–87. [CrossRef]
42. Hannigan, A.; Villarroel, N.; Roura, M.; LeMaster, J.; Basogomba, A.; Bradley, C.; MacFarlane, A. Ethnicity recording in health and social care data collections in Ireland: Where and how is it measured and what is it used for? *Int. J. Equity Health* **2019**, *19*, 2. [CrossRef]
43. Jorgensen, S.; Thorlby, R.; Weinick, R.M.; Ayanian, J.Z. Responses of Massachusetts hospitals to a state mandate to collect race, ethnicity and language data from patients: A qualitative study. *BMC Health Serv. Res.* **2010**, *10*, 352. [CrossRef]
44. Khunti, K.; Routen, A.; Banerjee, A.; Pareek, M. The need for improved collection and coding of ethnicity in health research. *J. Public Health* **2021**, *43*, e270–e272. [CrossRef]
45. Knox, S.; Bhopal, R.S.; Thomson, C.S.; Millard, A.; Fraser, A.; Gruer, L.; Buchanan, D. The challenge of using routinely collected data to compare hospital admission rates by ethnic group: A demonstration project in Scotland. *J. Public Health* **2020**, *42*, 748–755. [CrossRef] [PubMed]
46. Liu, L.; Tanjasiri, S.; Cockburn, M. Challenges in Identifying Native Hawaiians and Pacific Islanders in Population-Based Cancer Registries in the U.S. *J. Immigr. Minor. Health* **2011**, *13*, 860–866. [CrossRef] [PubMed]
47. Mathur, R.; Bhaskaran, K.; Chaturvedi, N.; Leon, D.A.; vanStaa, T.; Grundy, E.; Smeeth, L. Completeness and usability of ethnicity data in UK-based primary care and hospital databases. *J. Public Health* **2014**, *36*, 684–692. [CrossRef]
48. Pinto, A.D.; Glattstein-Young, G.; Mohamed, A.; Bloch, G.; Leung, F.H.; Glazier, R.H. Building a Foundation to Reduce Health Inequities: Routine Collection of Sociodemographic Data in Primary Care. *J. Am. Board Fam. Med.* **2016**, *29*, 348–355. [CrossRef] [PubMed]
49. Polubriaginof, F.C.G.; Ryan, P.; Salmasian, H.; Shapiro, A.W.; Perotte, A.; Safford, M.M.; Hripcsak, G.; Smith, S.; Tatonetti, N.R.; Vawdrey, D.K. Challenges with quality of race and ethnicity data in observational databases. *J. Am. Med. Inform. Assoc.* **2019**, *26*, 730–736. [CrossRef]
50. Ryan, R.; Vernon, S.; Lawrence, G.; Wilson, S. Use of name recognition software, census data and multiple imputation to predict missing data on ethnicity: Application to cancer registry records. *BMC Med. Inf. Decis. Mak.* **2012**, *12*, 3. [CrossRef]
51. Russell, A.M.; Bryant, L.; House, A. Identifying people with a learning disability: An advanced search for general practice. *Br. J. Gen. Pr.* **2017**, *67*, e842–e850. [CrossRef]
52. Saperstein, A. Capturing complexity in the United States: Which aspects of race matter and when? *Ethn. Racial Stud.* **2012**, *35*, 1484–1502. [CrossRef]
53. Shah, S.N.; Russo, E.T.; Earl, T.R.; Kuo, T. Measuring and Monitoring Progress Toward Health Equity: Local Challenges for Public Health. *Prev. Chronic Dis.* **2014**, *11*, E159. [CrossRef]
54. Siegel, B.; Sears, V.; Bretsch, J.K.; Wilson, M.; Jones, K.C.; Mead, H.; Hasnain-Wynia, R.; Ayala, R.K.; Bhalla, R.; Cornue, C.M.; et al. A Quality Improvement Framework for Equity in Cardiovascular Care: Results of a National Collaborative. *J. Healthc. Qual.* **2012**, *34*, 32–43. [CrossRef]
55. Smith, L.; Norman, P.; Kapetanstrataki, M.; Fleming, S.; Fraser, L.K.; Parslow, R.C.; Feltbower, R.G. Comparison of ethnic group classification using naming analysis and routinely collected data: Application to cancer incidence trends in children and young people. *BMJ Open* **2017**, *7*, e016332. [CrossRef]
56. Smylie, J.; Firestone, M. Back to the basics: Identifying and addressing underlying challenges in achieving high quality and relevant health statistics for indigenous populations in Canada. *Stat. J. IAOS* **2015**, *31*, 67–87. [CrossRef]
57. Tan-McGrory, A.; Bennett-AbuAyyash, C.; Gee, S.; Dabney, K.; Cowden, J.D.; Williams, L.; Rafton, S.; Nettles, A.; Pagura, S.; Holmes, L.; et al. A patient and family data domain collection framework for identifying disparities in pediatrics: Results from the pediatric health equity collaborative. *BMC Pediatr.* **2018**, *18*, 18. [CrossRef]
58. Thorlby, R.; Jorgensen, S.; Siegel, B.; Ayanian, J.Z. How Health Care Organizations Are Using Data on Patients' Race and Ethnicity to Improve Quality of Care. *Milbank Q.* **2011**, *89*, 226–255. [CrossRef]
59. Wang, K.R.; Nardini, H.G.; Post, L.; Edwards, T.; Nunez-Smith, M.; Brandt, C. Information Loss in Harmonizing Granular Race and Ethnicity Data: Descriptive Study of Standards. *J. Med. Internet Res.* **2020**, *22*, e14591. [CrossRef]
60. Webster, P.S.; Sampangi, S. Did We Have an Impact? Changes in Racial and Ethnic Composition of Patient Populations Following Implementation of a Pilot Program. *J. Healthc. Qual.* **2017**, *39*, e22–e32. [CrossRef]
61. Wei-Chen, L.; Veeranki, S.P.; Serag, H.; Eschbach, K.; Smith, K.D. Improving the Collection of Race, Ethnicity, and Language Data to Reduce Healthcare Disparities: A Case Study from an Academic Medical Center. *Perspect. Health Inf. Manag.* **2016**, *13*.
62. Wolff, M.; Wells, B.; Ventura-DiPersia, C.; Renson, A.; Grov, C. Measuring Sexual Orientation: A Review and Critique of US Data Collection Efforts and Implications for Health Policy. *J. Sex Res.* **2017**, *54*, 507–531. [CrossRef]

63. Zhang, X.Z.; Hailu, B.; Tabor, D.C.; Gold, R.; Sayre, M.H.; Sim, I.; Jean-Francoi, B.; Casnoff, C.A.; Cullen, T.; Thomas, V.A.; et al. Role of Health Information Technology in Addressing Health Disparities Patient, Clinician, and System Perspectives. *Med. Care* **2019**, *57*, S115–S120. [CrossRef]
64. Hutt, P.; Gilmour, S. Tackling Inequalities in General Practice: An Enquiry into the Qualtiy of General Practice in England. 2010. Available online: https://www.kingsfund.org.uk/sites/default/files/field/field_document/health-inequalities-general-practice-gp-inquiry-research-paper-mar11.pdf (accessed on 24 January 2022).
65. Scottish Government. Improving Data and Evidence on Ethnic Inequalities in Health: Initial Advice and Recommendations from the Expert Reference Group on Ethnicity and COVID-19. 2020. Available online: https://www.gov.scot/publications/expert-reference-group-on-covid-19-and-ethnicity-recommendations-to-scottish-government/ (accessed on 24 January 2022).
66. NHS England. Advancing Mental Health Equalities Strategy. 2020. Available online: https://www.england.nhs.uk/publication/advancing-mental-health-equalities-strategy/ (accessed on 24 January 2022).
67. NHS. NHS Mental Health Implementation Plan 2019/20–2023/24. 2019. Available online: https://www.longtermplan.nhs.uk/publication/nhs-mental-health-implementation-plan-2019-20-2023-24/ (accessed on 24 January 2022).
68. NHS Race and Health Observatory. Ethnic Health Inequalities and the NHS: Driving Progress in a Changing System. 2021. Available online: https://www.nhsrho.org/publications/ethnic-health-inequalities-and-the-nhs/ (accessed on 24 January 2022).
69. NHS England. Improving Identification of People with a Learning Disability: Guidance for General Practice. 2019. Available online: https://www.england.nhs.uk/publication/improving-identification-of-people-with-a-learning-disability-guidance-for-general-practice/ (accessed on 24 January 2022).
70. National Services Scotland. Measuring Use of Health Services by Equality Group. 2017. Available online: https://www.isdscotland.org/Health-Topics/Equality-and-Diversity/Publications/2017-06-27/2017-06-27-Measuring-Use-of-Health-Services-by-Equality-Group-Report.pdf (accessed on 24 January 2022).
71. Abouzeid, M.; Bhopal, R.S.; Dunbar, J.A.; Janus, E.D. The potential for measuring ethnicity and health in a multicultural milieu – the case of type 2 diabetes in Australia. *Ethn. Health* **2014**, *19*, 424–439. [CrossRef]
72. Cummins, C.; Winter, H.; Cheng, K.K.; Maric, R.; Silcocks, P.; Varghese, C. An assessment of the Nam Pehchan computer program for the identification of names of south Asian ethnic origin. *J. Public Health Med.* **1999**, *21*, 401–406. [CrossRef] [PubMed]
73. National Services Scotland. *Improving Data Collection for Equality and Diversity Monitoring: All Scotland Ethnicity Completeness in SMR01 and SMR00*; National Services Scotland: Glasgow, Scotland, 2011.
74. Iqbal, G.; Gumber, A.; Johnson, M.; Szczepura, A.; Wilson, S.; Dunn, J. Improving ethnicity data collection for health statistics in the UK. *Divers. Health Care* **2009**, *6*, 267–285.
75. NHS Digital. [MI] Ethnic Category Coverage. 2022. Available online: https://digital.nhs.uk/data-and-information/publications/statistical/mi-ethnic-category-coverage/current (accessed on 24 January 2022).
76. Hogberg, P.; Henriksson, G.; Borrell, C.; Ciutan, M.; Costa, G.; Georgiou, I.; Halik, R.; Hoebel, J.; Kilpelainen, K.; Kyprianou, T.; et al. Monitoring Health Inequalities in 12 European Countries: Lessons Learned from the Joint Action Health Equity Europe. *Int. J. Env. Res. Public Health* **2022**, *19*, 7663. [CrossRef] [PubMed]
77. Hosseinpoor, A.R.; Bergen, N.; Schlotheuber, A.; Boerma, T. National health inequality monitoring: Current challenges and opportunities. *Glob. Health Action* **2018**, *11*, 1392216. [CrossRef]

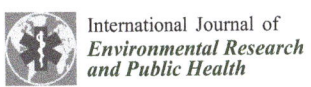

Article

Who Presents Where? A Population-Based Analysis of Socio-Demographic Inequalities in Head and Neck Cancer Patients' Referral Routes

Jennifer Deane [1], Ruth Norris [1], James O'Hara [1,2], Joanne Patterson [3] and Linda Sharp [1,*]

1. Newcastle University Centre for Cancer, Population Health Sciences Institute, Newcastle University, Newcastle-upon-Tyne NE1 4LP, UK
2. Freeman Hospital, Newcastle upon Tyne Hospitals, Newcastle-upon-Tyne NE7 7DN, UK
3. School of Health Sciences, Institute of Population Health, University of Liverpool, Liverpool L69 7ZX, UK
* Correspondence: linda.sharp@newcastle.ac.uk; Tel.: +44-191-208-6275

Abstract: Head and neck cancers (HNC) are often late stage at diagnosis; stage is a major determinant of prognosis. The urgent cancer referral pathway (two week wait; 2WW) within England's National Health Service aims to reduce time to diagnosis. We investigated factors associated with HNC route to diagnosis. Data were obtained from the English population-based cancer registry on 66,411 primary invasive HNCs (ICD C01-14 and C31-32) diagnosed 2006–2014. Multivariable logistic regression determined the likelihood of different diagnosis routes by patients' demographic and clinical characteristics. Significant socio-demographic inequalities were observed. Emergency presentations declined over time and 2WW increased. Significant socio-demographic inequalities were observed. Non-white patients, aged over 65, residing in urban areas with advanced disease, were more likely to have emergency presentations. White males aged 55 and older with an oropharynx cancer were more likely to be diagnosed via 2WW. Higher levels of deprivation were associated with both emergency and 2WW routes. Dental referral was more likely in women, with oral cancers and lower stage disease. Despite the decline over time in emergency presentation and the increased use of 2WW, socio-demographic variation is evident in routes to diagnosis. Further work exploring the reasons for these inequalities, and the consequences for patients' care and outcomes, is urgently required.

Keywords: head and neck cancer; routes to diagnosis; socio-demographic inequalities; healthcare inequalities; emergency presentation

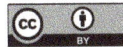

1. Introduction

The UK lags significantly behind other European and high human development countries with regards to cancer outcomes [1]. Evidence suggests that this is due, in part, to later-stage diagnosis [2], including relatively high proportions of cancers which are diagnosed on emergency presentation [3].

In general, cancer survival rates are strongly associated with stage at diagnosis; the earlier the stage the better the chance of survival [4]. Late-stage cancer at diagnosis may be the result of delays at various points across the diagnostic pathway; these delays can be in presentation (time from symptom onset to first presentation to primary care), primary care (time from first presentation to referral for specialist assessment), and secondary care (time from specialist referral to diagnosis) [5].

1.1. Routes to Diagnosis in Cancer

The Urgent Cancer Pathway, known as 2 Week Wait (2WW), was established in the English National Health Service (NHS) in 2000 [6]. A target of 14 days from the point of referral for suspected cancer symptoms, to the point of first assessment with a specialist at the hospital, was put in place. Whilst, in part, this pathway was intended to reduce patient anxiety around waiting for investigations into a possible cancer diagnosis, it was also hoped that it would shorten the primary care interval, allowing identification of cancers at an earlier stage, widening treatment options, and improving survival. A decline over time in the proportion of cancers which present as emergencies has been attributed, in part, to the introduction of this pathway [7,8].

1.2. Head and Neck Cancers

Head and neck cancer (HNC) is an umbrella term for malignant tumours arising in the oral cavity, larynx, pharynx, nose and salivary glands. HNC is now the 8th most common cancer and is responsible for 3% of all cancer diagnosis in the UK [9]. No effective, organised, HNC screening is in place (although there are country-specific and international events designed to increase awareness among healthcare practitioners (HCP) and the public such as head and neck cancer awareness weeks). Therefore, patients are generally diagnosed due to the presence of symptoms. Symptoms vary and include ear pain, persistent sore throat, a neck lump (enlarged lymph node), persistent mouth ulcers, and airway obstruction. Due to tumour location, patients may present symptomatically at a variety of different healthcare settings, including the GP practice, community Dental practice, a Dental hospital or, less commonly, a hospital emergency department [10].

1.3. Inequalities in HNC

Equity in healthcare systems is a marker for healthcare quality [11]. Care should be provided in a way that does not vary in quality due to sociodemographic or socio-economic status (SES). There are multiple inequalities relating to HNC in the UK. Incidence is strongly socio-economically patterned, with rates around 2–4 times higher in those resident in more deprived, compared to less deprived areas [9]. Around 60% of HNCs are diagnosed at a late stage [12] and the proportion diagnosed early is lowest in the most deprived areas [12]. Moreover, survival is also worse in those resident in more deprived areas [13,14].

Current knowledge on the route(s) patients take to receive a HNC diagnosis is limited; improved understanding of whether there are socio-demographic inequalities in this could help to highlight areas for improvement in service provision. We therefore undertook a population-based study investigating socio-demographic inequalities in HNC routes to diagnosis in England. Specifically, this study set out to establish whether there are socio-demographic inequalities in HNC patients diagnosed via (i) emergency versus primary care routes; (ii) 2WW versus any standard primary care routes; and (iii) dentists versus all other non-emergency routes.

2. Methods

2.1. Study Design and Setting

Registrations for all patients with a primary invasive HNC (ICD C01-14 and C31-32) diagnosed in England between 2006 and 2014 were abstracted from the National Cancer Registration Database (NCRD). Ethnical approval was obtained from the Yorkshire and the Humber South Yorkshire Research Ethics Committee on 16th November 2017 (Ref number 206040), and this population-based study is reported according to the Strengthening the Reporting of Observational Studies in Epidemiology (STROBE) guidance [15].

2.2. Data Sources and Linkage

The NCRD is a population-based cancer registry that seeks to systematically identify and record information on all newly diagnosed tumours in patients resident in England. The registry receives data from across the NHS which approximates to around 300,000 malignant tumour diagnoses annually [16]. Reporting of NHS hospital cancer data is mandatory. Each NCRD record is linked, using patient NHS number, to UK NHS Hospital Episode Statistics (HES) data to provide information on comorbidities and cancer treatments.

A "route to diagnosis" was assigned, by the National Cancer Registration and Analysis Service (NCRAS) to each cancer registration using a combination of data from the NCRD, HES, Cancer Waiting Times, and Cancer Screening programmes. The route to diagnosis refers to a sequence of interactions between the patient and the healthcare system which leads to the diagnosis of cancer [17]. Each registration is assigned one of eight main routes to diagnosis codes: GP referral; 2WW; emergency presentation; other outpatient, screen detected (not relevant for HNC); inpatient elective; death certificate only (DCO); and unknown. Within several of these main routes, there are (sub) routes which can be used to distinguish patients who were referred from different types of practitioners (e.g., 2WW (GP), 2WW (dentist), 2WW (other)). This route to diagnosis dataset has been used to document the diagnostic route for a range of cancers [18], but it has not been previously used to compare which HNC patients are present and are diagnosed through which routes.

2.3. Population

The population of interest was patients with an incident primary invasive HNC (n = 70,334). In instances where a patient had records for multiple primary tumours in the head and neck (n = 1308), a hierarchy determined which tumour record to retain for analysis. This was as follows: (i) the earliest diagnosed tumour; (ii) the earliest tumour referral date; (iii) the tumour marked as potentially positive for human papilloma virus (HPV), based on proxy information (morphology and subsite); and (iv) selected at random from the remaining tumours. Childhood tumours in patients aged <20 years old were excluded from the analysis. Cases with missing routes to diagnosis (n = 2243) and cases diagnosed only at the time of death (n = 98) were also then excluded. This left an analytical cohort of 66,411 patients (Figure 1).

2.4. Explanatory Variables

Explanatory variables of interest were as follows: age at diagnosis, sex, cancer site, deprivation category, period of diagnosis, ethnicity, urban/rural category, stage, grade and comorbidities. Age at diagnosis was categorised as 20–54, 55–64, 65–79 and 80+ years. Cancer sites were grouped as oral cavity (C02-C06; including palate), oropharynx (C01, C09, C10), larynx (C32) and other HNC (nasopharynx C11; hypopharynx C12, C13; salivary glands C07, C08; other sites C05, C07-C08, C11-C13; and non-specific sites C14, C31). Deprivation was an area-based measure of the income domain of the Index of Multiple Deprivation (IMD) [19] Quintile 1 includes the people resident in the least deprived and quintile 5 those resident in the most deprived areas; these refer to quintiles of the general population. Deprivation was used as a SES proxy measure. Period of diagnosis was grouped into 3-year time bands (2006–2008; 2009–2011; and 2012–2014). Ethnicity was classified as white, non-white (other ethnic group) and unknown (missing and unknown ethnicity). Urban/rural categorisation was based on areas of residence at diagnosis and was collapsed to either rural or urban [20]. Cancer summary stage was assigned using the TNM staging system (I–IV or other (unknown/missing)). Tumour grade was classified as 1 (low grade, undifferentiated)—4 (high grade, differentiated) and unknown (unknown/missing). A weighted comorbidity score based on the Charlson Comorbidity Index [21] reported the number of in-patient hospital admission for different relevant comorbidities recorded in the period 3 to 27 months before diagnosis (with the index cancer disregarded). Comorbidities were classified as none, 1 and 2+.

2.5. Outcome Variables

The outcome variables of interest were route to diagnosis. For the purpose of this analysis, the NCRD operationalisation of (sub)route to diagnosis was categorised as follows: (i) emergency presentation (comprising (sub)routes: A&E, emergency GP referral, emergency transfer, emergency admission or attendance); (ii) all primary care routes (that is, all routes which would have been initiated in primary care: GP referral, inpatient referral, outpatient (dentist and other referral), 2WW (dentist, GP and other)); (iii) 2WW (all urgent cancer referral routes: dentist, GP and other); (iv) standard care routes (that is, all non-urgent non-emergency, cancer referral routes: GP referral, inpatient referral, outpatient (other and dentist referral)); (v) dentist (all routes which started with a dentist: outpatient and 2WW); (vi) and all other non-emergency routes (referral routes which did not start with a dentist: GP referral, inpatient, outpatient (other referral) and 2WW (GP and other)) (Supplementary Figure S1).

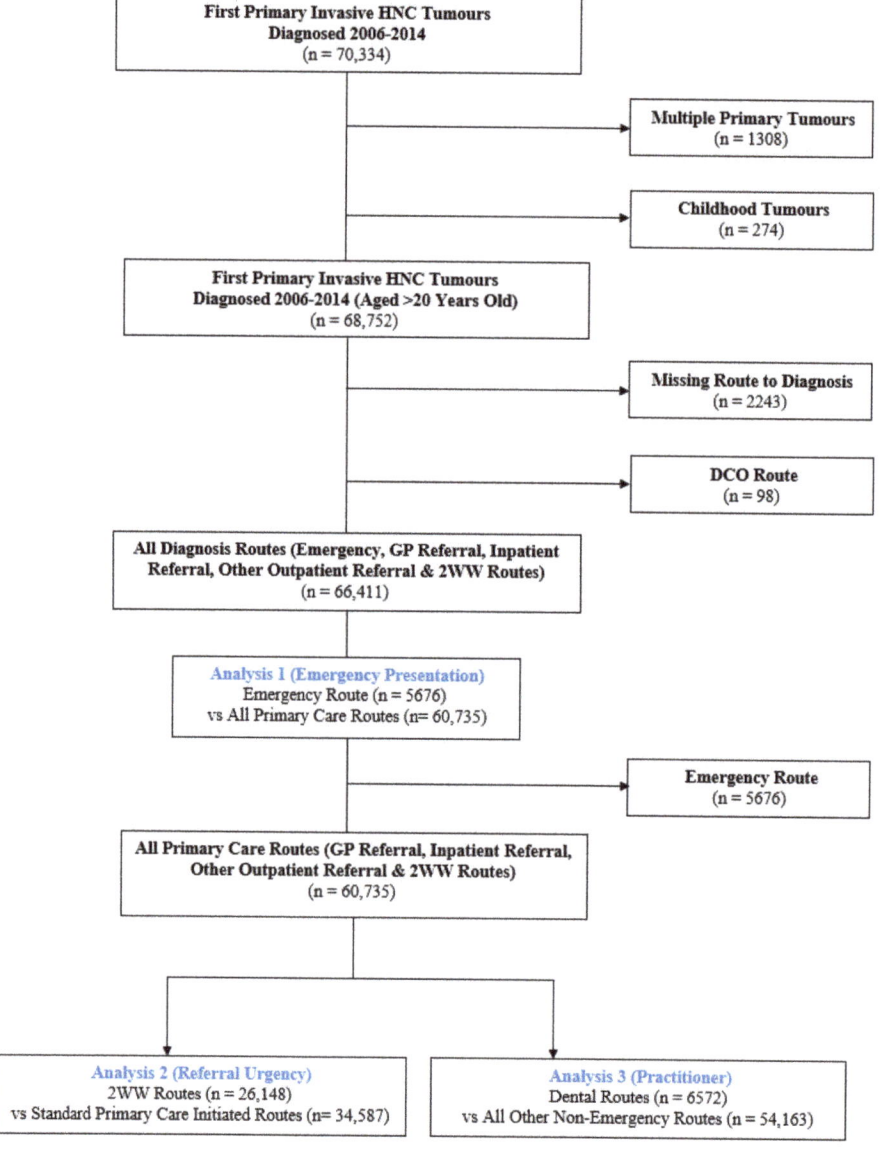

Figure 1. Flow diagram of the analytical cohorts for Analyses 1–3. Abbreviations: DCO: Death certificate only; GP: General practitioner; HNC: Head and neck cancer; 2WW: Two week wait.

2.6. Statistical Analyses

Three analyses were undertaken to explore the role of socio-demographics on route to diagnosis (Figure 1; Supplementary Figure S1). Analysis 1 included the whole analytical cohort (emergency presentation) and considered whether there was a difference in those patients presenting through the emergency route compared with all primary care routes (i.e., comparing categorisations (i) and (ii) above). Analysis 2 considered only patients coming through primary care routes (category (ii) above), and compared 2WW referral versus standard primary care-initiated routes (i.e., (iii) vs. (iv)). Analysis 3 again considered only patients coming through primary routes (category (ii) above), but this time compared dentist referral vs. all other non-emergency (non-dental) routes (i.e., categories (v) vs. (vi) above).

For each analysis, baseline descriptive statistics were reported for the analytic population along with chi-square tests of associations between socio-demographic and clinical variables with diagnosis route. Univariable and multivariable logistic regression models were then developed to assess the likelihood of diagnosis route by socio-demographic characteristics with and without adjustment for confounders. Any variables significant in univariate analyses (likelihood ratio tests (LRT) $p \leq 0.05$) were included in multivariable models. Models were reduced to contain only statistically significant variables (LRT $p \leq 0.05$). Model goodness-of-fit was assessed, and care taken to avoid multicollinearity. The Akaike Information Criterion (AIC) was used to differentiate between competing models. All final models had adequate fit. Odds ratios (ORs) and 95% confidence intervals (CIs) were reported. Stata V.15 [22] was used for all analyses.

3. Results

3.1. Patient Characteristics

In total, 66,411 patients were diagnosed with a first, invasive primary HNC between 2006 and 2014. HNC diagnoses increased over time. Almost two-thirds of patients were aged 55–79 at diagnosis (64.1%); almost 70% were male (69.6%); and more than 4 out of 5 were of white ethnicity (81.2%). Diagnosis was associated with deprivation: a higher proportion of patients were resident in the most deprived areas (24.5%) than in the least deprived areas (15.7%). Most patients resided in an urban area at the time of diagnosis (82.4%). The site distribution was as follows: oral cavity (34.1%), larynx (23.9%), oropharynx (22.8%) and other HNC (19.2%). At diagnosis, the most common summary stage was stage IV (19.6%) and grade 2 (37.8%); stage was not recorded for most cases. Referral via each route to diagnosis was as follows: emergency (8.5%); all primary care routes (91.5%); 2WW (39.4%); standard care routes (52.1%); dentist (9.9%); and all other routes (81.6%). Demographic and clinical characteristics of the population are shown in Table 1. A full breakdown by individual route to diagnosis can be viewed in Supplementary Table S1.

Table 1. Demographic and clinical characteristics of HNC diagnosed during 2006–2014.

	Overall (n = 66,411; 100%)
Age at Diagnosis	
20–54 years	15,259 (23.0)
55–64 years	19,459 (29.3)
65–79 years	23,092 (34.8)
80+ years	8601 (13.0)
Sex	
Male	46,241 (69.6)
Female	20,170 (30.4)
Cancer Site	
Oral Cavity [1]	22,620 (34.1)
Oropharynx	15,128 (22.8)
Larynx	15,885 (23.9)
Other [2]	12,778 (19.2)

Table 1. Cont.

	Overall (n = 66,411; 100%)
Deprivation Category	
IMD 1 (Least Deprived)	10,417 (15.7)
IMD 2	12,260 (18.4)
IMD 3	13,245 (19.9)
IMD 4	14,217 (21.4)
IMD 5 (Most Deprived)	16,272 (24.5)
Period of Diagnosis	
2006–2008	19,623 (29.5)
2009–2011	22,206 (33.4)
2012–2014	24,582 (37.0)
Ethnicity	
White	53,919 (81.2)
Non-White [3]	3032 (4.6)
Unknown [4]	9460 (14.2)
Urban/Rural Category	
Urban	54,704 (82.4)
Rural	11,707 (17.6)
Stage	
I	5301 (8.0)
II	3276 (4.9)
III	3526 (5.3)
IV	13,043 (19.6)
Other [5]	41,265 (62.1)
Grade	
1 (Low)	5589 (8.4)
2	25,074 (37.8)
3	17,851 (26.9)
4 (High)	603 (0.9)
Unknown [6]	17,294 (26.0)
Comorbidities [7]	
None	48,572 (73.1)
1	8690 (13.1)
2+	9149 (13.8)
Diagnosis Route [8]	
2WW [9]	26,148 (39.4)
Dentist [10]	6572 (9.9)
Emergency [11]	5676 (8.5)
All Other Non-Emergency Routes [12]	54,163 (81.6)
Standard Primary Care-Initiated Routes [13]	34,587 (52.1)
All Primary Care Routes [14]	60,735 (91.5)

[1] Includes palate; [2] Other cancer site refers to nasopharynx, hypopharynx, salivary glands, other sites and non-specific sites; [3] Non-white refers to other ethnic groups; [4] Unknown ethnicity refers to missing and unknown ethnicity; [5] Other stage refers to missing and unstageable tumours; [6] Unknown grade refers to unknown and missing tumour grades; [7] Measured using the Charlson Comorbidity Index; [8] Reported as a percentage of the analytical population (n = 66,411); [9] 2WW refers to 2WW (dentist), 2WW (GP) and 2WW (other); [10] Dentist refers to outpatient (dentist) and 2WW (dentist); [11] Emergency refers to A&E, emergency GP referral, emergency transfer, emergency admission or attendance; [12] All other non-emergency routes refers to GP referral, inpatient referral, outpatient (other referral), 2WW (GP) and 2WW (other). [13] Standard primary care-initiated routes refers to GP referral, inpatient referral, outpatient (other referral) and outpatient (dentist); [14] All primary care routes refers to GP referral, inpatient referral, outpatient (other referral), outpatient (dentist), 2WW (dentist), 2WW (GP) and 2WW (other) Abbreviations: GP: General practitioner; IMD: Index of multiple deprivation; 2WW: Two week wait.

3.2. Analysis 1: Emergency Presentation vs. All Primary Care Routes

In total, 8.5% of patients (n = 5676) were diagnosed through emergency presentation, compared to 91.5% identified through primary care (n = 60,735). The percentage of emergency presentations declined slightly over time from 9.6% in 2006–2008 to 7.9% in 2012–2014. In univariate analyses, several variables were associated with diagnosis through the emergency route. These were older age, being male, living in a more deprived area, having two or more comorbidities, non-white ethnic group, stage IV disease and higher-grade cancer (Table 2). Compared with oral cancers, cancers of the larynx and other HNCs were more likely to present through emergency routes.

Table 2. Likelihood (OR, 95% CI and p values) from logistic regression of emergency versus all primary care routes by socio-demographic and clinical characteristics for Analysis 1 (n = 66,411).

	Emergency [1] n = 5676 (8.5%)	All Primary Care Routes [2] n = 60,735 (91.5%)	Analysis 1: Emergency Presentation Emergency [1] vs. All Primary Care Routes [2]					
			Unadjusted			Adjusted		
			OR	95% CI	p Values [3]	OR	95% CI	p Values [3]
Age at Diagnosis					<0.001			<0.001
20–54 years	1061 (7.0)	14,198 (93.0)	1.00	-	-	1.00	-	-
55–64 years	1383 (7.1)	18,076 (92.9)	1.02	0.94–1.11	0.578	1.01	0.92–1.09	0.908
65–79 years	2006 (8.7)	21,086 (91.3)	1.27	1.18–1.38	<0.001	1.17	1.08–1.27	<0.001
80+ years	1226 (14.3)	7375 (85.7)	2.22	2.04–2.43	<0.001	2.00	1.82–2.19	<0.001
Sex					0.0215			
Male	4028 (8.7)	42,213 (91.3)	1.00	-	-	-	-	-
Female	1648 (8.2)	18,522 (91.8)	0.93	0.88–0.99	0.022	-	-	-
Cancer Site					<0.001			<0.001
Oral Cavity [4]	1316 (5.8)	21,304 (94.2)	1.00	-	-	1.00	-	-
Oropharynx	1024 (6.8)	14,104 (93.2)	1.18	1.08–1.28	<0.001	1.17	1.07–1.28	0.001
Larynx	1686 (10.6)	14,199 (89.4)	1.92	1.78–2.07	<0.001	1.92	1.78–2.07	<0.001
Other [5]	1650 (12.9)	11,128 (87.1)	2.40	2.22–2.59	<0.001	1.98	1.83–2.14	<0.001
Deprivation Category					<0.001			<0.001
IMD 1 (Least Deprived)	656 (6.3)	9761 (93.7)	1.00	-	-	1.00	-	-
IMD 2	808 (6.6)	11,452 (93.4)	1.05	0.94–1.17	0.371	1.06	0.96–1.19	0.254
IMD 3	1062 (8.0)	12,183 (92.0)	1.30	1.17–1.43	<0.001	1.28	1.15–1.42	<0.001
IMD 4	1319 (9.3)	12,898 (90.7)	1.52	1.38–1.68	<0.001	1.46	1.32–1.61	<0.001
IMD 5 (Most Deprived)	1831 (11.3)	14,441 (88.7)	1.89	1.72–2.07	<0.001	1.82	1.65–2.00	<0.001
Period of Diagnosis					<0.001			0.0001
2006–2008	1875 (9.6)	17,748 (90.4)	1.00	-	-	1.00	-	-
2009–2011	1850 (8.3)	20,356 (91.7)	0.86	0.80–0.92	<0.001	0.90	0.84–0.96	0.003
2012–2014	1951 (7.9)	22,631 (92.1)	0.82	0.76–0.87	<0.001	1.05	0.97–1.14	0.203
Ethnicity					<0.001			<0.001
White	4325 (8.0)	49,594 (92.0)	1.00	-	-	1.00	-	-
Non-White [6]	318 (10.5)	2714 (89.5)	1.34	1.19–1.52	<0.001	1.28	1.13–1.45	<0.001
Unknown [7]	1033 (10.9)	8427 (89.1)	1.41	1.31–1.51	<0.001	1.32	1.22–1.43	<0.001
Urban/Rural Category					<0.001			0.0286
Urban	4889 (8.9)	49,815 (91.1)	1.00	-	-	1.00	-	-
Rural	787 (6.7)	10,920 (93.3)	0.73	0.68–0.79	<0.001	0.91	0.84–0.99	0.030
Stage					<0.001			<0.001
I	105 (2.0)	5196 (98.0)	0.19	0.16–0.24	<0.001	0.18	0.15–0.23	<0.001
II	115 (3.5)	3161 (96.5)	0.35	0.29–0.42	<0.001	0.30	0.25–0.37	<0.001
III	214 (6.1)	3312 (93.9)	0.62	0.53–0.72	<0.001	0.55	0.47–0.64	<0.001
IV	1235 (9.5)	11,808 (90.5)	1.00	-	-	1.00	-	-
Other [8]	4007 (9.7)	37,258 (90.3)	1.03	0.96–1.10	0.415	0.87	0.80–0.94	0.001
Grade					<0.001			<0.001
1 (Low)	323 (5.8)	5266 (94.2)	1.00	-	-	1.00	-	-
2	1770 (7.1)	23,304 (92.9)	1.24	1.10–1.40	0.001	1.18	1.04–1.33	0.010
3	1424 (8.0)	16,427 (92.0)	1.41	1.25–1.60	<0.001	1.24	1.09–1.41	0.001
4 (High)	66 (10.9)	537 (89.1)	2.00	1.52–2.65	<0.001	1.45	1.09–1.93	0.012
Unknown [9]	2093 (12.1)	15,201 (87.9)	2.24	1.99–2.53	<0.001	1.74	1.54–1.98	<0.001
Comorbidities [10]					<0.001			<0.001
None	3586 (7.4)	44,986 (92.6)	1.00	-	-	1.00	-	-
1	878 (10.1)	7812 (89.9)	1.41	1.30–1.52	<0.001	1.29	1.19–1.40	<0.001
2+	1212 (13.2)	7937 (86.8)	1.92	1.79–2.05	<0.001	1.68	1.56–1.81	<0.001

[1] Emergency refers to A&E, emergency GP referral, emergency transfer, emergency admission or attendance; [2] All primary care routes refers to GP referral, inpatient referral, outpatient (dentist), outpatient (other referral), 2WW (dentist), 2WW (GP) and 2WW (other); [3] p values in bold are from LRT of the contribution of the variable to the model. Unbolded p values are from a test of whether the OR is different from 1; [4] Includes palate; [5] Other cancer site refers to nasopharynx, hypopharynx, salivary glands, other sites and non-specific sites; [6] Non-white refers to other ethnic groups; [7] Unknown refers to missing and unknown ethnicity; [8] Other stage refers to missing and unstageable tumours; [9] Unknown grade refers to unknown and missing tumour grades; [10] Measured using the Charlson Comorbidity Index. Abbreviations: A&E: Accident and emergency; CI: Confidence interval; IMD: Index of multiple deprivation; GP: General practitioner; LRT: likelihood ratio test; OR: Odds ratio: 2WW; Two week wait. Model adjusted for age at diagnosis, cancer site, deprivation category, period of diagnosis, ethnicity, urban/rural categorisation, stage, grade, and comorbidities.

Socio-demographic associations (apart from with sex) persisted in multivariable analyses and were statistically significant. Those aged 80 and over were almost twice as likely to be diagnosed through emergency presentation (80+ years old vs. 20–54 years old; multivariable odds ratio (mvOR) 2.00, 95% CI 1.82, 2.19). There was also a consistent trend of increased likelihood of emergency diagnosis as the level of deprivation increased. Those patients resident in the most deprived areas were 1.82 times more likely to come through an emergency route than those patients resident in the least deprived areas (IMD5 vs. IMD 1; mvOR 1.82, 95% CI 1.65, 2.00). Non-white patients were 1.28 times more likely to be diagnosed via emergency presentation than white patients (non-whites vs. white; mvOR 1.28, 95% CI 1.13, 1.45). Patients residing in rural areas were significantly less likely to be referred through an emergency route (rural vs. urban mvOR; 0.91, 95% CI 0.84, 0.99). In terms of clinical variables, patients diagnosed with a higher-grade cancer were 1.45 times more likely to present through emergency routes (high vs. low grade; mvOR 1.45, 95% CI 1.09, 1.93). Stage I cancers were 82% less likely than stage IV cancers to be diagnosed via emergency presentation (I vs. IV; mvOR 0.18, 95% CI 0.15, 0.23).

3.3. Analysis 2: 2WW vs. Standard Primary Care-Initiated Routes

Of HNC patients who were diagnosed through a route initiated in primary care, just over 40% came through the urgent 2WW pathway (n = 26,148; 43.1%). This proportion rose over time from 36.0% in 2006–2008 to 49.8% in 2012–2014. When comparing patients referred via 2WW rather than via other standard care routes, the variables associated with an increased likelihood of urgent referral in univariate analyses were as follows: being aged 55–64 years old male, and of white ethnicity; having a cancer of the oropharynx, stage III and IV disease, grade 3 tumours, no comorbidities and residing in an area of higher deprivation. There was no observed variation by urban/rural residence. In multivariable analysis, associations with stage and grade did not persist. Patients aged 55–64 years were more likely to be referred via the urgent 2WW pathway than younger patients (55–64 years vs. 20–54 years; mvOR 1.18, 95% CI 1.13, 01.24); more modest increased risks were seen for the two older age-groups. Compared to cancers of the oral cavity, cancers of the oropharynx were more likely to been referred via 2WW (mvOR 1.64, 95% CI 1.57, 1.71). Patients were 1.43 more than 40% more likely to be referred by 2WW pathways if they resided in the most deprived areas (IMD5 vs. IMD1; mvOR 1.43, 95% CI 1.35, 1.50). Being female was associated with a reduced likelihood of 2WW referral (mvOR 0.76, 95% CI 0.73, 0.79) as was being from a non-white ethnic group (non-white ethnic group vs. white; mvOR 0.57, 95%CI 0.52, 0.62) (Table 3).

3.4. Analysis 3: Dentist vs. All Other Non-Emergency Routes

Overall, 10.8% (n = 6572) of all HNC patients who followed a non-emergency route were referred via a dentist. This percentage rose slightly from 9.6% in 2006–2008 to 11.8% in 2012–2014. In the univariable analysis, when compared with referral via all other routes, dental referral was associated with older age, female gender, residence in a less deprived area and having an oral cancer. All variables apart from urban/rural category and comorbidities were statistically significant in the final model. In multivariable analyses, patients aged 65–79 years old were most likely to be referred via the dentist (65–79 vs. 20–54 years; mvOR 1.13, 95%CI 1.05, 1.22) as were female patients (mvOR 1.27, 95% CI 1.20, 1.34) and those from a non-white ethnic group (non-white vs. white; mvOR 1.26, 95%CI 1.12, 1.43). Residence in an area of increasing deprivation was associated with a reduced chance of dental referral when compared to all other routes (IMD 5 vs. IMD1; mvOR 0.71, 95%CI 0.65, 0.78). Patients with stage I cancer (stage I vs. stage IV; mvOR 1.19, 95%CI 1.07, 1.32) were more likely to be referred via dental routes. Diagnoses via dental referral when compared to all other routes also increased over time (2012–2014 vs. 2006–2008; mvOR 1.22, 95% CI 1.12, 1.32) (Table 4).

Table 3. Likelihood (OR, 95% CI and *p* values) from logistic regression of 2WW versus standard primary care-initiated routes by socio-demographic and clinical characteristics for Analysis 2 (n = 60,735).

	2WW [1] n = 26,148 (43.1%)	Standard Primary Care-Initiated Routes [2] n = 34,587 (56.9%)	Analysis 2: Primary Care 2WW [1] vs. Standard Primary Care-Initiated Routes [2]					
			Unadjusted			Adjusted		
			OR	95% CI	*p* Values [3]	OR	95% CI	*p* Values [3]
Age at Diagnosis					<0.001			<0.001
20–54 years	5983 (42.1)	8215 (57.9)	1.00	-	-	1.00	-	-
55–64 years	8415 (46.6)	9661 (53.4)	1.20	1.14–1.25	<0.001	1.18	1.13–1.24	<0.001
65–79 years	8888 (42.2)	12,198 (57.8)	1.00	0.96–1.04	0.983	1.07	1.02–1.12	0.005
80+ years	2862 (38.8)	4513 (61.2)	0.87	0.82–0.92	<0.001	1.06	1.00–1.13	0.062
Sex					<0.001			<0.001
Male	19,206 (45.5)	23,007 (54.5)	1.00	-	-	1.00	-	-
Female	6942 (37.5)	11,580 (62.5)	0.72	0.69–0.74	<0.001	0.76	0.73–0.79	<0.001
Cancer Site					<0.001			<0.001
Oral Cavity [4]	8462 (39.7)	12,842 (60.3)	1.00	-	-	1.00	-	-
Oropharynx	7653 (54.3)	6451 (45.7)	1.80	1.72–1.88	<0.001	1.64	1.57–1.71	<0.001
Larynx	6152 (43.3)	8047 (56.7)	1.16	1.11–1.21	<0.001	1.07	1.02–1.12	0.005
Other [5]	3881 (34.9)	7247 (65.1)	0.81	0.77–0.85	<0.001	0.81	0.77–0.85	<0.001
Deprivation Category					<0.001			<0.001
IMD 1 (Least Deprived)	3812 (39.1)	5949 (60.9)	1.00	-	-	1.00	-	-
IMD 2	4738 (41.4)	6714 (58.6)	1.10	1.04–1.16	0.001	1.11	1.05–1.17	<0.001
IMD 3	5242 (43.0)	6941 (57.0)	1.18	1.12–1.24	<0.001	1.21	1.14–1.28	<0.001
IMD 4	5649 (43.8)	7249 (56.2)	1.22	1.15–1.28	<0.001	1.26	1.19–1.33	<0.001
IMD 5 (Most Deprived)	6707 (46.4)	7734 (53.6)	1.35	1.28–1.43	<0.001	1.43	1.35–1.50	<0.001
Period of Diagnosis					<0.001			<0.001
2006–2008	6392 (36.0)	11,356 (64.0)	1.00	-	-	1.00	-	-
2009–2011	8494 (41.7)	11,862 (58.3)	1.27	1.22–1.33	<0.001	1.27	1.22–1.33	<0.001
2012–2014	11,262 (49.8)	11,369 (50.2)	1.76	1.69–1.83	<0.001	1.71	1.64–1.79	<0.001
Ethnicity					<0.001			<0.001
White	22,192 (44.7)	27,402 (55.3)	1.00	-	-	1.00	-	-
Non-White [6]	843 (31.1)	1871 (68.9)	0.56	0.51–0.60	<0.001	0.57	0.52–0.62	<0.001
Unknown [7]	3113 (36.9)	5314 (63.1)	0.72	0.69–0.76	<0.001	0.84	0.80–0.88	<0.001
Urban/Rural Category					0.504			-
Urban	21,478 (43.1)	28,337 (56.9)	1.00	-	-	-	-	-
Rural	4670 (42.8)	6250 (57.2)	0.99	0.95–1.03	0.504	-	-	-
Stage					<0.001			-
I	2035 (39.2)	3161 (60.8)	0.53	0.50–0.57	<0.001	-	-	-
II	1495 (47.3)	1666 (52.7)	0.74	0.69–0.80	<0.001	-	-	-
III	1733 (52.3)	1579 (47.7)	0.91	0.84–0.98	0.013	-	-	-
IV	6467 (54.8)	5341 (45.2)	1.00	-	-	-	-	-
Other [8]	14,418 (38.7)	22,840 (61.3)	0.52	0.50–0.54	<0.001	-	-	-
Grade					<0.001			-
1 (Low)	1921 (36.5)	3345 (63.5)	1.00	-	-	-	-	-
2	10,754 (46.1)	12,550 (53.9)	1.49	1.40–1.59	<0.001	-	-	-
3	8107 (49.4)	8320 (50.6)	1.70	1.59–1.81	<0.001	-	-	-
4	209 (38.9)	328 (61.1)	1.11	0.92–1.33	0.264	-	-	-
Unknown [9]	5157 (33.9)	10,044 (66.1)	0.89	0.84–0.95	0.001	-	-	-
Comorbidities [10]					<0.001			<0.001
None	19,688 (43.8)	25,298 (56.2)	1.00	-	-	1.00	-	-
1	3342 (42.8)	4470 (57.2)	0.96	0.92–1.01	0.105	0.93	0.88–0.98	0.004
2+	3118 (39.3)	4819 (60.7)	0.83	0.79–0.87	<0.001	0.80	0.76–0.85	<0.001

[1] 2WW refers to 2WW (dentist), 2WW (GP) and 2WW (other); [2] Standard primary care-initiated routes refers to GP referral, inpatient referral, outpatient (other referral) and outpatient (dentist); [3] *p* values in bold are from LRT of the contribution of the variable to the model. Unbolded *p* values are from a test of whether the OR is different from 1; [4] Includes palate; [5] Other cancer site refers to nasopharynx, hypopharynx, salivary glands, other sites and non-specific sites; [6] Non-White refers to other ethnic groups; [7] Unknown ethnicity refers to missing and unknown ethnicity; [8] Other stage refers to missing and unstageable tumours; [9] Unknown grade refers to unknown and missing tumour grades; [10] Measured using the Charlson Comorbidity Index. Abbreviations: CI: Confidence interval; IMD: Index of multiple deprivation; GP: General practitioner; LRT: Likelihood ratio tests; OR: Odds ratio; 2WW: Two week wait. Model adjusted for age at diagnosis, sex, cancer site, deprivation category, period of diagnosis, ethnicity, and comorbidities.

Table 4. Likelihood (OR, 95% CI and *p* values) from logistic regression of dentist versus all other non-emergency routes by socio-demographic and clinical characteristics for Analysis 3 (n = 60,735).

	Dentist [1] n = 6572 (10.8%)	All Other Non-Emergency Routes [2] n = 54,163 (89.2%)	Analysis 3: Practitioner Dentist [1] vs. All Other Non-Emergency Routes [2]					
			Unadjusted			Adjusted		
			OR	95% CI	*p* Values [3]	OR	95% CI	*p* Values [3]
Age at Diagnosis					<0.001			0.0106
20–54 years	1476 (10.4)	12,722 (89.6)	1.00	-	-	1.00	-	-
55–64 years	1784 (9.9)	16,292 (90.1)	0.94	0.88–1.02	0.119	1.04	0.97–1.13	0.283
65–79 years	2348 (11.1)	18,738 (88.9)	1.08	1.01–1.16	0.028	1.13	1.05–1.22	0.001
80+ years	964 (13.1)	6411 (86.9)	1.30	1.19–1.41	<0.001	1.06	0.96–1.16	0.256
Sex					<0.001			<0.001
Male	3636 (8.6)	38,577 (91.4)	1.00	-	-	1.00	-	-
Female	2936 (15.9)	15,586 (84.1)	2.00	1.90–2.11	<0.001	1.27	1.20–1.34	<0.001
Cancer Site					<0.001			<0.001
Oral Cavity [4]	5629 (26.4)	15,675 (73.6)	1.00	-	-	1.00	-	-
Oropharynx	456 (3.2)	13,648 (96.8)	0.09	0.08–0.10	<0.001	0.11	0.10–0.12	<0.001
Larynx	43 (0.3)	14,156 (99.7)	0.01	0.01–0.01	<0.001	0.01	0.01–0.01	<0.001
Other [5]	444 (4.0)	10,684 (96.0)	0.12	0.10–0.13	<0.001	0.13	0.11–0.14	<0.001
Deprivation Category					<0.001			<0.001
IMD 1 (Least Deprived)	1269 (13.0)	8492 (87.0)	1.00	-	-	1.00	-	-
IMD 2	1351 (11.8)	10,101 (88.2)	0.90	0.82–0.97	0.008	0.92	0.84–1.01	0.075
IMD 3	1354 (11.1)	10,829 (88.9)	0.84	0.77–0.91	<0.001	0.88	0.80–0.96	0.004
IMD 4	1297 (10.1)	11,601 (89.9)	0.75	0.69–0.81	<0.001	0.80	0.73–0.88	<0.001
IMD 5 (Most Deprived)	1301 (9.0)	13,140 (91.0)	0.66	0.61–0.72	<0.001	0.71	0.65–0.78	<0.001
Period of Diagnosis					<0.001			<0.001
2006–2008	1707 (9.6)	16,041 (90.4)	1.00	-	-	1.00	-	-
2009–2011	2202 (10.8)	18,154 (89.2)	1.14	1.07–1.22	<0.001	1.14	1.06–1.22	<0.001
2012–2014	2663 (11.8)	19,968 (88.2)	1.25	1.18–1.34	<0.001	1.22	1.12–1.32	<0.001
Ethnicity					<0.001			<0.001
White	5185 (10.5)	44,409 (89.5)	1.00	-	-	1.00	-	-
Non-White [6]	407 (15.0)	2307 (85.0)	1.51	1.35–1.69	<0.001	1.26	1.12–1.43	<0.001
Unknown [7]	980 (11.6)	7447 (88.4)	1.13	1.05–1.21	0.001	1.14	1.05–1.23	0.002
Urban/Rural Category					0.0004			-
Urban	5285 (10.6)	44,530 (89.4)	1.00	-	-	-	-	-
Rural	1287 (11.8)	9633 (88.2)	1.13	1.06–1.20	<0.001	-	-	-
Stage					<0.001			<0.001
I	904 (17.4)	4292 (82.6)	1.74	1.59–1.91	<0.001	1.19	1.07–1.32	0.001
II	361 (11.4)	2800 (88.6)	1.07	0.94–1.21	0.319	0.88	0.77–1.01	0.073
III	273 (8.2)	3039 (91.8)	0.74	0.65–0.85	<0.001	0.83	0.72–0.96	0.013
IV	1275 (10.8)	10,533 (89.2)	1.00	-	-	1.00	-	-
Other [8]	3759 (10.1)	33,499 (89.9)	0.93	0.87–0.99	0.027	0.89	0.82–0.96	0.005
Grade					<0.001			<0.001
1 (Low)	938 (17.8)	4328 (82.2)	1.00	-	-	1.00	-	-
2	3045 (13.1)	20,259 (86.9)	0.69	0.64–0.75	<0.001	0.86	0.79–0.94	0.001
3	1143 (7.0)	15,284 (93.0)	0.35	0.31–0.38	<0.001	0.62	0.56–0.68	<0.001
4 (High)	19 (3.5)	518 (96.5)	0.17	0.11–0.27	<0.001	0.54	0.33–0.87	0.011
Unknown [9]	1427 (9.4)	13,774 (90.6)	0.48	0.44–0.52	<0.001	0.88	0.79–0.97	0.009
Comorbidities [10]					0.204			-
None	4891 (10.9)	40,095 (89.1)	1.00	-	-	-	-	-
1	802 (10.3)	7010 (89.7)	0.94	0.87–1.01	0.111	-	-	-
2+	879 (11.1)	7058 (88.9)	1.02	0.95–1.10	0.594	-	-	-

[1] Dentist refers to outpatient (dentist) and 2WW (dentist); [2] All other non-emergency routes refers to GP referral, inpatient referral, outpatient (other referral), 2WW (GP) and 2WW (other); [3] *p* values in bold are from LRT of the contribution of the variable to the model. Unbolded *p* values are from a test of whether the OR is different from 1; [4] Includes palate; [5] Other cancer site refers to nasopharynx, hypopharynx, salivary glands, other sites, and non-specific sites; [6] Non-White refers to other ethnic groups; [7] Unknown ethnicity refers to missing and unknown ethnicity; [8] Other stage refers to missing and unstageable tumours; [9] Unknown grade refers to unknown and missing tumour grades; [10] Measured using the Charlson Comorbidity Index. Abbreviations: CI: Confidence interval; IMD: Index of multiple deprivation; GP: General practitioner; LRT: Likelihood ratio tests; OR: Odds ratio: Model adjusted for age at diagnosis, sex, cancer site, deprivation category, period of diagnosis, ethnicity, stage, and grade.

4. Discussion

To our knowledge, this is the first comprehensive analysis of routes to diagnosis for HNC in England. In this population-based study, significant socio-demographic inequalities were observed and were shown to vary across diagnosis routes.

There were some indications in the results of positive changes over time, most notably the increase in those picked up through the urgent cancer referral route (2WW). How-ever, there are several areas of concern. The analysis showed that there has been an in-crease over time in the number of HNCs diagnosed, although the distribution of HNC cancer subsites has changed with the predominant tumour site being the oropharynx in 2012–2014, rather than larynx which was most common in 2006–2008. This echoes trends re-ported elsewhere [23] and likely reflects changes in risk factors such as a reduction in smoking prevalence and an increase in HPV-related cancers [24]. Although overall the number of patients diagnosed through the emergency route is relatively small compared to some other cancers [25,26], there was a small increase in the number (albeit not the percentage) of emergency presentations over time. This is concerning as emergency cancer presentations may be considered, in some ways, as a "failure" of the system, and indicative of significant delays or barriers to presentation.

4.1. Emergency Route

Those that were diagnosed through the emergency route were more likely to present with advanced disease, which is consistent with patterns of other cancers in the UK and internationally [3]. In terms of socio-demographic characteristics, emergency presentations were more often patients from urban areas and areas of greater deprivation, from non-white ethnic groups, and over the age of 65.

The association between older age and emergency presentation is supported by previous research in all cancers in England where likelihood of emergency presentation rose significantly in those over 70 years [27]. Whilst it is known that advanced age is a risk factor for HNC, the vague or non-specific nature of some HNC symptoms may mean that symptoms are not recognised as being of concern or are perceived as "normal" aging. Previous research has shown that cancer awareness is lower in this age group than among younger people [28]. It has also shown that people, and in particular older adults, can be more reticent to seek help in primary care due to a fear of wasting clinicians' time, particularly when symptoms are vague [29,30]. This fear may then reduce the chances of a person seeking help from primary care, resulting in a delay to diagnosis and an increased likelihood of an emergency presentation.

There are a growing number of reports on healthcare experiences of ethnic minority groups in the UK and internationally; people from ethnic minorities more often experience significant barriers to accessing healthcare, and once within the system, more often report poor experiences (for example: [31–34]). Much of the recent work has focused on the experience with COVID-19; however, it seems plausible that barriers such as lack of trust, inappropriate services and discrimination impacted help-seeking prior to COVID-19 too [35]. The finding here that patients from non-white ethnic groups are more likely to be diagnosed after an emergency presentation adds further to this accumulating evidence base [36].

Older age, deprivation and being from an ethnic minority have all been associated with suboptimal health literacy [37,38]. Health literacy is the extent to which an individual has the capacity, knowledge, understanding and confidence to access, understand, evaluate, use and navigate health and social care information and services [39]. It includes the capacity to communicate, assert and enact health decisions [40]. It has been associated—in other clinical areas—with less use of preventive health services and greater use of emergency services [39]. Given the socio-demographic patterns observed here, future research exploring the role of health literacy in emergency cancer presentation (and, more generally, across the entire cancer diagnosis pathway) would be of value.

4.2. Urgent Cancer Referral (2WW)

Those patients diagnosed through the urgent cancer referral route, compared to other routes which commenced in primary care, were more likely to be white, male, aged 55 years and older, resident in areas of greater deprivation and to have a cancer of the oropharynx.

The 2WW pathway requires that a patient meets a list of referral criteria for urgent investigation of a suspected cancer. Compared to other HNC tumours, oropharyngeal cancer more often presents with a neck lump/swelling [41]. This may mean that it is more likely to be recognised as potentially concerning by patients and primary care clinicians than vague, less specific (and perhaps more benign-seeming) symptoms, thus triggering a 2WW referral far quicker. Previous research on multiple different cancers has shown that those with vague symptoms delay attending primary care take a median of 34 days longer to diagnosis than those with alarm symptoms [42]. Moreover, the stereotypical "traditional" HNC patient is an older deprived male (likely with tobacco and alcohol addiction problems) [43]. It is therefore possible that primary care staff may be more likely to have a higher index of suspicion of a potentially serious underlying condition around individuals who match this profile, and therefore refer them for urgent investigation.

Some research in Denmark suggests that GPs suspect cancer in more patients than they refer onto cancer specific pathways, and that those patients who reported vague symptoms are less likely to be referred [44]. This suggests the possibility that those who do not display what the GP considers to be clear symptoms of a potential HNC, despite a suspicion of cancer, may not be being referred through the 2WW pathway.

4.3. Dental Referral Route

Patients from ethnic minorities, women, and those from less deprived areas, were more likely to have been referred through a dentist than through other primary care routes. As might be expected, oral cavity cancers were more often diagnosed through this route, but it is noteworthy that dentists also referred patients who were diagnosed with cancers elsewhere in the head and neck.

The dental system in the UK involves payment at the point of treatment, in contrast to the rest of primary care which is free at point of treatment; moreover, not all dental costs are subsidised by the State. There are significant barriers to accessing NHS dental services, including financial difficulties, lack of availability of services (i.e., no appointments being available), or lack of services being offered in the local area [45]. Our finding that people from more deprived areas were less likely to be diagnosed through the dental route may be explained by the cost of accessing dental check-ups and treatment. While some of those on the lowest incomes are entitled to free dental care, this involves the completion of lengthy forms [46]. Research has shown that areas of deprivation have far less NHS dentists (so called "dental deserts") [47], suggesting that those who may be entitled to free dental care may not be able to access a dentist. This is concerning given that dentists provide a potential route for early diagnosis of some HNC.

The finding that women are more likely to have been diagnosed from a dentist referral is supported by previous research which has shown women are more likely to have made an NHS dental appointment [48]. The association between being from an ethnic minority and diagnosed through a dentist is more striking. It has been reported that people from all minority ethnicity groups have greater mistrust of dentists, are less likely to have visited a dentist and, of those who have visited, are more likely to have done so because of a specific issue rather than a routine checkup [46]. Often, research which focusses on ethnicity and health outcomes is confounded by SES, which may not be controlled for in the analysis. However, our finding was apparent after adjusting for the effects of deprivation. It is consistent with results from a small study in London, which found that once SES had been considered, Asian people were far more likely, than white people, to have visited the dentist [49]. This is an area which would benefit from further investigation.

4.4. Limitations

This study had several known limitations associated with analyses of routine cancer registry data. Routine data sometimes have a significant amount of missing information and in this dataset, levels of missingness for summary stage and ethnicity were high. For the latter, this meant we could not explore whether there were differences between different ethnic minority groups, and further research on this topic would be of value. For the former, care is needed in making inferences from our findings. Completeness of stage details has improved over time in registry data, so subsequent studies would be of value to confirm the findings here. We took the decision not to exclude patients with missing information as the data were unlikely to be missing completely at random, and exclusion may have introduced bias. In addition, information was not available on risk factors for HNC, such as HPV status (which was not routinely tested for during the study period), and tobacco and alcohol use; these could be associated with patient diagnostic route. The registry provided a proxy variable for inferred HPV status based on tumour site and morphology, but this was not used in the final analysis as it was not more informative than cancer site alone. It is also likely that analyses are subject to residual confounding from comorbidities; the Charlson Comorbidity Index is a crude measure of the number of comorbidities that a patient has and only includes particular conditions documented during hospital admissions in a specified time period [50], so likely underestimates true levels of comorbidity. However, as comorbidities increase with age, and age was also included in the models, any residual confounding is likely somewhat mitigated.

Another important factor is that this data are from 2006 to 2014. While cancer pathways in England have not changed in the intervening years, it is possible that the frequency with which different routes are followed, or variations between socio-demographic groups, may have changed in the intervening years. In particular, the impact of the COVID-19 pandemic had a significant impact on cancer services; in England, urgent referrals decreased dramatically, and it is estimated that there will be substantial increases in cancer deaths due to delays in diagnosis and treatment [51,52]. Research investigating whether the inequalities in route to cancer diagnosis reported here have persisted since 2014, leading up to, during, and following the pandemic should be a priority. The current analysis could usefully serve as a baseline for such future work. Finally, these results may not be generalisable to all healthcare systems outside of England which may differ in terms of processing of diagnosis routes.

5. Conclusions

In conclusion, this population-based analysis of English cancer registry data showed significant socio-demographic inequalities in HNC routes to diagnosis. In many instances, groups who are already experiencing higher risk of HNC are further disadvantaged by inequalities inherent within their route to diagnosis. Understanding the reasons for these inequalities is the first step to being able to improve and speed the pathways to HNC diagnosis; this, in turn, would reduce inequalities and optimise patients' clinical outcomes.

Supplementary Materials: The following supporting information can be downloaded at: https://www.mdpi.com/article/10.3390/ijerph192416723/s1, Figure S1: Route to diagnosis categorisation by each analysis, Table S1: Demographic and clinical characteristics of all individual HNC diagnosis routes during 2006–2014.

Author Contributions: Conceptualisation, L.S. and J.P.; Methodology, J.D. and L.S.; Formal analysis, J.D., L.S. and J.P.; Writing—original draft preparation, J.D. and R.N.; Writing review and editing, J.D., R.N., J.O., J.P. and L.S.; Supervision, L.S. and J.P.; Project administration, J.D.; Funding acquisition, L.S. All authors have read and agreed to the published version of the manuscript.

Funding: This research was conducted as part of JD's PhD, funded by Newcastle University. RN was funded by a grant from Cancer Research UK (A25618).

Institutional Review Board Statement: The study was conducted in accordance with the Declaration of Helsinki, and approved by the Institutional Review Board (or Ethics Committee) of Yorkshire and the Humber—South Yorkshire Research Ethics Committee (protocol code 206040; 16th November 2017).

Informed Consent Statement: Patient consent was waived due to only receiving pseudonymised data.

Data Availability Statement: The data used in this study were released to the authors for the purpose of this analysis; the authors are not permitted to share it. Interested individuals may apply for dataset including registrations of head and neck cancer over the study period from the current data controllers, NHS Digital.

Acknowledgments: This study was possible as a result of routine data collection by the NHS as part of standard cancer care and support. The data are collated and maintained by the NCRAS, previously part of PHE. Special mention is also noted to colleagues at the Office for Data Re-lease for their help during the data application process.

Conflicts of Interest: The authors declare no conflict of interest. The funders had no role in the design of the study; in the collection, analyses, or interpretation of data; in the writing of the manuscript; or in the decision to publish the results.

Abbreviations

AIC: Akaike information criterion; CI(s): Confidence intervals; DCO: Death certificate only; GP: General practitioner; HES: Hospital Episode Statistics; HNC: Head and neck cancer; HPV: Human papilloma virus; IMD: Index of Multiple Deprivation; LRT: Likelihood ratio test; NCRAS: National Cancer Registration and Analysis Service; NCRD: National Cancer Registration Database; NCWT: National cancer waiting time; NHS: National Health Service; ODR: Office for Data Release; OR(s): Odds ratio(s); SES: socio-economic status; STROBE: Strengthening the Reporting of Observational Studies in Epidemiology; UK: United Kingdom; 2WW: Two week wait.

References

1. Abdel-Rahman, M.; Stockton, D.; Rachet, B.; Hakulinen, T.; Coleman, M.P. What if cancer survival in Britain were the same as in Europe: How many deaths are avoidable? *Br. J. Cancer* **2009**, *101* (Suppl. S2), S115–S124. [CrossRef] [PubMed]
2. Thomson, C.; Forman, D. Cancer survival in England and the influence of early diagnosis: What can we learn from recent EUROCARE results? *Br. J. Cancer* **2009**, *101* (Suppl. S2), S102–S109. [CrossRef] [PubMed]
3. McPhail, S.; Swann, R.; Johnson, S.A.; Barclay, M.E.; Elkader, H.; Alvi, R. Risk factors and prognostic implications of diagnosis of cancer within 30 days after an emergency hospital admission (emergency presentation): An International Cancer Benchmarking Partnership (ICBP) population-based study. *Lancet Oncol.* **2022**, *23*, 587–600. [CrossRef]
4. McPhail, S.; Johnson, S.; Greenberg, D.; Peake, M.; Rous, B. Stage at diagnosis and early mortality from cancer in England. *Br. J. Cancer* **2015**, *112* (Suppl. S1), S108–S115. [CrossRef]
5. Walter, F.; Webster, A.; Scott, S.; Emery, J. The Andersen Model of Total Patient Delay: A systematic review of its application in cancer diagnosis. *J. Health Serv. Res. Policy* **2012**, *17*, 110–118. [CrossRef] [PubMed]
6. Department of Health. The NHS Cancer Plan. London. Available online: www.thh.nhs.uk/documents/_Departments/Cancer/NHSCancerPlan.pdf (accessed on 25 October 2022).
7. Herbert, A.; Abel, G.A.; Winters, S.; McPhail, S.; Elliss-Brookes, L.; Lyratzopoulos, G. Cancer diagnoses after emergency GP referral or A&E attendance in England: Determinants and time trends in Routes to Diagnosis data, 2006–2015. *Br. J. Gen. Pract.* **2019**, *69*, e724–e730. [CrossRef] [PubMed]
8. Herbert, A.; Winters, S.; McPhail, S.; Elliss-Brookes, L.; Lyratzopoulos, G.; Abel, G.A. Population trends in emergency cancer diagnoses: The role of changing patient case-mix. *Cancer Epidemiol.* **2019**, *63*, 101574. [CrossRef] [PubMed]
9. Cancer Research UK. Head and Neck Cancer Incidence Statistics. Available online: https://www.cancerresearchuk.org/health-professional/cancer-statistics/statistics-by-cancer-type/head-and-neck-cancers (accessed on 25 October 2022).
10. Bannister, M.; Vallamkondu, V.; Ah-See, K. Emergency presentations of head and neck cancer: A modern perspective. *J. Laryngol. Otol.* **2016**, *130*, 571–574. [CrossRef]
11. Agency for Healthcare Research and Quality. Six Domains of Health Care Quality. Available online: https://www.ahrq.gov/talkingquality/measures/six-domains.html (accessed on 30 March 2020).
12. NHS Digital. Case-Mix Adjusted Percentage of Cancers Diagnosed at Stages 1 and 2 by CCG in England. 2019. Available online: https://digital.nhs.uk/data-and-information/publications/statistical/case-mix-adjusted-percentage-cancers-diagnosed-at-stages-1-and-2-by-ccg-in-england (accessed on 10 October 2022).

13. Macmillan Cancer Support/National Services Scotland. Deprivation and Survival from Head and Neck Cancer in Scotland. February 2017. Available online: https://www.macmillan.org.uk/_images/Head-and-neck-Cancer-Survival-and-Deprivation-Brief_tcm9-308831.pdf (accessed on 10 October 2022).
14. Ingarfield, K.; McMahon, A.D.; Hurley, K.; Toms, S.; Pring, M.; Thomas, S.J.; Waylen, A.; Pawlita, M.; Waterboer, T.; Ness, A.R.; et al. Inequality in survival of people with head and neck cancer: Head and Neck 5000 cohort study. *Head Neck* **2021**, *43*, 1252–1270. [CrossRef] [PubMed]
15. Von Elm, E.; Altman, D.G.; Egger, M.; Pocock, S.J.; Gøtzsche, P.C.; Vandenbroucke, J.P. STROBE Initiative. The Strengthening the Reporting of Observational Studies in Epidemiology (STROBE) statement: Guidelines for reporting observational studies. *Ann. Intern. Med.* **2007**, *147*, 573–577. [CrossRef]
16. Henson, K.E.; Elliss-Brookes, L.; Coupland, V.H.; Payne, E.; Vernon, S.; Rous, B.; Rashbass, J. Data Resource Profile: National Cancer Registration Dataset in England. *Int. J. Epidemiol.* **2020**, *49*, 16-16h. [CrossRef]
17. Elliss-Brookes, L.; McPhail, S.; Ives, A.; Greenslade, M.; Shelton, J.; Hiom, S.; Richards, M. Routes to diagnosis for cancer—Determining the patient journey using multiple routine data sets. *Br. J. Cancer* **2012**, *107*, 1220–1226. [CrossRef] [PubMed]
18. Public Health England. Routes to Diagnosis 2006–2016 Workbook, Version 2.1a. Available online: http://www.ncin.org.uk/publications/routes_to_diagnosis (accessed on 24 October 2022).
19. Department for Communities and Local Government. The English Index of Multiple Deprivation (IMD) 2015—Guidance. Available online: https://assets.publishing.service.gov.uk/government/uploads/system/uploads/attachment_data/file/464430/English_Index_of_Multiple_Deprivation_2015_-_Guidance.pdf (accessed on 28 August 2021).
20. Office for National Statistics. The 2011 Rural-Urban Classification for Small Area Geographies: A User Guide and Frequently Asked Questions (v1.0). Available online: https://assets.publishing.service.gov.uk/government/uploads/system/uploads/attachment_data/file/239478/RUC11user_guide_28_Aug.pdf (accessed on 26 October 2022).
21. Charlson, M.E.; Pompei, P.; Ales, K.L.; MacKenzie, C.R. A new method of classifying prognostic comorbidity in longitudinal studies: Development and validation. *J. Chronic Dis.* **1987**, *40*, 373–383. [CrossRef]
22. StataCorp. *Stata Statistical Software: Release 15*; StataCorp LLC: College Station, TX, USA, 2017.
23. Jakobsen, K.K.; Grønhøj, C.; Jensen, D.H.; Schmidt Karnov, K.K.; Klitmøller Agander, T.; Specht, L.; von Buchwald, C. Increasing incidence and survival of head and neck cancers in Denmark: A nation-wide study from 1980 to 2014. *Acta Oncol.* **2018**, *57*, 1143–1151. [CrossRef] [PubMed]
24. Sturgis, E.; Cinciripini, P.M. Trends in head and neck cancer incidence in relation to smoking prevalence. An emerging epidemic of human papillomavirus-associated cancers? *Cancer* **2007**, *110*, 1429–1435. [CrossRef] [PubMed]
25. Tsang, C.; Bottle, A.; Majeed, A.; Aylin, P. Cancer diagnosed by emergency admission in England: An observational study using the general practice research database. *BMC Health Serv. Res.* **2013**, *14*, 308. [CrossRef] [PubMed]
26. McPhail, S.; Elliss-Brookes, L.; Shelton, J.; Ives, A.; Greenslade, M.; Vernon, S.; Morris, E.J.; Richards, M. Emergency presentation of cancer and short-term mortality. *Br. J. Cancer* **2013**, *1109*, 2027–2034. [CrossRef]
27. Kmietowicz, Z. One in three cases of cancer in patients over 70 are diagnosed at emergency admission. *BMJ* **2012**, *345*, e6402. [CrossRef]
28. Forbes, L.J.; Simon, A.E.; Warburton, F.; Boniface, D.; Brain, K.E.; Dessaix, A.; Donnelly, C.; Haynes, K.; Hvidberg, L.; Lagerlund, M.; et al. International Cancer Benchmarking Partnership Module 2 Working Group. Differences in cancer awareness and beliefs between Australia, Canada, Denmark, Norway, Sweden and the UK (the International Cancer Benchmarking Partnership): Do they contribute to differences in cancer survival? *Br. J. Cancer* **2013**, *108*, 292–300. [CrossRef] [PubMed]
29. Smith, L.K.; Pope, C.; Botha, J.L. Patients' help-seeking experiences and delay in cancer presentation: A qualitative synthesis. *Lancet* **2005**, *366*, 825–831. [CrossRef]
30. Cromme, S.K.; Whitaker, K.L.; Winstanley, K.; Renzi, C.; Smith, C.F.; Wardle, J. Worrying about wasting GP time as a barrier to help-seeking: A community-based, qualitative study. *Br. J. Gen. Pract.* **2016**, *66*, e474–e482. [CrossRef] [PubMed]
31. Pinder, R.J.; Ferguson, J.; Møller, H. Minority ethnicity patient satisfaction and experience: Results of the National Cancer Patient Experience Survey in England. *BMJ Open* **2016**, *6*, e011938. [CrossRef] [PubMed]
32. Sze, M.; Butow, P.; Bell, M.; Vaccaro, L.; Dong, S.; Eisenbruch, M.; Jefford, M.; Girgis, A.; King, M.; McGrane, J.; et al. Migrant health in cancer: Outcome disparities and the determinant role of migrant specific variables. *Oncologist* **2015**, *20*, 523–531. [CrossRef] [PubMed]
33. Smedley, B.D.; Stith, A.Y.; Nelson, A.R. Unequal treatment: Confronting racial and ethnic disparities in health care. *N. Engl. J. Med.* **2003**, *349*, 1296. [CrossRef]
34. National Cancer Patient Experience Survey 2021 National Report (Quantitative). Available online: https://www.ncpes.co.uk/wp-content/uploads/2022/07/CPES21_Standard-National-Report_JK-PF-NG_RM_BA_SH_280622_FINAL.pdf (accessed on 10 October 2022).
35. Public Health England. Beyond the Data: Understanding the Impact of COVID-19 on BAME Groups. Available online: https://assets.publishing.service.gov.uk/government/uploads/system/uploads/attachment_data/file/892376/COVID_stakeholder_engagement_synthesis_beyond_the_data.pdf (accessed on 15 October 2022).
36. Razai, M.S.; Kankam, H.K.N.; Majeed, A.; Esmail, A.; Williams, D.R. Mitigating ethnic disparities in covid-19 and beyond. *BMJ* **2021**, *372*, m4921. [CrossRef] [PubMed]

37. Rowlands, G.; Protheroe, J.; Winkley, J.; Richardson, M.; Seed, P.T.; Rudd, R. A mismatch between population health literacy and the complexity of health information: An observational study. *Br. J. Gen. Pract.* **2015**, *65*, e379–e386. [CrossRef] [PubMed]
38. NHS Scotland. The Health Literacy Place. Available online: http://www.healthliteracyplace.org.uk/ (accessed on 15 October 2022).
39. Public Health Literacy. Improving Health Literacy to Reduce Health Inequalities. Available online: https://www.gov.uk/government/publications/local-action-on-health-inequalities-improving-health-literacy (accessed on 15 October 2022).
40. NHS England. National Health Literacy Toolkit. Available online: https://www.england.nhs.uk/personalisedcare/health-literacy/ (accessed on 10 October 2022).
41. Macmillan Cancer Support. Available online: https://www.macmillan.org.uk/cancer-information-and-support/head-and-neck-cancer/signs-and-symptoms-of-oropharyngeal-cancer (accessed on 29 September 2022).
42. Neal, R.D.; Din, N.U.; Hamilton, W.; Ukoumunne, O.C.; Carter, B.; Stapley, S.; Rubin, G. Comparison of cancer diagnostic intervals before and after implementation of NICE guidelines: Analysis of data from the UK General Practice Research Database. *Br. J. Cancer* **2014**, *110*, 584–592. [CrossRef]
43. Doximity Network OP-ED. Oral Cavity Cancer: Time to Re-Think Stereotypes. Available online: https://opmed.doximity.com/articles/oral-cavity-cancer-time-to-re-think-stereotypes (accessed on 20 October 2022).
44. Jensen, H.; Torring, M.L.; Olesen, F.; Overgaard, J.; Vedsted, P. Cancer suspicion in general practice, urgent referral and time to diagnosis: A population-based GP survey and registry study. *BMC Cancer* **2014**, *14*, 636. [CrossRef]
45. UK Government. Available online: https://www.gov.uk/government/publications/inequalities-in-oral-health-in-england/inequalities-in-oral-health-in-england-summary (accessed on 17 October 2022).
46. Marshman, Z.; Nower, K.; Wright, D. *Oral Health and Access to Dental Services from People from Black and Minority Ethnic Groups. A Race Equality Foundation Briefing Paper*; Better Health Briefing 29; Race Equality Foundation: London, UK, 2013.
47. Local Government Association. Available online: http://pas.gov.uk/about/news/nhs-dental-deserts-persist-rural-and-deprived-communities-lga-analysis#:~{}:text=Analysis%20of%20data%2C%20collected%20by%20the%20Care%20Quality,proportion%20of%20residents%20in%20rural%20areas.%20More%20items (accessed on 20 October 2022).
48. Hill, K.B.; Chadwick, B.; Freeman, R.; O'Sullivan, I.; Murray, J.J. Adult Dental Health Survey 2009: Relationships between dental attendance patterns, oral health behaviour and the current barriers to dental care. *Br. Dent. J.* **2013**, *214*, 25–32. [CrossRef] [PubMed]
49. Al-Haboubi, M.; Klass, C.; Jones, K.; Bernabé, E.; Gallagher, J.E. Inequalities in the use of dental services among adults in inner South East London. *Eur. J Oral Sci.* **2013**, *121 Pt 1*, 176–181. [CrossRef]
50. Schneeweiss, S.; Maclure, M. Use of comorbidity scores for control of confounding in studies using administrative databases. *Int. J. Epidemiol.* **2000**, *29*, 891–898. [CrossRef] [PubMed]
51. Lai, A.G.; Pasea, L.; Banerjee, A.; Hall, G.; Denaxas, S.; Chang, W.H.; Katsoulis, M.; Williams, B.; Pillay, D.; Noursadeghi, M.; et al. Estimated impact of the COVID-19 pandemic on cancer services and excess 1-year mortality in people with cancer and multimorbidity: Near real-time data on cancer care, cancer deaths and a population-based cohort study. *BMJ Open* **2020**, *10*, e043828. [CrossRef] [PubMed]
52. Maringe, C.; Spicer, J.; Morris, M.; Purushotham, A.; Nolte, E.; Sullivan, R.; Rachet, B.; Aggarwal, A. The impact of the COVID-19 pandemic on cancer deaths due to delays in diagnosis in England, UK: A national, population-based, modelling study. *Lancet Oncol.* **2020**, *21*, 1023–1034. [CrossRef] [PubMed]

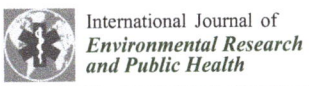

International Journal of
Environmental Research and Public Health

Article

A Qualitative Evaluation of a *Health Access Card* for Refugees and Asylum Seekers in a City in Northern England

Malcolm Moffat [1,*], Suzanne Nicholson [2], Joanne Darke [3], Melissa Brown [1], Stephen Minto [4], Sarah Sowden [1] and Judith Rankin [1]

1 Population Health Sciences Institute, Newcastle University, Newcastle upon Tyne NE2 4AX, UK
2 Newcastle City Council, Public Health Team, Civic Centre, Newcastle upon Tyne NE1 8QH, UK
3 UK Health Security Agency North East, Health Protection Team, Civic Centre, Newcastle upon Tyne NE1 8QH, UK
4 Northumbria Healthcare NHS Foundation Trust, One-to-One Centre Shiremoor, Brenkley Avenue, Shiremoor, Newcastle upon Tyne NE27 0PR, UK
* Correspondence: malcolm.moffat@newcastle.ac.uk

Citation: Moffat, M.; Nicholson, S.; Darke, J.; Brown, M.; Minto, S.; Sowden, S.; Rankin, J. A Qualitative Evaluation of a *Health Access Card* for Refugees and Asylum Seekers in a City in Northern England. *Int. J. Environ. Res. Public Health* **2023**, *20*, 1429. https://doi.org/10.3390/ijerph20021429

Academic Editor: Paul B. Tchounwou

Received: 28 October 2022
Revised: 3 January 2023
Accepted: 10 January 2023
Published: 12 January 2023

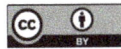

Copyright: © 2023 by the authors. Licensee MDPI, Basel, Switzerland. This article is an open access article distributed under the terms and conditions of the Creative Commons Attribution (CC BY) license (https://creativecommons.org/licenses/by/4.0/).

Abstract: Refugees and asylum seekers residing in the UK face multiple barriers to accessing healthcare. A *Health Access Card* information resource was launched in Newcastle upon Tyne in 2019 by Newcastle City Council, intended to guide refugees and asylum seekers living in the city, and the professional organisations that support them, to appropriate healthcare services provided locally. The aim of this qualitative evaluation was to explore service user and professional experiences of healthcare access and utilisation in Newcastle and perspectives on the *Health Access Card*. Eleven semi-structured interviews took place between February 2020 and March 2021. Participants provided diverse and compelling accounts of healthcare experiences and described cultural, financial and institutional barriers to care. Opportunities to improve healthcare access for these population groups included offering more bespoke support, additional language support, delivering training and education to healthcare professionals and reviewing the local support landscape to maximise the impact of collaboration and cross-sector working. Opportunities to improve the *Health Access Card* were also described, and these included providing translated versions and exploring the possibility of developing an accompanying digital resource.

Keywords: refugee; asylum seeker; health access; health information; intervention

1. Introduction

In 2021, more than 89,000,000 people worldwide were forcibly dispersed from their homes as a result of persecution, conflict, violence, human rights violations or events seriously disturbing public order [1]. This included more than 27,000,000 refugees (people who have fled war, violence, conflict or persecution and have crossed an international border to find safety in another country) and more than 4,000,000 asylum seekers (a refugee whose request for sanctuary has yet to be processed) [2,3]. A total of 56,495 people applied for asylum in the UK in 2021, and of the 14,572 applications that were processed 4083 (28%) were refused [4]. A refused asylum seeker refers to a person whose asylum claim has not been granted following initial review. By the end of 2021, 100,564 asylum seekers in the UK were still awaiting an initial decision on their asylum application [4]. Mass migration on this scale has the potential to significantly impact on healthcare provision in host countries. Research suggests that displaced migrants face multiple barriers, both structural and political, to accessing healthcare in their host countries, potentially leading to unmet need and poor-quality care [5]. Although the 1951 Convention relating to the Status of Refugees and its 1967 Protocol does not explicitly define refugees' right to healthcare, there is a more modern appreciation that access to healthcare should be regarded as a fundamental right for people seeking asylum, as is reflected in the International Organization for Migration's

2019 Migration Governance Indicators and in the United Nation's Sustainable Development Goals [6–8]. Indeed, the UN Global Compact on Refugees states that "in line with national health care laws, policies and plans, and in support of host countries, States and relevant stakeholders will contribute resources and expertise to expand and enhance the quality of national health systems to facilitate access by refugees and host communities" [9].

In the UK, the National Health Service (NHS) is a comprehensive healthcare system providing care that is free at the point of access to all UK residents. Asylum seekers awaiting review and people who have been granted refugee status in the UK are entitled to free access to all elements of NHS care. Although some restrictions are placed on the NHS care that refused asylum seekers are entitled to use, access to primary care, Accident and Emergency and 111 services (telephone triage and advice) is free and universal. People who have been refused asylum may also use services providing treatment for specific infectious diseases, sexually transmitted diseases and treatment for conditions caused by torture, female genital mutilation and/or domestic/sexual violence. Access to health visitors, school nursing and family planning services should also be freely available to this population, as should end of life care services [10].

Despite these entitlements, it is known that refugees, asylum seekers and those whose asylum application has been refused are often inappropriately denied free UK NHS care, while some individuals may not seek it due to a lack of awareness [11]. Dominant themes that emerge from qualitative studies describing barriers to care among these populations include language barriers and inadequate access to interpreter services; limited understanding of the structure and function of the NHS; difficulty meeting the costs of dental care, prescription fees, and transport to appointments; an absence of timely and culturally sensitive mental health services, properly equipped to deal with the esoteric needs of these populations; and perceived feelings of discrimination relating to ethnicity, religion and immigration status alongside concerning professional attitudes [12–14]. This tension, between the expectation that people seeking asylum in the UK should have access to comprehensive healthcare and the reality of the often inadequate and incomplete care that many of them actually receive, has been at the heart of efforts to improve healthcare access in these populations. However, although barriers to care are well-documented, research examining the impact of interventions intended to address and overcome them is limited: a 2021 study explored qualitative perspectives on a pre-departure medical health assessment (MHA) for refugees accepted for resettlement prior to arrival in the UK, and the Doctors of the World Safe Surgeries initiative has championed improved access to primary care services for socially excluded groups including refugees and asylum seekers [15,16]. A systematic review published in 2021 explored primary care interventions delivered primarily in North American settings and found a lack of evaluations of community-focused approaches that might be expected to be particularly beneficial in these communities [17]. Evaluations of health information resources for these populations are seldom reported. With potentially more discriminatory changes to refugee and asylum seeker policy in the post-Brexit era, and with the passing of the Nationality and Borders Bill in 2022 that effectively criminalises asylum seekers who arrive in the UK via unregistered routes, an understanding of the challenges faced by these populations in accessing healthcare and of the opportunities offered by approaches that look to address some of these barriers is more important than ever.

In response to reports that new entrants to the North East of England (including refugees and asylum seekers) were struggling to navigate the local healthcare system, Newcastle City Council's (NCC) Public Health team, in collaboration with the Health and Race and Equality Forum (HAREF), Newcastle Council for Voluntary Services (NCVS) and the Regional Refugee Forum, developed and launched a *Health Access Card* for refugees and asylum seekers in 2019. Professional representatives from these and other organisations as well as refugees and asylum seekers living in Newcastle co-produced the resource, and 5000 copies of a folded, pocket-sized card were distributed to a number of key providers in healthcare and third sector organisations. The cards were made available in facilities commonly accessed by members of these communities (such as GP practice waiting areas and community centres), and cards were also shared with professional staff in a number of organisations to be given out in person. It was intended that the card would be used by refugees and asylum seekers themselves, and also by professionals as an adjunct to conversations concerning healthcare access. An online pdf of the card is available to view at https://cdn.cityofsanctuary.org/uploads/sites/35/2019/05/Newcastle-Health-Access-Card-2.pdf, (accessed on 4 October 2019).

The aim of this qualitative evaluation was to explore perspectives on the impact and usefulness of the *Health Access Card* through semi-structured interviews with service users and professionals based in Newcastle, and to propose improvements and changes that could be considered for future iterations of the card. A secondary objective was to use these conversations as an opportunity to explore service user and professional perspectives on refugee and asylum seeker healthcare access and on barriers to care in Newcastle more generally.

2. Methods

Service users with refugee or asylum/failed asylum status and professional staff who work with these groups in Newcastle upon Tyne were invited to take part in a 30–40 min semi-structured interview with a researcher from Newcastle University. There were no exclusion criteria for participation if these basic eligibility criteria were met. Previous familiarity with the *Health Access Card* was not a prerequisite to participation. Participants were recruited through partner organisations including HAREF, the Action Foundation, Refugee Voices and NCC. Researchers had intended to recruit service user participants in person, by attending community group sessions and approaching potential participants with information about the study: this approach was not feasible following the implementation of COVID-19 lockdowns in March 2020, and potential service user participants were approached instead by staff in partner organisations. Although it was originally intended that professional participants would take part in focus group discussions, semi-structured interviews were undertaken instead in view of in-person group meetings being prohibited. Participants were provided with a study information leaflet to read prior to undertaking the interview and were asked to sign a consent form to confirm their participation. The information leaflet was only available in English, but interpreters were offered in circumstances where a potential participant who did not speak English expressed an interest in taking part in the study. Ultimately, interpreting services were not used—interviews with service users were conducted in English with their agreement. Two topic guides were prepared (for interviews with service user and professional participants), exploring participant perspectives on how the *Health Access Card* had been used, on the design and content of the card, and on how the card might be improved. Participants were also asked to describe their or their clients'/patients'/friends' experiences of healthcare in Newcastle, and to consider barriers to good care and opportunities to improve the healthcare offer for refugees and asylum seekers living in the city. Topic guides are included in the Supplementary Materials.

The first two interviews were conducted face to face; subsequent interviews took place online on the Microsoft Teams platform or by phone in view of COVID-19 lockdown restrictions. All interviews were conducted by MM; interviews were audio-recorded with participant consent and anonymised transcripts were produced by MM, MB and SM. Interview data were coded by MM using NVivo 12 software, and a thematic analysis of emergent themes was carried out. Thematic analysis is a flexible and intuitive method of qualitative analysis that involves examining multiple data outputs for recurring patterns and motifs that can be organised into themes [18]. Codes and emerging themes and subthemes from a sample of transcripts were also discussed by the research steering group (involving all authors). Illustrative quotations are provided, and we assign a P (professional) and SU (Service User) number for each quotation.

Ethical approval for the study was granted by Newcastle University Faculty of Medical Sciences (ref: 1847/18699/2019).

3. Results

Eleven participants took part in this qualitative evaluation between February 2020 and March 2021. Participant characteristics are described in Table 1.

Table 1. Participant characteristics.

Study ID	Role	Age	Gender	Ethnicity
P (professional) 1	Third sector support worker	-	Female	White British
P2	Third sector support worker	-	Female	White British
P3	Third sector support worker	-	Female	White British
P4	Local authority support worker	-	Female	White British
P5	GP	-	Male	White British
P6	Third sector support officer	-	Male	White British
P7	Third sector organisation trustee	-	Female	Middle Eastern
P8	Local authority support worker	-	Female	White British
SU (service user) 1	Service user (refugee status)	Late 20s	Male	Pakistani
SU2	Service user (refugee status)	Mid 30s	Female	Eastern European
SU3	Service user (refugee status)	Late teens	Female	Indian

Three themes and associated subthemes emerged from the participant interview data (see Figure 1).

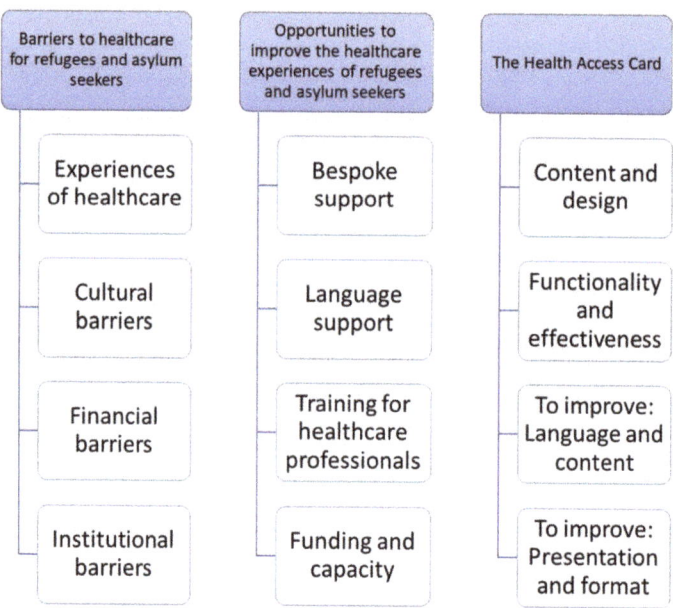

Figure 1. Themes and subthemes from interviews with service users and professionals around the Health Access Card.

4. Barriers to Healthcare for Refugees and Asylum Seekers

4.1. Experiences of Healthcare

Where participants described positive experiences of using healthcare services in Newcastle, either their own experiences or those of friends, relatives or clients, these often related to interactions with individual clinical staff who had delivered tailored and compassionate care. GPs in particular were commended for some of their work with asylum seekers and refugees, and one professional participant highlighted the role that health visitors and midwives had played in arranging comprehensive care for their patients/clients. Referral to appropriate mental health support was mentioned as an example of good care:

> "We've had a few clients who have moved from the East end of the city over to the West end, and they won't change their GP because the GP they've got is great, they love their GP and they're wonderful and they don't want to change, so, and that GP has been quite happy to still have that person registered with them … " (P1)

> "Health visitors and midwives are absolutely fantastic with this client group, yeah they really go above and beyond to try to help them as much as they can, so yeah I would say that's been really good, and I've done lots of joint working with midwives and health visitors … " (P7)

Participants also described the important work done by third sector organisations in supporting refugees and asylum seekers to understand their healthcare rights, to access appropriate services, and to have recourse to non-NHS lifestyle and wellbeing support:

> "The [support organisation], that's for LBGT support for refugees and asylum seekers, I think, yeah it is it's on the bottom of the card, I suppose it's not physical health but more mental health support but they've been really good to work with, both for the [clients] and we've found them really helpful as well … " (P3)

However, largely positive experiences of healthcare for refugees and asylum seekers were not necessarily replicated in different settings or for friends/family/clients, representing inconsistent care for this population group. One service user also described frustrations when initially trying to navigate the NHS system due to unfamiliarity with UK healthcare, but these frustrations were allayed when they became more aware of NHS practices:

> "At the start I was confused, but once I got used to the system it seems alright … first time when I went to the emergency for example … I used to wait really long time [and would think] oh my goodness what's that, but then I realised how the system works, how the patients are looked after … but yeah, it was alright … " (SU2)

All participants described direct or indirect awareness of refugees and asylum seekers in Newcastle having poor healthcare experiences and/or struggling to access the healthcare services and support that they needed. Several participants described negative experiences of accessing or utilising healthcare services that were related to language challenges. In particular, access to interpreters and translated literature was inconsistent and frequently inadequate, and these problems were exacerbated during the COVID-19 pandemic:

> "[The client] tried to ring up to get another prescription for, I think it was sleeping pills to help her because she struggles with anxiety and they said they can't, they can't have a meeting with her, the GP can't see her because they're not doing face to face [due to COVID-19 restrictions] and they don't have someone to be an interpreter so she'll just have to wait until after this." (P3)

Negative experiences of mental health management, and of accessing appropriate mental health support, were commonly reported, and these, again, were likely exacerbated by the pandemic:

> "I've got this client whose daughter is having quite severe psychotic episodes, she was admitted to hospital, she was, I don't know if it's like a young person's mental health team or something, she was under their care for a few weeks, and now nothing's happened, they haven't kind of followed up with anything, and she's had another quite serious episode in school where she was quite dangerous to other people, and I think she's just been, well I think they feel like she's been left … " (P7)

Several participants described how they or their clients/patients were treated differently by healthcare services, often in terms of presenting complaints not being appropriately investigated/explored or of being expected to wait longer for review/access to services because of their asylum seeker/refugee status:

"They feel like that because they don't understand, so they think because they are aliens [healthcare professionals] are reacting to them like that ... "they don't help us because we are foreigners"" (SU1)

Experiences of problems in accessing appropriate and timely dental care were also widely reported:

"It's always been dental care that they've had most problems with, so a lot of the dentists that they go to register with tell them that they've got to pay, even if they've got an HC2, I think for some of the dental practices maybe there's a misunderstanding with some of them ... " (P1)

Poor experiences relating to the restrictions placed on free access to healthcare services for refugees and asylum seekers were also described:

"That lady I mentioned before who had the miscarriage, she was destitute at the time that happened and she got charged for the work they did when she had to be taken in for the miscarriage, and the letters are quite brutal in that they say that if you don't pay this within three months we will inform the Home Office and it will affect your claim, so people really panic and she found that really upsetting, having just gone through what she went through, and I went through Doctors of the World and they said yes the charges would stand currently." (P1)

4.2. Cultural Barriers

All participants described inadequate language support as a significant barrier to care. Often, this related to difficulties in accessing services due to problems arranging appointments or understanding what services were available; in other circumstances it related to interpreters not being offered or provided, or the standard of interpreter being inconsistent or inadequate; and sometimes it related to service users being sent or provided with literature/information about their care in a language that they were unable to understand:

"We've had one learner who's sent me pictures of a letter from a consultant at a hospital to his GP, which he's been copied into, and it's all in English, he doesn't speak any English, so he hasn't received any kind of translated version of it, and it's talking, I mean I know those letters do talk in third person, I saw so-and-so, but it's really important the stuff that it's talking about, and describing that there was a communication barrier and that she's booked him in for a MRI scan anyway but she doesn't know how much he understands ... " (P3)

Cultural variation in the way in which service users understood and interpreted health and illness was also reported as a barrier to accessing care in a UK context. This was considered particularly important in the context of service users' often-extensive mental health needs:

"I'm the only one who's accessed those services [counselling], because my family doesn't believe in mental health that much, like now they do but back then they didn't ... " (SU3)

"A lot of people come from cultures where mental health wouldn't be something that was even recognised as an issue, so being able to describe that in the first place [is a barrier] ... " (P4)

For a number of participants, limited understanding of and familiarity with the UK healthcare system and its practices and procedures in terms of referrals, waiting times, etc., was seen as a barrier to refugees and asylum seekers accessing healthcare services. Where service users were perceived to access services inappropriately as a result of this, there was a feeling that this fuelled stigmatising and divisive rhetoric directed at these communities:

> "Another barrier is the assumption that people leaving their home and living here are used to the system, they assume that it's the same everywhere but it isn't, they'd be really frustrated if they went to my country for example and tried to access, which is not stressful for me as I understand it . . . " (SU2)

4.3. Financial Barriers

Financial barriers to healthcare experienced by refugees and asylum seekers in Newcastle were commonly described. In some cases, this related to access to specific services for which failed asylum seekers would not be eligible for free care; in other cases, it related to the costs associated with, for example, travelling to an appointment, or, during COVID-19 lockdowns, paying for a supermarket delivery to reduce the likelihood of exposure to the virus in a public space:

> "A lot of [clients] are saying "oh well we walked for two hours to get here, if we'd paid for the bus we wouldn't have enough food for the day" so I think in terms of weighing up often it would be prioritising is it important enough to go to the doctors, more important than buying food for the week . . . " (P3)

4.4. Institutional Barriers

Participants described institutional barriers to care that were rooted in NHS structures and in healthcare professionals' attitudes and behaviours. These barriers arose not only in relation to healthcare professionals' limited awareness of the healthcare rights and entitlements of these population groups, but also in relation to the professional understanding of the particular healthcare backgrounds of refugees and asylum seekers, many of whom have considerable mental and physical health needs arising from histories of trauma and/or torture:

> "I've worked with lots of people over the years who've kind of been in and out of various medical appointments talking about physical symptoms when actually it's turned out, you know talking about headaches talking about stomach aches talking about different things, and again some if that is their way of describing it with the language and the cultural barriers, and some of that is I think the practitioners' awareness of the particular needs of this population and that actually, you know, lots of people have experienced trauma and persecution and different things and actually for you to be aware of that, if people are coming in with headaches or different things, just explore some of that stuff . . . " (P4)

5. Opportunities to Improve the Healthcare Experiences of Refugees and Asylum Seekers

5.1. Bespoke Support

Several participants proposed offering more individualised and bespoke healthcare support to refugees and asylum seekers in Newcastle, particularly upon arrival in the city as they begin to navigate the local health and care system for the first time. Offering this population the opportunity to visit healthcare premises under the supervision of a supportive and knowledgeable guide (from the client's accommodation provider or from a third sector/local authority organisation) was particularly well-supported:

> "Actually the most useful part was when a visitor came to my home and he actually took me and my husband to the places and he was speaking English but he tried to show how the places looked like, I didn't understand everything he said but it gave me the idea how to get used to the system, so he actually took us to the places and, yeah, tried really hard to explain . . . " (SU2)

Additional, targeted mental health support was identified as a particular priority:

> "I think like there's more work to be done around people's mental health, really. Like a lot more work. It's such a huge area for our clients and for a lot of people, it's a really difficult thing to manage and to deal with and talk about." (P2)

5.2. Language Support

Developing services that embed appropriate language support in every part of the healthcare pathway was identified as an opportunity to improve the healthcare experiences of these populations:

> "it's [the client's] right to be able to understand that information, so just having translated documents, and then people who understand the barriers that people might be experiencing when they're trying to access a service, would be really useful . . . " (P3)

5.3. Training for Healthcare Professionals

Supporting healthcare staff to be more aware of the healthcare needs and personal circumstances of refugees and asylum seekers was identified as a priority opportunity by a number of participants. Good experiences of care almost always involved compassionate and understanding professionals, recognising and addressing the sometimes-unique needs of these population groups. Facilitating a better understanding of refugee and asylum seeker healthcare entitlement, among healthcare administrators as well as clinicians, was seen as an opportunity to improve care pathways, and potentially to encourage more empathy towards service users who have arrived in the UK in challenging circumstances. There was also a feeling that unconscious biases among healthcare staff should be challenged:

> "I think it's always a training issue. The more the surgery buys into training staff appropriately, the more awareness of someone's situation and know what to pick up on, the work that these surgeries have been doing is great, because you know there's a commitment there isn't there and their staff are going to have that level of training and you know they're kind of signed up to being welcoming to people and so, the more of that stuff that gets done the better, really." (P2)

5.4. Funding and Capacity

Several participants discussed the context in which healthcare access work with refugees and asylum seekers in Newcastle was currently funded and delivered and praised the role of the third sector in trying to support these populations' needs in a difficult economic climate. Trying to integrate and co-ordinate some of this work across the city's various networks was proposed as a local albeit imperfect response to ongoing challenges, in the absence of more comprehensive support from central government:

> "Because of various factors in Newcastle including years of you know austerity and funding cuts that have meant that lots of services that were previously there for asylum seekers and refugees are kind of contracted because of that, they [the voluntary sector] have been picking up asylum seekers much earlier in their journey so they've been picking up people who are just arriving in Newcastle, they've been picking up people who have been here and they haven't had their decisions yet and actually they've got lots of work around integration at those earliest levels around school access and health access and different things . . . " (P4)

6. The *Health Access Card*

6.1. Content and Design

Several participants commented favourably on the content of the information provided on the *Health Access Card*, mentioning in particular the useful information on the range of services available in an emergency situation and on how to access other services such as dentists and opticians:

"Having that information on there that we can like point to, and make sure that people are informed and know how to use the kind of UK system of healthcare is really useful as well . . . " (P3)

"I think the information about the services is crucial, what service is provided at what time, and how, is important . . . " (SU3)

However, one professional participant observed that the section on maternity care was potentially misleading, and should be revised and expanded:

"I think what I'd like to see in there is something about midwives and health visitors as well, because clients don't always realise that when you're pregnant it's a midwife you would see most rather than your GP, so I think that section could be improved . . . " (P1)

The bright colours and effective use of images on the card was welcomed by participants:

"It gives, like, images in its own self telling people that this is the thing you need to read if you're looking for an optician or a dentist because there's a picture of the glasses or a tooth, or the mother with the baby for pregnancy . . . so I think it's easier in a graphical way . . . " (SU3)

However, participants also felt that a lot of text on a small card might be off-putting to some people, and that the size of the card might result in it being missed or dismissed:

"There is a lot of information on there now, obviously it's quite dense, there is a lot of writing on there, so anybody, even if they do speak reasonably good English anybody where English isn't a first language, it's probably going to be quite daunting." (P5)

"It doesn't really look like something important, so . . . when you make something small, it doesn't look big, the best way to say it . . . they don't make [you] take it serious[ly] . . . " (SU1)

6.2. Functionality and Distribution

Participants commented favourably on the functionality of the card, with professionals reflecting on the usefulness of the resource as a signposting tool when having discussions about healthcare with clients and service users describing the card as compact and user-friendly. For several participants, if a client or friend expressed a particular healthcare need, the *Health Access Card* was a useful physical adjunct to verbal descriptions of what was available:

"Clients in [name of charity], yes, some of them ask us how can I access this kind of healthcare, so I just gave it to them and, you know, point them to try this . . . " (SU1)

However, for some professional participants, the fact that the card was only available in English was a barrier to them and their clients/patients using it more widely, and for one service user participant, the card was a poor substitute for the more bespoke and personalised support that a support worker might give.

Professional participants also described challenges in making the resource available to its target population—if they showed a service user the card, it would often be the first time they had seen it, and there was a feeling, among professionals and service users, that the card should be made available immediately upon arrival in Newcastle to maximise its usefulness. Professional participants rarely used the card in their own practice.

"Frankly, when I came into the country, I wanted something like this, the only thing was there was nothing at that time . . . now I know these places where I have to go." (SU3)

"Most of the time when I've used it it's been the first time that someone has seen it, I've never given it out and someone's already had one or known about it." (P3)

6.3. To Improve: Language and Content

Participants recommended making the card available in other languages. Some participants also suggested that, if translated versions were not feasible, including a sentence or two in the most commonly used languages in this population that directed service users to translation and interpreting services would be beneficial:

> "Another thing is, yeah, the best option would be if it is translated into as many languages as possible … " (SU2)

One service user also cautioned against using abbreviations and acronyms that might not be familiar to people new to the UK/NHS:

> "I don't know what a GP is for example, I would add an explanation of this abbreviation … it's still complicated, it's still really hard for me, everywhere abbreviations are used and it assumes that you know about it … " (SU2)

Participants also emphasised the importance of including information on the card that was directly relevant to the experiences of refugees and asylum seekers, in particular with regards to bespoke services (including services that promoted physical and mental wellbeing as well as healthcare services) and to accessing interpreters if and when required:

> "Maybe if there were specific projects that were aimed at refugees they might be more accessible than just the general link to the website." (P3)

> "Something about certain organisations that are working with people from a similar [refugee and asylum] background … so that they can tell them about the Health Access Card more properly, so that they can take them to the GP services because I know they have, like, health care champions … " (SU3)

Participants were also keen for the card to provide some additional guidance on the nature and structure of the UK healthcare system:

> "In our countries doctors do not work like this so we just go to doctor and you can meet them right away, it's like a drop-in, you just go there and it's not ten minutes, so you can share whatever the problem is for as long as you want, but there are some different systems and they are expecting that to happen here but I've seen a lot of people, you know, complaining about how doctors are working." (SU1)

6.4. To Improve: Presentation and Format

Including more pictures on the card, to aid comprehension among service users with limited understanding of English, was suggested by several participants:

> "I think we need to make more use of images in explaining something, because images, you know, they're international, and there's a lot more graphic designers out there who can do, who can explain something graphically with a picture that people get the concept of … " (P1)

> "I would like a bit more pictures, something more visual, rather than lots of writing I would add a bit more of this kind of pictures … maybe I would add a bit, for example a tiny map, for example there is not many A&E department in Newcastle … " (SU2)

Several participants proposed making the card available online as a digital resource, which would make it easier to provide translated versions and could include expanded content and links to other online resources:

> "Maybe consider having an expanded version of the cards available online, so you could have less text on the actual card. You could say, actually you can find more information on this website … " (P5)

However, although it was suggested that the hardware required to access online resources was often available in these communities, reliable and consistent Wi-Fi access/data provision could be challenging:

> "The majority of patients, do have [internet] access, but you, of course, there are patients that don't either have devices or don't have data or Wi-Fi, so whenever you are providing service online you do have make sure that is also available in other formats as well." (P5)

7. Discussion

Participants in this study described diverse accounts of the healthcare experiences of refugees and asylum seekers in Newcastle. Good experiences tended to occur on account of healthcare and other support professionals providing compassionate, personalised care, but these experiences were not consistent. Negative experiences often related to challenges in accessing care in a language that service users were able to understand, difficulties navigating an unfamiliar healthcare system, and frustrations around the availability of dental care in particular. Related to these experiences, barriers to healthcare among these populations included inadequate language support, cultural unfamiliarity with NHS structures and processes, financial barriers (including the costs of travel to healthcare premises as well as the costs of accessing health and wellbeing services themselves), and inconsistent and often-poor understanding of refugee and asylum seeker healthcare needs and entitlements among healthcare professionals. Opportunities to address some of these barriers included offering more bespoke healthcare support to refugees and asylum seekers (particularly to new arrivals to the city), embedding language support at every stage of NHS care pathways, enabling healthcare professionals to better-understand refugee and asylum seeker care needs through additional training, and working with the range of excellent third sector organisations in Newcastle to co-ordinate the important services that they provide.

The Newcastle *Health Access Card* was found to be an effective and user-friendly resource for refugees and asylum seekers in the Newcastle upon Tyne that presents helpful content in a well-designed format. The information describing emergency/urgent care services and dental provision was especially welcome, and study participants appreciated the engaging use of bright colours and graphics. Professional participants described the card as a useful *aide memoire* during conversations about healthcare with service users. However, there was a sense that the information on the card describing services that are targeted at the refugee and asylum seeker population could be expanded, and that not making the card available in non-English translations was a barrier to it being utilised more widely. It was also suggested that the density of text on the card might be off-putting to service users with limited English language skills, and that the card had not necessarily reached the service users who might benefit most from having sight of it. Recommendations for policy and practice for future versions of the *Health Access Card* include for it to be made available in other languages and to avoid abbreviations/acronyms where possible; to consider reducing the volume of text and replacing some of this with additional pictures and graphics; to expand the content describing third sector support available to these population groups; and to explore the possibility of launching a more interactive, digital resource as an alternative to the paper version.

These findings should represent a call to action for those responsible for healthcare policy and practice in the Newcastle upon Tyne to tackle the barriers to healthcare experienced by refugees and asylum seekers and to spearhead the development of inclusive, culturally sensitive and responsive services in light of the professional and service user experiences described above, but they come at a time of political turmoil and economic uncertainty. Although the war in Ukraine and the resurgence of the Taliban in Afghanistan has inspired a compassionate and generous response to refugees and asylum seekers among many parts of the UK public, media portrayals of these populations remain provocative, and it is likely that public and overt efforts to improve access to healthcare services for these groups in particular, at a time of waiting list and workforce crises in the NHS, would be highly contentious [19].

In this challenging context, a population approach cognisant of the importance of the wider determinants of health is more important than ever. A 2019 study examining refugee integration in Newcastle highlighted the social barriers to integration in a post-austerity (and pre-COVID) context, and in many instances these barriers to integration also represent barriers to effective access to healthcare resources [20]. The mental health experiences of asylum seekers in Newcastle last appeared in the research literature seventeen years ago, and many of the barriers and experiences described in 2005 are repeated in this study [21].

The author of that paper also highlights the important role that social and economic circumstances play in determining (mental) health and wellbeing. An ethnopsychiatric approach to identifying and treating mental health presentations among migrant populations, that positions mental health in its appropriate cultural context, offers a more nuanced and patient-centred response to the significant burden of mental health need described in this paper, but delivering services of this nature places demands on providers that may, in the current UK healthcare climate, be unachievable [22].

The opportunity described in this study, to map and integrate the range of services currently provided by a range of local authority, NHS and third sector organisations, so as to better understand the comprehensiveness of current support and to deliver a more joined-up and consistent offer to refugees and asylum seekers, is persuasive in this context—as in other populations, people who are economically secure and socially connected are more likely to have better health and better healthcare access. Healthcare providers should facilitate and participate in these interdisciplinary conversations and should review how the support that they offer to these populations can be improved. This may include relatively minor changes such as ensuring that clinic letters describing management plans and test results are offered in translated versions, and upskilling patient-facing and administrative staff to be more aware of these patients' complex medical histories and healthcare entitlements. For those involved in developing health information resources for refugees and asylum seekers, this study demonstrates that there is an appetite for digital resources among these population groups, and previous research has identified a positive role for, for example, social media in supporting refugee youth to navigate and understand health systems in host countries [23]. The findings of the study also suggest that a resource that simply describes available services is potentially of less value than one that guides service users to third sector and other organisations that are able to provide more personalized and bespoke healthcare access support.

The period during which this study was undertaken, coinciding with the onset of the COVID-19 pandemic in February/March 2020 and with qualitative data collection continuing during UK lockdowns in the months that followed, served to shine a light on refugee healthcare access during crisis situations. The move away from face to face/in-person care exacerbated the barriers to healthcare already experienced by these populations, and in many instances removed meaningful access to support networks that previously would have looked to enable links to healthcare services. This had a harmful impact on service users' physical and, in particular, mental health, and services were slow to respond to a rapidly evolving situation. These findings are in keeping with the research evidence presented elsewhere [24]. However, the shift to online provision of some services also served to act as impetus to providers and support groups to improve their clients' digital access capabilities, and this, if sustained, offers healthcare organisations an opportunity to reconsider the means by which they engage with refugees and asylum seekers, and to look to overcome some of the barriers to care described above. The more specific experiences of refugees and asylum seekers in relation to health protection policies implemented to manage the pandemic response—including testing, quarantining and care and support for people required to isolate—were not explored in this study, but it is known that the accommodation given to vulnerable populations during the COVID-19 pandemic often fell short of providing a safe environment that was conducive to good population health management [25]. It is known anecdotally that similar challenges were faced by asylum seekers housed in temporary accommodation in Newcastle, and these experiences should be explored and documented and should inform the work of local authority and health protection practitioners in the event of future public health emergencies.

The strengths of this study include the range of professional partners involved in the research design and recruitment, the diverse sample of professional participants working in various important roles, the in-depth exploration of stories and experiences using semi-structured interviews, and the robust thematic analysis involving several members of the research team. The study has significant limitations—due to pandemic restrictions and the impact of these on recruitment, only three service participants were able to participate in semi-structured interviews, and those that did participate spoke good English and were well-established in Newcastle with settled refugee status, potentially unrepresentative of those with the most acute and urgent healthcare access needs. Several important voices, such as those of asylum seekers awaiting a Home Office decision and those of children, were not explored in this study. It is known, for example, that unaccompanied refugee minors are more likely to present with PTSD and other mental health conditions than children arriving in a host country with parents/other adult carers: the healthcare access experiences of this population are unlikely to be adequately represented in the findings of the current study [26]. Participants also had very limited experience of using the *Health Access Card* themselves or, in the case of professional participants, in their own practice, and while this is perhaps indicative of some of the challenges associated with the effective dissemination of the card, it makes any discussion of how the resource was used and the impact that it may have had impossible in the context of the current study.

8. Conclusions

This study sheds light on the impact of a simple but potentially wide-reaching health information resource for population groups that experience multiple complex barriers to healthcare, with important recommendations as to how the resource might be improved and expanded. It is the first study to consider the physical and mental healthcare needs of refugees and asylum seekers in Newcastle and the first to evaluate a bespoke healthcare access resource targeted at these groups, and the findings described herein are likely to be generalizable to over settings. It explores service user perspectives on barriers to healthcare alongside professional voices with extensive experience of the local and regional health and social care system, and the emerging themes complement the existing literature and offer an expanded exploration of cultural and language barriers in an urban UK context.

By virtue of the period during which interviews were conducted, the study was also able to consider refugee and asylum seeker healthcare experiences in the context of the COVID-19 pandemic. The healthcare access needs and experiences of refugees and asylum seekers newly arrived in the city who do not speak English are likely to be more extensive and complex, and future research should prioritise hearing these voices, as well as exploring the experiences of children and, in particular, unaccompanied minors. Researchers should also explore the healthcare access experiences of Ukrainian refugees, a group that was welcomed into Britain in large numbers as part of a national "Homes for Ukraine" scheme following Russia's invasion of Ukraine in 2022, but which we anecdotally know has faced similar healthcare access challenges to those described above.

Supplementary Materials: The following supporting information can be downloaded at: https://www.mdpi.com/article/10.3390/ijerph20021429/s1, Supplementary Materials: Service user and professional participant topic guides.

Author Contributions: Conceptualisation: M.M., S.N., J.D., M.B., S.M., S.S. and J.R.; Methodology: M.M., S.N., J.D., M.B., S.M., S.S. and J.R.; Formal Analysis, M.M.; Investigation: M.M.; Resources: M.M., S.N. and J.D.; Data Curation: M.M., M.B. and S.M.; Writing—Original Draft Preparation: M.M.; Writing—Review and Editing: M.M., S.N., J.D., M.B., S.M., S.S. and J.R.; Visualisation: M.M.; Supervision: S.S. and J.R.; Project Administration: M.M., S.N. and J.D. All authors have read and agreed to the published version of the manuscript.

Funding: This research received no external funding. J.R. and S.S. are part-funded by the National Institute of Health and Care Research (NIHR) Applied Research Collaboration (ARC) North-East and North Cumbria (NIHR200173). S.S. is supported by Health Education England (HEE) and the National Institute for Health Research (NIHR) through an Integrated Clinical Academic Lecturer Fellowship (Ref CA-CL-2018-04-ST2-010) and RCF funding, NHS North of England Care System Support (NECS).

Institutional Review Board Statement: The study was conducted according to the guidelines of the Declaration of Helsinki and approved by the Ethics Committee of Newcastle University Faculty of Medical Sciences (protocol code 1847/18699/2019; date of approval 14 February 2020).

Informed Consent Statement: Informed consent was obtained from all subjects involved in the study.

Data Availability Statement: The data presented in this study are available on request from the corresponding author. The data are not publicly available due to participant confidentiality.

Acknowledgments: The authors acknowledge the generous contribution of the research participants and of the organisations in Newcastle that supported with recruitment to this study.

Conflicts of Interest: The authors declare no conflict of interest.

References

1. UNHCR (United Nations High Commissioner for Refugees). Available online: www.unhcr.org/uk/figures-at-a-glance.html (accessed on 23 October 2022).
2. UNHCR. Available online: www.unhcr.org/refugees.html (accessed on 23 October 2022).
3. UNHCR. Available online: www.unhcr.org/asylum-seekers.html (accessed on 23 October 2022).
4. Home Office (UK Government). Available online: www.gov.uk/government/statistics/immigration-statistics-year-ending-december-2021/how-many-people-do-we-grant-asylum-or-protection-to#data-tables (accessed on 23 October 2022).
5. Luiking, M.L.; Heckemann, B.; Ali, P.; Dekker-van Doorn, C.; Ghosh, S.; Kydd, A.; Watson, R.; Patel, H. Migrants' Healthcare Experience: A Meta-Ethnography Review of the Literature. *J. Nurs. Scholarsh.* **2019**, *51*, 58–67. [CrossRef] [PubMed]
6. UNHCR. The 1951 Convention Relating to the Status of Refugees and its 1967 Protocol. Available online: https://www.unhcr.org/uk/about-us/background/4ec262df9/1951-convention-relating-status-refugees-its-1967-protocol.html (accessed on 2 December 2022).
7. IOM (International Organization for Migration). Migration Governance Indicators: A Global Perspective. 2019. Available online: https://publications.iom.int/books/migration-governance-indicators-global-perspective (accessed on 2 December 2022).
8. United Nations Foundation. Available online: https://unfoundation.org/what-we-do/issues/sustainable-development-goals/?gclid=Cj0KCQiA4aacBhCUARIsAI55maGlLKpdsKowwJEfZs0QO2FzDyPXi-QP-K2Rw-XfwGNb9he9wQO-jl8aAgynEALw_wcB (accessed on 2 December 2022).
9. UNHCR. Global Compact on Refugees. Available online: https://www.unhcr.org/5c658aed4 (accessed on 2 December 2022).
10. OHID (Office for Health Improvement and Disparities, UK Government). Available online: www.gov.uk/guidance/nhs-entitlements-migrant-health-guide (accessed on 23 October 2022).
11. Khanom, A.; Alanazy, W.; Couzens, L.; Evans, B.A.; Fagan, L.; Fogarty, R.; John, A.; Khan, T.; Kingston, M.R.; Moyo, S.; et al. Asylum seekers' and refugees' experiences of accessing health care: A qualitative study. *BJGP Open* **2021**, *5*. [CrossRef] [PubMed]
12. Kang, C.; Tomkow, L.; Farrington, R. Access to primary health care for asylum seekers and refugees: A qualitative study of service user experiences in the UK. *Br. J. Gen. Pract.* **2019**, *69*, e537–e545. [CrossRef] [PubMed]
13. Pollard, T.; Howard, N. Mental healthcare for asylum-seekers and refugees residing in the United Kingdom: A scoping review of policies, barriers, and enablers. *Int. J. Ment. Health Syst.* **2021**, *15*, 60. [CrossRef] [PubMed]
14. McKnight, P.; Goodwin, L.; Kenyon, S. A systematic review of asylum-seeking women's views and experiences of UK maternity care. *Midwifery* **2019**, *77*, 16–23. [CrossRef] [PubMed]
15. Dunn, T.J.; Browne, A.; Haworth, S.; Wurie, F.; Campos-Matos, I. Service Evaluation of the English Refugee Health Information System: Considerations and Recommendations for Effective Resettlement. *Int. J. Env. Res. Public Health* **2021**, *18*, 10331. [CrossRef] [PubMed]
16. Bates, E. Safe surgeries: How Doctors of the World are helping migrants access healthcare. *BMJ* **2019**, *364*, 188. [CrossRef] [PubMed]
17. PIqbal, M.; Walpola, R.; Harris-Roxas, B.; Li, J.; Mears, S.; Hall, J.; Harrison, R. Improving primary health care quality for refugees and asylum seekers: A systematic review of interventional approaches. *Health Expect* **2022**, *25*, 2065–2094. [CrossRef] [PubMed]
18. Kiger, M.E.; Varpio, L. Thematic analysis of qualitative data: AMEE Guide No. 131. *Med. Teach.* **2020**, *42*, 846–854. [CrossRef] [PubMed]
19. Cooper, G.; Blumell, L.; Bunce, M. Beyond the 'refugee crisis': How the UK news media represent asylum seekers across national boundaries. *Int. Comm. Gaz.* **2021**, *83*, 195–216. [CrossRef]
20. Flug, M.; Hussein, J. Integration in the Shadow of Austerity—Refugees in Newcastle upon Tyne. *Soc. Sci.* **2019**, *8*, 212. [CrossRef]
21. Crowley, P. The mental health needs of adult asylum seekers in Newcastle upon Tyne. *J. Public Ment. Health* **2005**, *4*, 17. [CrossRef]
22. Caroppo, E.; Muscelli, C.; Brogna, P.; Paci, M.; Camerino, C.; Bria, P. Relating with migrants: Ethnopsychiatry and psychotherapy. *Ann. Ist. Super. Sanita* **2009**, *45*, 331–340. [PubMed]
23. Pottie, K.; Ratnayake, A.; Ahmed, R.; Veronis, L.; Alghazali, I. How refugee youth use social media: What does this mean for improving their health and welfare? *J. Public Health Pol.* **2020**, *41*, 268–278. [CrossRef] [PubMed]

24. Fu, L.; Lindenmeyer, A.; Phillimore, J.; Lessard-Phillips, L. Vulnerable migrants' access to healthcare in the early stages of the COVID-19 pandemic in the UK. *Public Health* **2022**, *203*, 36–42. [CrossRef] [PubMed]
25. Guma, T.; Blake, Y.; Maclean, G.; Sharapov, K. *Safe Environment? Understanding the Housing of Asylum Seekers and Refugees during the COVID-19 Outbreak*; Final Report; Edinburgh Napier University: Edinburgh, UK, 2022.
26. Bamford, J.; Fletcher, M.; Leavey, G. Mental Health Outcomes of Unaccompanied Refugee Minors: A Rapid Review of Recent Research. *Curr. Psychiatry Rep.* **2021**, *23*, 46. [CrossRef] [PubMed]

Disclaimer/Publisher's Note: The statements, opinions and data contained in all publications are solely those of the individual author(s) and contributor(s) and not of MDPI and/or the editor(s). MDPI and/or the editor(s) disclaim responsibility for any injury to people or property resulting from any ideas, methods, instructions or products referred to in the content.

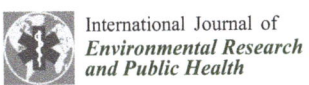

Protocol

Understanding the Lives of Aboriginal and Torres Strait Islander Women with Traumatic Brain Injury from Family Violence in Australia: A Qualitative Study Protocol

Michelle S. Fitts [1,2,3,*], Jennifer Cullen [4,5], Gail Kingston [6], Yasmin Johnson [1], Elaine Wills [1] and Karen Soldatic [1,7]

1. Institute for Culture and Society, Western Sydney University, Parramatta, NSW 2751, Australia
2. Menzies School of Health Research, Charles Darwin University, Alice Springs, NT 0871, Australia
3. Australian Institute of Tropical Health and Medicine, James Cook University, Cairns, QLD 4878, Australia
4. Synapse Australia, Brisbane, QLD 3356, Australia
5. College of Healthcare Sciences, James Cook University, Cairns, QLD 4878, Australia
6. Townsville Hospital and Health Service, Townsville, QLD 4814, Australia
7. School of Social Sciences, Western Sydney University, Parramatta, NSW 2751, Australia
* Correspondence: m.fitts@westernsydney.edu.au; Tel.: +61-8-8959-5387

Abstract: Globally, there is growing recognition of the connection between violence and head injuries. At present, little qualitative research exists around how surviving this experience impacts everyday life for women, particularly Aboriginal and Torres Strait Islander women. This project aims to explore the nature and context of these women's lives including living with the injury and to identify their needs and priorities during recovery. This 3-year exploratory project is being conducted across three Australian jurisdictions (Queensland, Northern Territory, and New South Wales). Qualitative interviews and discussion groups will be conducted with four key groups: Aboriginal and Torres Strait Islander women (aged 18+) who have acquired a head injury through family violence; their family members and/or carers; and hospital staff as well as government and non-government service providers who work with women who have experienced family violence. Nominated staff within community-based service providers will support the promotion of the project to women who have acquired a head injury through family violence. Hospital staff and service providers will be recruited using purposive and snowball sampling. Transcripts and fieldnotes will be analysed using narrative and descriptive phenomenological approaches. Reflection and research knowledge exchange and translation will be undertaken through service provider workshops.

Keywords: women; traumatic brain injury; violence; Australia; Aboriginal and Torres Strait Islander; care systems

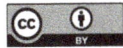

1. Introduction

Exposure to violence has serious health outcomes for women [1], with the elimination of violence against women and children a recognised national priority in Australia [2,3]. Due to the recurrent nature of family violence [4], women are vulnerable to sustaining injuries that impact upon the functioning of their brain. Traumatic brain injury (TBI) is defined as damage to, or alteration of, brain function due to a blow or force to the head [5]. A subset of acquired brain injury (ABI), the experience of TBI is unique and can consist of various short- and long-term cognitive impacts as well as psychological and physical consequences. These changes can include memory loss, difficulty with motivation, lack of insight, sensory and perceptual problems, posttraumatic epilepsy, fatigue and sleep difficulties, mood changes, and anxiety [6–9]. Even mild TBI is a risk factor for the development of early onset dementia and other chronic health conditions [10]. Although there has been growing recognition of the intersection between family violence and head injury both in Australia and worldwide [11,12], this has yet to translate into significant research action to listen to the voices of Aboriginal and Torres Strait Islander women who have acquired a head injury or been diagnosed with a TBI connected to family violence. The development of new knowledge is critical for informing robust, evidence-based family violence, disability and health policy, and practice.

Indigenous women in Australia and other settler nations such as Aotearoa New Zealand and the United States of America experience higher levels of violence than their non-Indigenous counterparts. Compared to other Australian women, Aboriginal and Torres Strait Islander women are more likely to be hospitalised due to violence and die due to injuries sustained from violence [13–15]. Concerningly, Aboriginal and Torres Strait Islander women in remote and very remote areas are more likely to be hospitalised for family violence than their urban counterparts (26.5 versus 2.8 per 1000) [13]. Violence against Aboriginal and Torres Strait Islander women is perpetuated by men of all cultural backgrounds including non-Indigenous men. In response to these high rates of violence, Aboriginal and Torres Strait Islander community leaders have led actions to prevent and address family violence [16,17]. Such trends are similarly reflected in assault-related head injury presentations [5,18]. One study found Aboriginal and Torres Strait Islander women are hospitalised with a head injury due to assault (1999–2005) 69 times the rate of other Australian women [5]. Factors such as alcohol are associated with TBI experienced by Indigenous peoples [19]. However, further research to understand the potential contribution of alcohol with TBI occurrence is warranted [20]. Incomplete and inaccurate data collection, together with the underreporting of violence by survivors of violence, also suggests that the published rates are, at best, an indication of the extent of violence experienced by women [21–23].

The terms domestic violence, family violence, and intimate partner violence are often used to describe violence against women. Although these terms are used interchangeably, the preferred term for Aboriginal and Torres Strait Islander communities tends to be family violence, as it encapsulates the extended nature of Aboriginal and Torres Strait Islander families and the kinship relationship within which a range of forms of violence occur [24]. For Aboriginal and Torres Strait Islander communities, family violence is a complex issue and must be seen in the context of wide-scale colonisation involving oppression, dispossession, massacres, the removal of children, and the loss of linguistic and cultural authority combined with the direct consequences of these policies on Aboriginal and Torres Strait Islander communities. Impacts include intergenerational trauma, economic and housing stress, unemployment as well as alcohol and other drug misuse [25–27].

Despite Aboriginal and Torres Strait Islander women experiencing high rates of head injury connected to family violence [5], research to document and examine their lived experiences remains scarce. Two reviews of TBI research with Indigenous populations identified a lack a studies investigating the lived experiences of Indigenous women in Aotearoa New Zealand, Australia, Canada, and the United States of America with head injury connected to violence [19,28]. Since then, two large scale Australian studies, 'The transition from hospital to home' (2016–2018; Queensland and Northern Territory) and 'Healing Right Way' (2017–2021; Western Australia), focused only on the transition period of Aboriginal and Torres Strait Islander peoples, which consists of hospital admission through to discharge and return to community and country [29–31]. Culturally responsive community rehabilitation models and resources were developed and implemented from these works [32,33]. Despite these promising advancements, the research area has narrowly focused on those patients who accessed hospital care alone. Thus, the models of rehabilitation developed are general in nature and may not recognise the unique issues that emerge when TBI is a direct outcome of family violence. Women who live with an acquired head injury as a result of family violence may not access health care, with fear shaping their daily lives and ability to seek help and access resources [34]. Other barriers to accessing health care include marginalisation, shame and stigma, and worries about confidentiality in tight-knit communities [31,35,36].

Study Aims

Although there are distinct bodies of literature examining family violence and TBI that demonstrate Aboriginal and Torres Strait Islander women experience high rates of both phenomena, the intersectionality of TBI and family violence has been overlooked [34]. Appropriate, effective, and equitable access to service providers that support and address the unmet needs and priorities of these women and their families has the potential to reduce the high incidence of head injury rates experienced by women and improve their health and well-being across their life course. With the increased recognition of both family violence and TBI in national initiatives [2], it is now critical to document and understand the beliefs, perceptions, and experiences of Aboriginal and Torres Strait Islander women with acquired head injury in the context of family violence. The aims of this project are to:

- Document the nature and context of the lives of Aboriginal and Torres Strait Islander women who are living with the consequences of a head injury caused through family violence.
- Map and compare populations of Aboriginal and Torres Strait Islander women living with a head injury and key issues for these populations across the three contrasting locations.
- Enrich the theoretical and applied understandings of the growing TBI population of Aboriginal and Torres Strait women and their experiences of change and reconstruction of self-identity after a head injury acquired through family violence.
- Develop outputs (such as resources) and a rigorous theoretical framework to inform government (national, state, local level) policies and programs.

2. Methods

2.1. Setting

This project will be undertaken at three sites in three Australian jurisdictions (Queensland, Northern Territory, and New South Wales). Family violence research demonstrates recognition of the heterogeneity in the experiences of survivors and service providers across regional and remote areas [37]. Therefore, the involvement of the three locations will help to better understand the effects of social and geographical isolation on the ability of women to disclose, report, and seek help about family violence. In addition, these sites were selected to understand the impact of different programs, policies, and geography for women who live with head injury and the services who support them. Together, this will allow for a comparative analysis and close examination of three different jurisdictions. The population of project location 1 is approximately 25,000, with an Aboriginal and Torres Strait population of 4361 (17.6%). The population of project location 2 is approximately 230,000 with 18,008 (7.9%) of residents identifying as Aboriginal and/or Torres Islander [38]. In project location 3, approximately 1.4% ($n = 13{,}426$) of the total population ($n = 936{,}433$) identify as Aboriginal and/or Torres Strait Islander.

2.2. Conceptual and Theoretical Innovation

This project will draw upon socially-embedded phenomenology to develop a richer and more sophisticated understanding of the way acquired head injury disrupts a person's embodied being in the world. Exploration of the social creation of impairment through inequality, deconstructing the cultural construction of impairment, and analysing the personal significance of impairment identities is required to build upon existing research knowledge [39]. While previous TBI studies have made important contributions to understanding disability through TBI, under the medical model, there is a strong focus on outcomes that are valued within a Western framework. Indeed, under the medical model, the emphasis is on 'fixing' the impairment, so that people can 'function' in society as active participants (such as returning to employment) [40]. A general assumption is made that illnesses and disabilities are universal and invariant to the cultural and social contexts in which they exist [41]. In turn, the research and guidance for workforces who support these women are limited, with the intersections of cultural identity potentially complicating what is already a complex issue. Within this project, an understanding of how different intersectionalities [42] such as gender, cultural belonging, and geographical location contribute to the women's experiences of services and systems after acquiring a head injury through family violence will be explored.

2.3. Research Governance

Aligning with the national research guidelines [43], the project will ensure Aboriginal and Torres Strait Islander peoples are involved in all aspects of the project. An advisory group consisting of members that represent a selection of service providers, community groups and hospitals participating in the project as well as representatives from national disability advocacy groups will meet twice a year (by teleconference). A critically reflective process will be completed at each site, entailing ongoing adjustments to the research process and incorporating iterative feedback into the research approach undertaken at each site [44,45]. This will enable the process to be locally guided to ensure that processes are responsive to local community requirements and local cultural protocols across the project, and simultaneously draw out comparative and contrasting aspects across each of the sites to inform a comprehensive interpretative analysis of the findings [46]. Individual advisors including Aboriginal and Torres Strait Islander women with lived experience of violence-related TBI will also help guide the project.

2.4. Definition of Traumatic Brain Injury

There is not one consistent definition used to define a TBI [47]. The inclusion criteria for the project are broad to include women with different severity levels of TBI. The project will define mild TBI (which can also be referred to as a head injury) as trauma to the head that is severe enough to cause neurological symptoms (including sensitivity to light, headache, and nausea). A moderate to severe TBI can be identified by one of the following: (1) loss of conscious for any duration, OR (2) post-traumatic amnesia > 24 h, OR (3) injury verified on a computerized tomography (CT) scan or magnetic resonance imaging (MRI). All major hospitals in the three project locations have CT and MRI facilities. The broad criteria also account for the suite of factors that can reduce accessibility to health care and specialist services following a TBI for women living in regional and remote communities [48,49].

2.5. Participants and Recruitment

The participants are outlined in Table 1. Aligning with the qualitative nature of the project, a non-probability sampling approach will be adopted, and no sample size calculation will be carried out [50]. The sampling aims to include information-rich cases and achieve in-depth understanding of the phenomena being explored rather than striving to meet a specific (statistically determined) sample size [51]. Sampling aims to reach a diverse range of participants (including age and location) and achieve data saturation across themes. The sample size of each group has also been determined by practical considerations including timeframes of qualitative fieldwork and reasonable workload requests for service providers who will support the recruitment of women who have experienced a head injury through family violence.

2.5.1. Women Who Have Experienced a Head Injury through Family Violence

To preserve the safety of women, the research team will work closely with frontline service providers and community groups within each project site to purposefully sample women who fit the criteria. The broad inclusion criteria for this study are women who: (1) identify as Aboriginal and Torres Strait Islander; (2) are aged 18+; and (3) have experienced a head injury (or been diagnosed with a TBI) as a direct consequence of family violence. The recruitment of women will continue until data saturation is reached [52]. Frontline service providers are well-equipped to identify potential participants, with some service providers (such as legal and health services) having access to medical discharge summaries that confirm whether their patient or client would meet the study criteria. Other services have active risk management plans and communication strategies in place with their clients, which makes them well-equipped to have knowledge and awareness of the different factors that may place each client at greater or lesser risk to participate in the study. Nominated service staff (such as women's groups coordinators, medical practitioners, case workers, and lawyers) will identify patients or clients who meet the eligibility criteria. Once a clinician has identified a patient that meets the eligibility criteria, a member of the research team will be notified. To ensure consent is conducted in an appropriate manner, the research team member will approach the patient or client with the assistance of an Aboriginal Interpreter Translator (where necessary) to explain the study fully. Potential participants will be provided with written information about the study, a short video about the project, face-to-face discussion with a research team member, and given an opportunity to ask questions about the project. To support nominated staff from service providers to identify women who meet the criteria, TBI education sessions will be delivered to participating service providers by two Aboriginal and Torres Strait Islander educators from a national brain injury organisation [53]. Aboriginal Interpreter Translators will also be employed to assist with data collection.

Table 1. Summary of participants, sampling, recruitment, and data collection.

Participant Group	Examples	Sampling and Recruitment Method	Data Collection
Women who have experienced a head injury (or diagnosed TBI) as a result of family violence	Women (aged 18+) who have experienced a head injury (or diagnosed TBI) as a direct result of family violence	Convenience sampling via key staff within community-based service providers and community groups. Purposive sampling, as required, to include underrepresented groups (such as young women)	Individual interview or small group discussion
Family members or caregivers of women	May include grandmother, parent, sister, guardian	Women who have experienced a head injury (or diagnosed TBI) as a direct result of family violence will be asked to nominate a family member or caregiver to participate in the project	Individual interview or small group discussion
Hospital staff	Aboriginal Liaison Officers, Aboriginal Leadership staff, specialists, and allied health staff	Purposive and snowball sampling	Individual interview or small group discussion
Community-based service providers	Family violence, legal and justice, health and community groups	Purposive and snowball sampling	Individual interview or small group discussion
Workshops	Community leaders, service providers, hospital staff, national advocacy group, and policymakers	A selection of service provider and hospital staff will be directly invited to take part in a one-day workshop	Workshop discussion

2.5.2. Family Members and Carers

Women who have experienced a head injury through family violence will be asked to nominate a family member or carer (aged 18+) to take part in an interview. Family members and carers can nominate to take part in an interview or small discussion group. Women with acquired head injury related to family violence can participate in the study without nominating a family member or carer.

2.5.3. Hospital Staff

Direct invitations will be made to hospital staff and a 'snowballing' approach will also be used for recruitment, where participants will be able to recommend other staff to approach. A variety of disciplines will be targeted with the aim to include individuals who have lived experience of working with women who present to the hospital with head injury connected to family violence, their families, and perpetrators of family violence, and those who provide medical treatment to women who have sustained a head injury. Potential staff that will participate in an interview for the project include Indigenous hospital liaison officers, Aboriginal health workers, specialists, nurses, occupational therapists, physiotherapists and social workers.

2.5.4. Service Professionals, Community Groups, and National Advocacy Groups

Frontline workers, community-based groups, and advocacy groups will be invited to participate in an individual interview or small discussion group. Frontline workers will represent primary health care (both Aboriginal community-controlled and government), the legal and justice sector (including magistrates, lawyers, victims support), housing and crisis accommodation, disability support services, and family violence services. Examples of community groups include women's and Elder groups. Representatives from national and regional disability and brain injury advocacy groups will also be invited to participate in an individual interview. This previously used approach [54] involves the selection of experts based on their knowledge and experience of the core research issue [55]. Prioritising contact with Aboriginal and Torres Strait Islander community groups and organisations, a list of potential participants will be developed by the research team. Sampling will occur through the networks of the research team and a 'snowballing' approach, with participants asked to recommend other relevant individuals and agencies to participate in the research [51]. As presented in Table 2, the interview protocol for service professionals aims to understand the delivery and practice of service models as well as to understand the knowledge of service professionals related to TBI and family violence.

Table 2. Overview of the interview and discussion group topics.

Participant Group	Topics
Women who have experienced a head injury (or diagnosed TBI) as a direct result of family violence	• Day to day living and challenges during the post-discharge period • How women maintain roles involving taking care of family and cultural responsibilities • How women re-construct their identity and life post-injury • Motivation to engage with services and reconnect with life, community engagement, managing issues, and ability to build relationships with family, friends, and service networks • Priorities, milestones, and outcomes that are important to women to achieve post-injury
Family members and carers	• Day to day living during the post-discharge period for women, families and carers • Challenges of caring for someone who has acquired a head injury connected to family violence • Service and systems accessed by women, families, and carers • Barriers and enablers for women, families, and carers to access services
Hospital staff	• Experiences of women accessing hospital care and post-discharge processes • Support for women in hospital and post-discharge including referral pathways • Enablers and barriers for women to access hospital and health care • Suggestions for improvements within services, systems, and policies
Community-based service providers	• Service programs and the delivery of services • Barriers and enablers for women to access services • Challenges for service providers in terms of service delivery and sustainability • Suggestion for reform and improvements for policy and service delivery

2.6. Data Collection

Interviews and discussion groups will be conducted by Aboriginal and non-Indigenous research team members. A semi-structured interview guide covering the topics listed in Table 2 will be used, but questions will also be informed by observations and new topics raised by the participant. Participants will have the opportunity to 'tell their story'. These methods have been rigorously applied in previous research with Aboriginal and Torres Strait Islander women and are drawn upon here as they can: (a) capture grounded subjective experiences and practices occurring locally and (b) effectively support the participation of highly marginalised groups who have a diverse range of skills, knowledge, and educational attainment [56]. Yarning is also a feature of Aboriginal and Torres Strait Islander convention for passing on information through informal conversations, reflecting the oral traditions that support the transmission of knowledge among Aboriginal and Torres Strait Islander peoples [57]. The interview guide was developed through a multi-phase process involving - aligning the interview questions with research questions, receiving feedback on the interview schedules, and piloting of the interview schedules [58].

2.7. Workshops

Once data have been collected from across all studies, service providers will be invited to participate in one-day workshops. Based on participatory models of qualitative research methods, discussion questions will be designed to elicit in-depth information about the existing knowledge and gather information and recommendations for the next steps in research, practice, and knowledge dissemination. Breakout groups will include at least one representative from different types of service providers and community groups to achieve triangulation of the data. Session summaries of the workshops with services will be presented to the collective group at each location to identify key themes and prioritise next steps. Discussions will be recorded in written and audio formats.

2.8. Data Analysis

All audio recorded interviews, discussion groups, and workshops will be transcribed verbatim. Transcripts, fieldnotes, and observations will be managed with NVivo 12 [59]. The transcripts will be analysed using a combination of narrative and descriptive phenomenological analyses. The aim of descriptive phenomenology is to describe particular phenomena, or the appearance of things, as lived experience [60]. The process is inductive and descriptive and seeks to record experiences from the viewpoint of the individual who had them without imposing a specific theoretical or conceptual framework on the study prior to collecting data [61]. The narrative analysis will focus on sense-making and Aboriginal and Torres Strait Islander women's changing identity and role post TBI from family violence. The two methodological approaches complement each other in terms of gaining knowledge of 'breadth' (narrative identity) and 'depth' (lived experiences), giving some support for a philosophical position that shows a person as both an active and passive agent, constructively making sense of their narrative identity as well as being constructed by their lived experiences. A constant comparative technique will be employed to systematically organise, compare, and understand the similarities and differences across the different participating groups and field sites, critically enriching the analysis and providing a substantive basis for theoretical extrapolation and affording critical points of comparative analysis across each of the locations.

2.9. Ethics

Ethics approval for this research has been obtained from the Central Australian Human Research Ethics Committee (CA-21-4160), Western Sydney University Human Research Ethics Committee (H14646), Townsville Hospital and Health Service Human Research Ethics Committee (HREC/QTHS/85271 and HREC/QTHS/88044), and the Aboriginal Health and Medical Research Council of New South Wales Human Research Ethics Committee (1922/22).

2.10. Consent

Participants will provide voluntary written informed consent. For women who experience severe impairment or are under a guardianship order, consent from a proxy for research participation from a person responsible for the person (such as a carer or guardian) will be sought. Participants may withdraw from the study at any time before dissemination of the findings, except for the discussion group participants, as it will be difficult to identify individual voices in the recording and transcript. Discussion group participants will be informed of this before consenting to the study. Participants will not be deceived in any way about the study objectives. All information regarding the study will be provided verbally and in writing prior to the interview. To minimise the risk of stigmatisation of potential participants and to ensure information regarding the study is understood fully by the participants, a flipchart that uses images and plain, easy English to describe key aspects of the project (e.g., what is a brain injury, reasons for the study, and participant rights) as well as video resources developed in a previous TBI study will be used [33].

2.11. Potential Benefits and Risks

Self-awareness plays an essential role in TBI rehabilitation and can impact motivation, safety, and rehabilitation goals during recovery [62]. Through self-exploration of their lived experiences, some participants may be able to fully explore their experiences, more fully explore their circumstances, and may also gain a new perspective. However, the recall of traumatic experiences by women and their family members may also cause discomfort or distress. Drawing upon the guidelines for working with women who have experienced family violence, all decisions within the research process will be driven by an awareness of the safety and ethical considerations [63–65]. Several strategies will be implemented to minimise any potential risk, and to identify the different levels of risk, of the women being identified as participating in the study. Promotion and recruitment through only service providers recognises the importance of recruiting women that are already connected with one or more of the participating services with access to ongoing support. Service providers have an existing awareness of the current life circumstances of the women referred to the project (e.g., if women are living in a high-risk environment). Existing connections between services and women who have experienced family members will also enable the research team to complete immediate referrals (with permission of the participant) back to the service for support should the women disclose that they are at risk of violence or have been identified by other community members as participating in the study. Other safeguards implemented for the safety and well-being of women and carers/support persons who take part in the study include the organisation of an experienced counsellor when interviews and discussion groups are conducted, and follow-up contact with each participant shortly after data collection.

2.12. Dissemination

A dissemination plan implemented within the project will ensure that the research findings and dissemination activities are controlled by Aboriginal and Torres Strait Islander peoples and service providers and ensure that the findings are disseminated throughout the course of the project in appropriate formats for the stakeholders. Stakeholders include research participants, government and non-government service providers, the health and legal sectors, state/territory and federal policymakers, the academic community, and advocacy groups. Findings will be disseminated through conference presentations and peer-review publications. Further dissemination activities will be determined in partnership with advisory groups and other service providers through the recommendations made in the workshops. Some of the expected dissemination formats include:

- Research translation workshops with services and hospital representatives as well as community presentations. Project partner policy papers for use by advocates involved in the project.
- Incorporating art, visual media, and other media to present essential information for community members about the key findings.
- Translating all findings into easy English versions of the final report.

While this study will directly inform policy and practice within Queensland, the Northern Territory, and New South Wales, the findings will be disseminated to other relevant states/territory service providers, government ministers, and advocacy groups beyond these jurisdictions to ensure that an applicable national-level strategy can be shared. Publications will adhere to the CONSolIDated critERia for strengthening the reporting of health research involving Indigenous Peoples (the CONSIDER statement) [66] as well as the Consolidated Criteria for Reporting Qualitative Research [67].

3. Conclusions

This qualitative project will comprehensively explore and document the strengths, challenges, and nuances in the day to day lives of Aboriginal and Torres Strait Islander women with an acquired head injury connected to family violence. Through partnerships with key services, the evidence generated will enable service providers that work with these women to better develop and tailor their services, programs, and workforce to support Aboriginal and Torres Strait Islander women and their families. The evidence may also help to inform resource allocation and provide vital information for governments to support the planning and development of equitable, holistic, appropriate care, and support that reflects the needs and priorities of Aboriginal and Torres Strait Islander Australian women experiencing head injury in the context of family violence. The evidence generated from this project is a critical step in addressing the unacceptable rates of head injury as a result of family violence among Aboriginal and Torres Strait Islander women.

Author Contributions: Conceptualisation, M.S.F.; Methodology, M.S.F., K.S., J.C. and G.K. Writing, original draft, M.S.F.; Writing–review and editing, K.S., J.C., G.K., Y.J. and E.W.; Funding acquisition, M.S.F. All authors have read and agreed to the published version of the manuscript.

Funding: This work was supported by the Australian Research Council via a Discovery Early Career Research Award for M Fitts (#210100639). The funders have no role in the study design, data collection and analysis, decision to publish or preparation of the manuscript. The views expressed in this publication are those of the authors and do not necessarily reflect the views of the funders.

Institutional Review Board Statement: The Central Australian Human Research Ethics Committee (CA-21-4160), Western Sydney University Human Research Ethics Committee (H14926), Townsville Hospital and Health Service Human Research Ethics Committee (HREC/QTHS/85271 and HREC/QTHS/88044), and the Aboriginal Health and Medical Research Council of New South Wales Human Research Ethics Committee (1922/22) have approved the study. Approval has also been received from Aboriginal, legal and health services, research committees, and boards. Dissemination will occur through stakeholder reports, workshops, presentations, peer-reviewed journal articles, and conference papers. Further dissemination will be determined in partnership with the project advisory group.

Informed Consent Statement: Not applicable.

Data Availability Statement: Not applicable.

Acknowledgments: The authors thank all study sites for their participation in the project including Elders, community leaders, advocates and service providers who are supporting the project. The authors would also like to thank the members of the advisory group and individual advisors for their advice on the study.

Conflicts of Interest: The authors declare no conflict of interest.

References

1. World Health Organization. *Preventing Intimate Partner and Sexual Violence against Women: Taking Action and Generating Evidence*; World Health Organization: Geneva, Switzerland, 2010.
2. Australian Government. *National Plan to End Violence against Women and Children 2022–2032*; Australian Government: Canberra, Australia, 2022. Available online: https://www.dss.gov.au/sites/default/files/documents/10_2022/national_plan_accessible_version_for_website.pdf (accessed on 20 October 2022).
3. Fitz-Gibbon, K.; Meyer, S.; Gelb, K.; McGowan, J.; Wild, S.; Batty, R.; Segrave, M.; Maher, J.M.M.; Pfitzner, N.; McCulloch, J.; et al. *National Plan Stakeholder Consultation: Final Report*; Monash University: Clayton, Australia, 2022.
4. Zieman, G.; Bridwell, A.; Cárdenas, J.F. Traumatic Brain Injury in Domestic Violence Victims: A Retrospective Study at the Barrow Neurological Institute. *J. Neurotrauma* **2017**, *34*, 876–880. [CrossRef] [PubMed]
5. Jamieson, L.M.; Harrison, J.E.; Berry, J.G. Hospitalisation for head injury due to assault among Indigenous and non-Indigenous Australians, July 1999–June 2005. *Med. J. Aust.* **2008**, *188*, 576–579. [CrossRef]
6. Langlois, J.A.; Rutland-Brown, W.; Wald, M.M. The epidemiology and impact of traumatic brain injury: A brief overview. *J Head Trauma Rehabil.* **2006**, *21*, 375–378. [CrossRef] [PubMed]
7. St. Ivany, A.; Schminkey, D. Intimate Partner Violence and Traumatic Brain Injury: State of the Science and Next Steps. *Fam. Community Health* **2016**, *39*, 129–137. [CrossRef] [PubMed]
8. Baxter, K.; Hellewell, S.C. Traumatic Brain Injury within Domestic Relationships: Complications, Consequences and Contributing Factors. *J. Aggress. Maltreat.* **2019**, *28*, 660–676. [CrossRef]
9. Xu, T.; Yu, X.; Ou, S.; Liu, X.; Yuan, J.; Huang, H.; Yang, J.; He, L.; Chen, Y. Risk factors for posttraumatic epilepsy: A systematic review and meta-analysis. *Epilepsy Behav.* **2016**, *67*, 1–6. [CrossRef] [PubMed]
10. Snowden, T.M.; Hinde, A.K.; Reid, H.M.O.; Christie, B.R. Does Mild Traumatic Brain Injury Increase the Risk for Dementia? A Systematic Review and Meta-Analysis. *J. Alzheimers Dis.* **2020**, *78*, 757–775.

11. Commonwealth of Australia. *Statement from Delegates—2021 National Summit on Women's Safety*; Commonwealth of Australia: Canberra, Australia, 2021. Available online: https://az659834.vo.msecnd.net/eventsairaueprod/production-regonsite-public/e626677d4b4c4a5ebfe33a68b05bdd6b (accessed on 20 October 2022).
12. Haag, H.L.; Jones, D.; Joseph, T.; Colantonio, A. Battered and Brain Injured: Traumatic Brain Injury Among Women Survivors of Intimate Partner Violence—A Scoping Review. *TVA* **2019**, *23*, 1270–1287. [CrossRef]
13. Australian Institute of Health and Welfare. *Family, Domestic and Sexual Violence in Australia: Continuing the National Story 2019 (Cat. no. FDV 3)*; Australian Institute of Health and Welfare: Canberra, Australia, 2019.
14. Chan, A.; Payne, J. *Homicide in Australia: 2008–09 to 2009–10 National Homicide Monitoring Program Annual Report*; Australian Government: Canberra, Australia, 2013.
15. Nancarrow, H. Legal Responses to Intimate Partner Violence: Gendered Aspirations and Racialised Realities. Doctoral Thesis, Griffith University, Brisbane, Australia, 2016.
16. Campbell, S.; Corbo, M.; Egan, R. Resilience in the Alice Springs Town Camps. In *Promoting Resilience: Responding to Adversity, Vulnerability, and Loss*; Thompson, N., Cox, G., Eds.; Routledge: New York, NY, USA, 2020; pp. 95–100.
17. Brown, C.; Homan, S.; Simpson, C.; Leung, L. *Rante-Rante Ampe Marle and Urreye: "Safe, Respected and Free from Violence" Projects Evaluation*; Australia's National Research Organisation for Women's Safety (ANROWS): Canberra, Australia, 2021. Available online: https://www.anrows.org.au/project/safe-respected-and-free-from-violence-an-evaluation-of-primary-prevention-projects/ (accessed on 20 October 2022).
18. Katzenellenbogen, J.M.; Atkins, E.; Thompson, S.C.; Hersh, D.; Coffin, J.; Flicker, L.; Hayward, C.; Ciccone, N.; Woods, D.; Greenland, M.E.; et al. Missing Voices: Profile, Extent, and 12-Month Outcomes of Nonfatal Traumatic Brain Injury in Aboriginal and Non-Aboriginal Adults in Western Australia Using Linked Administrative Records. *H Head Trauma Rehabil.* **2018**, *33*, 412–423. [CrossRef]
19. Lakhani, A.; Townsend, C.; Bishara, J. Traumatic brain injury amongst indigenous people: A systematic review. *Brain Inj.* **2017**, *31*, 1718–1730. [CrossRef]
20. Esterman, A.; Thompson, F.; Fitts, M.; Gilroy, J.; Fleming, J.; Maruff, P.; Clough, A.; Bohanna, I. Incidence of emergency department presentations for traumatic brain injury in Indigenous and non-Indigenous residents aged 15–64 over the 9-year period 2007–2015 in North Queensland, Australia. *Inj. Epidemiol.* **2018**, *5*, 40. [CrossRef] [PubMed]
21. Cripps, K. Indigenous family violence: A statistical challenge. *Injury* **2008**, *39*, S25–S35. [CrossRef] [PubMed]
22. Cunneen, C. *Alternative and Improved Responses to Domestic and Family Violence in Queensland Indigenous Communities*; Queensland Government: Brisbane, Australia, 2009.
23. Adams, R.; Hunter, Y. Surviving justice: Family violence, sexual assault and child sexual assault in remote Aboriginal communities in NSW. *Indig. Law Bull.* **2007**, *7*, 26–28.
24. Day, A.; Jones, R.; Nakata, M.; McDermott, D. Indigenous Family Violence: An Attempt to Understand the Problems and Inform Appropriate and Effective Responses to Criminal Justice System Intervention. *Psychiatry Psychol. Law* **2012**, *19*, 104–117. [CrossRef]
25. Nancarrow, H. In search of justice for domestic and family violence: Indigenous and non-Indigenous Australian women's perspectives. *Theor. Criminol.* **2006**, *10*, 87–106. [CrossRef]
26. Cheers, B.; Binell, M.; Coleman, H.; Gentle, I.; Miller, G.; Taylor, J.; Weetra, C. Family violence: An Australian Indigenous community tells its story. *Int. Soc. Work* **2006**, *49*, 51–63. [CrossRef]
27. Bryant, C. *Identifying the Risks for Indigenous Violent Victimisation. Brief 6. Written for Indigenous Justice Clearinghouse*; Australian Institute of Criminology: Canberra, Australia, 2009.
28. Levack, W.M.M.; Kayes, N.M.; Fadyl, J.K. Experience of recovery and outcome following traumatic brain injury: A metasynthesis of qualitative research. *Disabil. Rehabil.* **2010**, *32*, 986–999. [CrossRef]
29. Bohanna, I.; Fitts, M.S.; Bird, K.; Fleming, J.; Gilroy, J.; Esterman, A.; Maruff, P.; Clough, A. The Transition from Hospital to Home: Protocol for a Longitudinal Study of Australian Aboriginal and Torres Strait Islander Traumatic Brain Injury (TBI). *Brain Impair.* **2018**, *19*, 246–257. [CrossRef]
30. Armstrong, E.; Hersh, D.; Katzenellenbogen, J.M.; Coffin, J.; Thompson, S.; Ciccone, N.; Hayward, C.; Flicker, L.; Woods, D.; McAllister, M. Study Protocol: Missing Voices—Communication Difficulties after Stroke and Traumatic Brain Injury in Aboriginal Australians. *Brain Impair.* **2015**, *16*, 145–156. [CrossRef]
31. Fitts, M.S.; Bird, K.; Gilroy, J.; Fleming, J.; Clough, A.R.; Esterman, A.; Maruff, P.; Fatima, Y.; Bohanna, I. A Qualitative Study on the Transition Support Needs of Indigenous Australians Following Traumatic Brain Injury. *Brain Impair.* **2019**, *20*, 137–159. [CrossRef]
32. Armstrong, E.; McCoy, K.; Clinch, R.; Merritt, M.; Speedy, R.; McAllister, M.; Heine, K.; Ciccone, N.; Robinson, M.; Coffin, J. The development of aboriginal brain injury coordinator positions: A culturally secure rehabilitation service initiative as part of a clinical trial. *Prim. Health Care Res. Dev.* **2021**, *22*, e49. [CrossRef] [PubMed]
33. Bohanna, I.; Fitts, M.; Bird, K.; Fleming, J.; Gilroy, J.; Clough, A.; Esterman, A.; Maruff, P.; Potter, M. The Potential of a Narrative and Creative Arts Approach to Enhance Transition Outcomes for Indigenous Australians Following Traumatic Brain Injury. *Brain Impair.* **2019**, *20*, 160–170. [CrossRef]
34. Costello, K.; Greenwald, B.D. Update on domestic violence and traumatic brain injury: A narrative review. *Brain Sci.* **2022**, *12*, 122. [CrossRef] [PubMed]

35. Haag, H.; Sing, G.; Sokoloff, S.; Cullen, N.; MacGregor, N.; Samsa, S.; Broekstra, S.; Colantonio, A. Women Survivors of Intimate Partner Violence & Traumatic Brain Injury: Addressing Service & Knowledge Gaps. *Arch. Phys. Med. Rehabil.* **2019**, *100*, e32.
36. Fiolet, R.; Tarzia, L.; Hameed, M.; Hegarty, K. Indigenous Peoples' Help-Seeking Behaviors for Family Violence: A Scoping Review. *Trauma Violence Abus.* **2021**, *22*, 370–380. [CrossRef] [PubMed]
37. Blagg, H.; Bluett-Boyd, N.; Williams, E. *Innovative Models in Addressing Violence against Indigenous Women: State of Knowledge Paper*; Australia's National Research Organisation for Women's Safety Limited (ANROWS): Alexandria, Australia, 2015.
38. Australian Bureau of Statistics. Census 2016—Census Community Profiles. 2016. Available online: https://www.abs.gov.au/websitedbs/D3310114.nsf/Home/2016%20Census%20Community%20Profiles (accessed on 12 August 2022).
39. Sherry, M. A sociology of impairment. *Disabil. Soc.* **2016**, *31*, 729–744. [CrossRef]
40. Mitra, S. The Capability Approach and Disability. *J. Disabil. Policy Stud.* **2006**, *16*, 236–247. [CrossRef]
41. Conrad, P.; Barker, K.K. The Social Construction of Illness: Key Insights and Policy Implications. *J. Health Soc. Behav.* **2010**, *51* (Suppl. 1), S67–S79. [CrossRef]
42. Crenshaw, K. Mapping the Margins: Intersectionality, Identity Politics, and Violence against Women of Color. *Stanford Law Rev.* **1991**, *43*, 1241–1299. [CrossRef]
43. National Health and Medical Research Council (NHMRC). *National Statement on Ethical Conduct in Human Research (Updated 2018)*; Commonwealth of Australia: Canberra, Australia, 2007.
44. Zurba, M.; Maclean, K.; Woodward, E.; Islam, D. Amplifying Indigenous community participation in place-based research through boundary work. *Prog. Hum. Geogr.* **2019**, *43*, 1020–1043. [CrossRef]
45. Louis, R.P. Can You Hear us Now? Voices from the Margin: Using Indigenous Methodologies in Geographic Research. *Geogr. Res.* **2007**, *45*, 130–139.
46. Gilroy, J.; Donelly, M.; Colmar, S.; Parmenter, T. Twelve factors that can influence the participation of Aboriginal people in disability services. *Aust. Indig. Health Bull.* **2016**, *16*.
47. Lansdell, G.T.; Saunders, B.J.; Eriksson, A.; Bunn, R. Strengthening the Connection Between Acquired Brain Injury (ABI) and Family Violence: The Importance of Ongoing Monitoring, Research and Inclusive Terminology. *J. Fam. Violence* **2021**, *37*, 367–380. [CrossRef]
48. Fitts, M.; Cullen, J.; Kingston, G.; Johnson, Y.; Wills, E.; Soldatic, K. Moving research translation into research design: A disability case study with regional and remote Aboriginal and Torres Strait Islander communities and service providers in Australia. *Health Sociol. Rev.* **2023**; in press.
49. Fitts, M.S.; Cullen, J.; Kingston, G.; Wills, E.; Soldatic, K. "I Don't Think It's on Anyone's Radar": The Workforce and System Barriers to Healthcare for Indigenous Women Following a Traumatic Brain Injury Acquired through Violence in Remote Australia. *Int. J. Environ. Res. Public Health* **2022**, *19*, 14744. [CrossRef]
50. Palinkas, L.A.; Horwitz, S.M.; Green, C.A.; Wisdom, J.P.; Duan, N.; Hoagwood, K. Purposeful Sampling for Qualitative Data Collection and Analysis in Mixed Method Implementation Research. *Adm. Policy Ment. Health* **2013**, *42*, 533–544. [CrossRef]
51. Patton, M. *Qualitative Evaluation and Research Methods*, 2nd ed.; SAGE Publications: Newbury Park, CA, USA, 1990.
52. Guest, G.; Bunce, A.; Johnson, L. How Many Interviews Are Enough? An Experiment with Data Saturation and Variability. *Field Methods* **2006**, *18*, 59–82. [CrossRef]
53. Synapse Australia. Australia's Brain Injury Organisation. Available online: https://synapse.org.au/ (accessed on 20 October 2022).
54. Fitts, M.; Soldatic, K. Disability income reform and service innovation: Countering racial and regional discrimination. *Glob. Media J.* **2018**, *12*, 13.
55. Liamputtong, P. *Qualitative Research Methods*, 5th ed.; Oxford University Press: Docklands, Australia, 2019.
56. Grench, S.; Soldatic, K. Indigenous research methodologies. In *Disability in the Global South: The Critical Handbook*; Grech, S., Soldatic, K., Eds.; Springer: New York, NY, USA, 2015.
57. Bessarab, D.; Ng'andu, B. Yarning About Yarning as a Legitimate Method in Indigenous Research. *Int. J. Crit. Indig.* **2010**, *3*, 37–50. [CrossRef]
58. Castillo-Montoya, M. Preparing for Interview Research: The Interview Protocol Refinement Framework. *Qual. Rep.* **2016**, *21*, 811–831. [CrossRef]
59. Q.S.R International. NVivo Qualitative Data Analysis Software. 2021. Available online: https://www.qsrinternational.com/nvivo-qualitative-data-analysis-software/home (accessed on 20 October 2022).
60. Streubert, H.J. Philosophical Dimensions of Qualitative Research. In *Qualitative Research in Nursing: Advancing the Humanistic Imperative*; Streubert, J., Carpenter, D.R., Eds.; Lippincott: Philadelphia, PA, USA, 1995.
61. Polit, D.F.; Beck, C.T. *Nursing Research: Principles and Methods*, 7th ed.; Lippincott Williams & Wilkins: Philadelphia, PA, USA, 2004.
62. Robertson, K.; Schmitter-Edgecombe, M. Self-awareness and traumatic brain injury outcome. *Brain Inj.* **2015**, *29*, 848–858. [CrossRef] [PubMed]
63. Thomas, S.N.; Weber, S.; Bradbury-Jones, C. Using Participatory and Creative Methods to Research Gender-Based Violence in the Global South and With Indigenous Communities: Findings from a Scoping Review. *TVA* **2022**, *23*, 342–355. [CrossRef] [PubMed]
64. Ellsberg, M.; Potts, A. *Ethical Considerations for Research and Evaluation on Ending Violence against Women and Girls: Guidance Paper Prepared by the Global Women's Institute (GWI) for the Department of Foreign Affairs and Trade*; Department of Foreign Affairs and Trade: Canberra, Australia, 2018.

65. World Health Organization (WHO). *Ethical and Safety Recommendations for Intervention Research on Violence against Women. Building on Lessons from the WHO Publication 'Putting Women First: Ethical and Safety Recommendations for Research on Domestic Violence against Women*; WHO: Geneva, Switzerland, 2016.
66. Huria, T.; Palmer, S.C.; Pitama, S.; Beckert, L.; Lacey, C.; Ewen, S.; Smith, L.T. Consolidated criteria for strengthening reporting of health research involving indigenous peoples: The CONSIDER statement. *BMC Res. Methodol.* **2019**, *19*, 173. [CrossRef] [PubMed]
67. Tong, A.; Sainsbury, P.; Craig, J. Consolidated criteria for reporting qualitative research (COREQ): A 32-item checklist for interviews and focus groups. *Int. J. Qual. Health Care* **2007**, *19*, 349–357. [CrossRef]

Disclaimer/Publisher's Note: The statements, opinions and data contained in all publications are solely those of the individual author(s) and contributor(s) and not of MDPI and/or the editor(s). MDPI and/or the editor(s) disclaim responsibility for any injury to people or property resulting from any ideas, methods, instructions or products referred to in the content.

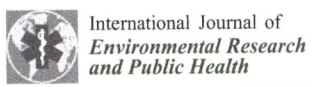

Article

Race and Ethnic Differences in the Protective Effect of Parental Educational Attainment on Subsequent Perceived Tobacco Norms among US Youth

Edward Adinkrah [1,*], Babak Najand [2] and Angela Young-Brinn [1,2]

[1] Department of Family Medicine, Charles R Drew University of Medicine and Science, Los Angeles, CA 90059, USA
[2] Marginalization-Related Diminished Returns, Los Angeles, CA 90059, USA
* Correspondence: edwardadinkrah@cdrewu.edu

Abstract: Background: Although parental educational attainment is known to be associated with a lower prevalence of behaviors such as tobacco use, these effects are shown to be weaker for Black than White youth. It is important to study whether this difference is due to higher perceived tobacco use norms for Black youth. Aim: To study the association between parental educational attainment and perceived tobacco use norms overall and by race/ethnicity among youth in the US. Methods: The current study used four years of follow-up data from the Population Assessment of Tobacco and Health (PATH-Youth) study conducted between 2013 and 2017. All participants were 12- to 17-year-old non-smokers at baseline and were successfully followed for four years (n = 4329). The outcome of interest was perceived tobacco use norms risk at year four. The predictor of interest was baseline parental educational attainment, the moderator was race/ethnicity, and the covariates were age, sex, and parental marital status at baseline. Results: Our linear regressions in the pooled sample showed that higher parental educational attainment at baseline was predictive of perceived disapproval of tobacco use at year four; however, this association was weaker for Latino than non-Latino youth. Our stratified models also showed that higher parental educational attainment was associated with perceived tobacco use norms for non-Latino but not for Latino youth. Conclusion: The effect of high parental educational attainment on anti-tobacco norms differs between Latino and non-Latino youth. Latino youth with highly educated parents remain at risk of tobacco use, while non-Latino youth with highly educated parents show low susceptibility to tobacco use.

Keywords: population groups; risk behavior; perceived tobacco use norms; ethnic groups; academic achievement

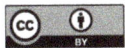

1. Introduction

Youth is associated with heightened risk behaviors, including tobacco use [1]. However, socioeconomic status (SES) indicators such as parental educational attainment may lower youth risk-taking behaviors such as tobacco use [2]. Some of the many mechanisms that may explain the lower behavioral and health risk of high SES youth are social norms and beliefs that are not favorable toward tobacco (also called perceived tobacco use norms) [3], which are under the influence of peers, families [4], and other factors such as availability of tobacco in the areas, tobacco ads, and prevalence of tobacco use in the community, neighborhood, school, and family and friends [5].

However, the protective effects of parental educational attainment on youth risk behaviors such as tobacco use may differ between diverse racial and ethnic groups of youth [6]. In addition, according to a phenomenon called marginalization-related diminished returns (MDRs) [7–16], due to racism and social stratification, resources and assets may be associated with lower levels of economic, behavioral, developmental, and health outcomes for marginalized and racialized groups than White individuals [17,18].

Research has indicated that race may alter how SES influences health and behavioral problems such as tobacco use [19–29]. The association between parental educational attainment and a wide range of health problems varies between racial/ethnic groups of youth [30–32]. Fuller Rowell showed that the association between youth educational attainment and health is racialized [30–32]. Under racism and discrimination, high educational attainment may be linked to more distress and discrimination for Black than White youth [30–32]. Education gains may be linked to worse mental health for Black youth who live in a social context that may impose a higher level of psychological tax for their educational success or chronic poverty from childhood [30–32]. At all SES levels, Black students are discriminated against [33,34], and high SES Black youth attend worse schools than White youth [35]. Similarly, high-SES Black youth have family members who are more likely to be substance users than high-SES White youth [36]. When high-SES Black youth move to high-SES neighborhoods and schools (that are predominantly White), they become even more exposed [37,38] and vulnerable [39] to discrimination. As the education system differently treats Black and White youth [40,41], health gain due to education is weaker for Blacks than Whites [30–32].

According to the marginalization-related diminished returns (MDRs), SES resources and even non-economic resources may generate fewer behavioral, developmental, and health outcomes for marginalized and racialized groups such as Blacks and Latinos than non-Latino Whites [17,18]. While most of this literature is generated on the effects of SES on health outcomes for adults [16,19,21,23,29,42–44], non-SES factors such as self-efficacy may also be associated with lower health gain for Black than White individuals [45]. Similarly, positive affect [46,47] and happiness [48–50] may generate less health for Blacks than Whites. We explain this phenomenon through racism and societal inequalities: Even when SES and other resources are available, societal and environmental conditions such as social stratification, segregation, racism, and discrimination make it more difficult for Black and Latino than non-Latino White families and individuals to secure outcomes. In this view, what makes a large change for Whites may generate smaller real-life changes for Black individuals [45,51].

As shown by systematic reviews, behaviors such as tobacco consumption are under influence of cognitive elements such as perceived tobacco norms [52]. According to theories such as Theory of Planned Behavior (TPB) [52] and Theory of Reasoned Action (TRA) [53], perceived norms predict behaviors such as tobacco use. Perceived norms are different than actual norms and can be defined as what individuals think are the norms of their group [54]. For example, even when actual norms can be low, perceived norms can be high. Thus perceived norms are what people think is the norm, while actual norm is the reality of the society [55]. Cognitive elements such as perceived tobacco norms can be used as a marker of tobacco susceptibility and vulnerability [56].

Built on the MDRs literature on tobacco use risk [57,58], we conducted this study with two aims: the first was to test the association between parental educational attainment and perceived tobacco use norms overall. The second aim was to test the variation of this association by race. Our first hypothesis was that overall, high parental educational attainment is associated with lower perceived tobacco use norms in youth. Our second hypothesis was that this inverse association would be weaker for Latinos and Blacks than non-Latinos and Whites.

2. Methods

For this study, we conducted a secondary analysis of the first four years of the Population Assessment of Tobacco and Health (PATH-Youth) study data. The PATH-Youth is the state-of-the-art study of tobacco use of US youth. Data collection was performed between 2013 (baseline) and 2017 (follow up). Youth PATH data are publicly available to all individuals. This data set is fully de-identified and can be accessed here: https://www.icpsr.umich.edu/web/NAHDAP/studies/36231 (accessed on 12 October 2022).

In the PATH study, participants are selected randomly. Stratified and clustered random samples were selected from all US states. Eligibility for inclusion in the current analysis were non-institutionalized members of US households, aged between 12 and 17 at baseline, having follow-up data for years (baseline and follow-up data), and being Latino or non-Latino White or Black. Participants were all never smoker at baseline. A total number of 4596 youth were entered who had and follow-up data for four years.

Study variables in this analysis included race, ethnicity, parental educational attainment, parental marital status, age, sex/gender, and perceived tobacco use norms. Age was a dichotomous variable 0 for lower than 15 and 1 for 15 and above. Gender was 1 for males and 0 for females. Parental educational attainment was the independent variable with five levels, and perceived tobacco use norms were the outcome. Both parental educational attainment and perceived tobacco use norms were treated as continuous measures. Perceived tobacco use norms were self-reported and measured using the following binary indicators: (a) People who are important to you: Their views on tobacco use in general, (b) People who are important to you: Their views on smoking cigarettes, (c) People who are important to you: Their views on using e-cigarettes or other electronic nicotine products, (d) People who are important to you: Their views on smoking traditional cigars, cigarillos, or filtered cigars, (e) People who are important to you: Their views on smoking shisha or hookah tobacco, (f) People who are important to you: Their views on using snus, and (g) People who are important to you: Their views on other types of smokeless tobacco. Each item was on a 1 (very positive) to 5 (very negative) response scale. The range of total scores was between 1 and 5, with a higher score indicating higher perceived tobacco use norms.

Parental educational attainment. Parental educational attainment was a five-level variable as below: 1 = "Some high school," 2 = "Completed high school," 3 = "Some college," 4 = "Completed college," 5 = "Graduate or professional school after college." This variable was a continuous variable.

Parental marital status. Parental marital status was a dichotomous variable that reflected married parents and any other condition (divorced, not married, partnered, etc.).

Race. Race was self-identified, treated as a nominal variable, and the moderator variable (White and Black). Race was the effect modifier (moderator). In this study race was a social rather than a biological variable. White was defined as a person having origins in any of the original peoples of Europe, the Middle East, or North Africa. Black or African American was defined as a person having origins in any of the Black racial groups of Africa. We used race as an effect modifier because MDRs theory suggests that due to racism and social stratification, returns of SES indicators such as parental education tend to be weaker for racialized groups.

Ethnicity. Ethnicity was self-identified as non-Latino, or Latino. We defined Latino as "a person of Cuban, Mexican, Puerto Rican, South or Central American, or other Spanish culture or origin regardless of race".

Data Analysis

Data analysis was performed using SPSS 24. SPSS was used for univariate, bivariate, and multivariable analysis. Univariate was descriptive statistics such as mean (standard deviation [SD]) and frequency (%). Bivariate included the Spearman correlation test. With the outcome being perceived tobacco use norms score at age 4, the predictor variable was parental educational attainment, and the moderators (effect modifiers) were race and ethnicity, and age, sex, and parental marital status as the covariates, six linear regression models were applied for multivariable modeling. *Model 1* and *Model 2* were run in the pooled sample. *Model 3* and *Model 4* were performed on non-Latino and Latino youth. *Model 5* and *Model 6* were performed on White and Black youth. *Model 1* did not have, and *Model 2* had the interaction term between race/ethnicity and parental education, our predictor variable. *Model 5* and *Model 6* were not shown because there were no race differences in associations. *Model 7* to *Model 10* were performed in race × ethnic groups. *Model 11* and 12 were performed by sex/gender. B, SE, 95% CI, and *p* were reported from each model.

3. Results

3.1. Descriptive Data

A total number of 4815 youth were entered who had and follow-up data for four years. Descriptive data are reported in Table 1.

Table 1. Descriptive data overall and by race in youth (*n* = 4329).

	All		Non-Latino White		Non-Latino Black		Latino White		Latino Black	
	n 4596	%	n 2507	%	n 757	%	n 966	%	n 99	%
12–14	4433	96.5	2427	96.8	714	94.3	938	97.1	96	97.0
15–18	163	3.5	80	3.2	43	5.7	28	2.9	3	3.0
Sex/Gender										
Female	2199	47.8	1201	47.9	367	48.5	455	47.1	49	49.5
Male	2384	51.9	1303	52.0	385	50.9	510	52.8	47	47.5
Marital Status of the Parents										
Not Married	1653	36.0	665	26.5	470	62.1	364	37.7	69	69.7
Married	2943	64.0	1842	73.5	287	37.9	602	62.3	30	30.3
Parental educational attainment (1–5)	2.7963	1.25674	3.2110	1.17118	2.6222	1.16380	2.1460	1.14105	2.2828	1.16969
Perceived tobacco use norms (1–5)	4.2577	0.80773	4.2525	0.81754	4.1477	0.87378	4.3365	0.73895	4.2225	0.83277

3.2. Pooled Sample Models

Table 2 presents the summary of linear regressions for *Model 1* and *Model 2* that were fitted to the pooled sample. As this model shows, higher parental educational attainment was associated with lower perceived tobacco use norms; however, this association was stronger for non-Latino than Latino youth. White and Black youth did not show difference in the slope of the effect of parental educational attainment on outcome.

Table 2. Pooled Sample models in US youth.

	Unstandardized B	Unstandardized Std. Error	Standardized Beta	Lower Bound	Upper Bound	Sig.
Model 1 (All, Main Effects)						
Race (Black)	−0.071	0.032	−0.036	−0.134	−0.009	0.025
Ethnicity (Latino)	0.175	0.031	0.095	0.115	0.236	0.000
Male	0.039	0.025	0.024	−0.010	0.087	0.117
Age	−0.029	0.067	−0.007	−0.160	0.102	0.664
Parental Educational Attainment (1–5)	0.106	0.011	0.165	0.085	0.126	0.000
Model 2 (All, M1 + Race Interaction)						
Race (Black)	−0.014	0.078	−0.007	−0.166	0.138	0.857
Ethnicity (Latino)	0.179	0.031	0.097	0.118	0.240	0.000
Male	0.039	0.025	0.024	−0.010	0.087	0.118
Age	−0.030	0.067	−0.007	−0.161	0.101	0.653
Parental Educational Attainment (1–5)	0.110	0.012	0.171	0.087	0.133	0.000
Parental educational attainment (1–5) × Race (Black)	−0.021	0.026	−0.031	−0.073	0.030	0.418
Model 2 (All, M1 + Ethnicity Interaction)						
Race(Black)	−0.053	0.032	−0.026	−0.115	0.010	0.099
Male	0.486	0.067	0.263	0.354	0.618	0.000
Age	0.037	0.025	0.023	−0.012	0.085	0.136
Married Parents	−0.029	0.067	−0.007	−0.160	0.102	0.663
Parental educational attainment (1–5)	0.137	0.012	0.214	0.113	.161	0.000
Parental educational attainment (1–5) × Ethnicity (Latino)	−0.129	0.025	−0.176	−0.178	−0.080	0.000

Outcome: Perceived tobacco use norms Score; Data: Population Assessment of Tobacco and Health (PATH).

3.3. Ethnic Stratified Models

Table 3 presents the summary of linear regressions for *Model 3* and *Model 4* that were fitted to White and Black youth, respectively. As these models show, higher parental educational attainment was associated with a lower perceived tobacco use norms for non-Latino but not for Latino youth.

Table 3. Stratified models in non-Latino and Latino youth.

	Unstandardized B	Unstandardized Std. Error	Standardized Beta	Lower Bound	Upper Bound	Sig.
Model 3 (Non-Latino)						
Race (Black)	−0.042	0.035	−0.022	−0.111	0.026	0.228
Male	0.018	0.029	0.011	−0.039	0.075	0.538
Age	−0.044	0.076	−0.010	−0.193	0.104	0.556
Parental educational attainment (1–5)	0.138	0.012	0.201	0.113	0.162	0.000
Model 4 (Latino)						
Race (Black)	−0.114	0.081	−0.044	−0.273	0.044	0.158
Male	0.094	0.046	0.063	0.003	0.185	0.044
Age	0.041	0.144	0.009	−0.242	0.324	0.776
Parental educational attainment (1–5)	0.008	0.020	0.013	−0.031	0.048	0.677

Outcome: Perceived tobacco use norms Score; Data: Population Assessment of Tobacco and Health (PATH).

3.4. Race × Ethnic Interactional Stratified Models

As shown by *Models 5 to 8* performed in race by ethnic intersectional groups, parental education was associated with higher perceived tobacco use norms score in non-Latino Whites and non-Latino Blacks. This association was not significant for Latino White and Latino Black individuals (Table 4).

Table 4. Models in race × ethnicity groups.

	Unstandardized B	Unstandardized Std. Error	Standardized Beta	Lower Bound	Upper Bound	Sig.
Model 5 (Non-Latino White)						
Age	−0.070	0.090	−0.015	−0.247	0.107	0.438
Male	0.023	0.032	0.014	−0.040	0.085	0.475
Parental educational	0.164	0.014	0.236	0.138	0.191	0.000
Model 6 (Non-Latino Black)						
Age	0.025	0.137	0.007	−0.244	0.293	0.856
Male	0.047	0.063	0.027	−0.077	0.172	0.456
Parental educational	0.093	0.027	0.124	0.040	0.147	0.001
Model 7 (Latino White)						
Age	0.100	0.141	0.023	−0.178	0.377	0.481
Male	0.132	0.048	0.089	0.039	0.225	0.006
Parental educational	0.005	0.021	0.008	−0.036	0.046	0.805
Model 8 (Latino Black)						
Age	−0.387	0.464	−0.085	−1.308	0.535	0.407
Male	−0.403	0.162	−0.255	−0.724	−0.082	0.015
Parental educational	0.030	0.067	0.045	−0.104	0.164	0.655

Outcome: Perceived tobacco use norms Score; Data: Population Assessment of Tobacco and Health (PATH).

3.5. Sex/Gender Stratified Models

Due to low sample size, interaction between race or ethnicity with parental education did not show significance in our male or female youth. Table 5 shows the summary of these findings.

Table 5. Stratified models in male and female youth.

	Unstandardized B	Std. Error	Standardized Beta	Lower Bound	Upper Bound	Sig.	Unstandardized B	Std. Error	Standardized Beta	Lower Bound	Upper Bound	Sig.
Females												
Race (Black)	−0.022	0.044	−0.011	−0.109	0.064	0.610	0.120	0.106	0.060	−0.088	0.328	0.257
Ethnicity (Hispanic)	0.181	0.040	0.102	0.102	0.260	0.000	0.186	0.044	0.099	0.100	0.271	0.000
Age	−0.125	0.092	−0.029	−0.305	0.055	0.172	−0.099	0.095	−0.023	−0.286	0.087	0.297
Parent eucation	0.114	0.014	0.178	0.086	0.142	0.000	0.133	0.017	0.206	0.101	0.166	0.000
Parent eucation × Race (Black)							−0.052	0.036	−0.076	−0.123	0.018	0.147
Males												
Race (Black)	−0.078	0.044	−0.037	−0.164	0.007	0.073	−0.053	0.110	−0.026	−0.269	0.163	0.630
Ethnicity (Hispanic)	0.213	0.040	0.119	0.135	0.291	0.000	0.215	0.043	0.113	0.131	0.299	0.000
Age	0.053	0.088	0.012	−0.119	0.225	0.547	0.062	0.091	0.014	−0.116	0.240	0.496
Parent eucation	0.108	0.014	0.167	0.080	0.135	0.000	0.109	0.016	0.166	0.077	0.140	0.000
Parent eucation × Race (Black)							−0.009	0.038	−0.012	−0.083	0.065	0.811

Outcome: Perceived tobacco use norms Score; Data: Population Assessment of Tobacco and Health (PATH).

4. Discussion

The current study was performed with two main aims: one to evaluate the overall association between parental educational attainment and perceived tobacco use norms in US youth, and two to test variation in this association by race and ethnicity. The first aim showed an inverse association between parental educational attainment and perceived tobacco use norms overall. The second aim showed moderation by ethnicity not race. This protective association was weaker for Latino than non-Latino youth. This association did not differ between Black and White youth.

The inverse association between parental educational attainment and perceived tobacco use norms is in line with theories of fundamental causes, social determinants, social status, status syndrome, and several other models that explain the lower risk of high SES populations and individuals. Due to Jim Crow, historical racism, the legacy of slavery, social stratification, and segregation, Black-White differences in living conditions sustain across all levels of socioeconomic inequalities [59–62]. According to ecological theories, individuals who live in proximity to low SES neighborhoods, peers, schools, families, and friends will have a higher risk, including tobacco use risk [63]. However, many mechanisms may explain why low SES is associated with race, peer risk, and poor neighborhoods.

There are multiple studies that show racial and ethnic variation in the association between SES, health, and behaviors, with weaker associations in racial and ethnic minorities than non-Latino White youth [64]. There are also studies showing weaker associations between SES and tobacco risk in Black and Latino than non-Latino White individuals [16,19–23,25–29,65]. However, we are unaware of any past studies on racial and ethnic differences in the association between parental educational attainment and perceived tobacco use norms.

There are several studies on racial and ethnic variation in health-behavior association [30–32]. One of their studies showed that Black and Native American adolescents pay greater social costs with academic success than Whites; however, this is seen in high-achieving schools with a smaller percentage of Black students [32]. In another study, they showed that the effects of educational attainment were weaker for Black than for whites, and only 8% of this difference was due to covariates. Analyses yielded consistent results. They concluded that the effects of educational attainment on inflammation levels are stronger for whites than for racial and ethnic minorities [31].

Most past research is conducted on Black, not Latino individuals. Our observation of a weaker association between parental educational attainment and perceived tobacco use norms in Latino than non-Latino youth is also in line with many previous publications on the MDRs. According to marginalization-related diminished returns, resources and assets generate fewer economic, behavioral, developmental, and health outcomes for marginalized groups than for White individuals. While most of this literature is generated on SES effects among adults, there are some studies showing that a sense of mastery, agency, and self-efficacy may be associated with lower health for Black than White individuals [45]. Similarly, positive affect [46,47], happiness [48–50], and a sense of health [66–68] may generate more life expectancy for Whites than Blacks [45,51]. The positive association between SES and John Henryism is also suggestive of the health risks that may be the price of success for Black individuals [69–73]. Hudson has published on the high costs of success for Black youth and young adults [70,74,75].

This study expanded the MDRs literature, which is written on tobacco use [57,58]. Previous work has shown that SES –tobacco use is racialized [57,58]. A study showed that education–tobacco knowledge is also racialized in the US [76]. This finding may be because high-SES White youth attend better schools than high-SES Black youth [35]. In addition, there are many challenges in the daily lives of Black youth in US schools [33,34]. Racial differences in the returns of education may be because of anti-Black discrimination at schools [33,34] or neighborhoods [37,38].

Our study is not without methodological limitations. First, all variables were self-report. Thus, our results may be affected by reporting bias and social desirability. Second, our variables were measured from youth. Norms could be measured from the social network of the youth. We did not measure many potential confounders, such as drug availability at home or neighborhood conditions, such as proximity to tobacco outlets. In addition, this was a study with an imbalanced sample size (larger n for non-Latino and White than Latino and Black youth). However, our main inference was based on pooled sample analysis with interaction rather than stratified models, which have differential power. Our study explored sex differences in the relationship between parental educational attainment and youth's perceived tobacco use norms, however, the sample size was inadequate for race by sex by parental education interaction term. Despite these limitations, the major contribution of this study is to document MDRs for perceived tobacco use norms for the first time. We are not aware of any previous studies that suggest perceived tobacco use norms may have a role in higher-than-expected tobacco use of Black and Latino youth with highly educated parents.

Future research is needed on the social and environmental causes of the observed MDRs. Future research should test the role of advertisement exposure, the prevalence of smokers, as well as other contextual factors at school and neighborhood that may weaken the effect of parental educational attainment for ethnic minority youth. The role of high-risk peers, family, friends, proximity to tobacco outlets, and other contextual conditions should be tested in future multi-level research.

5. Conclusions

To conclude, although overall, high parental educational attainment is associated with lower perceived tobacco use norms, this inverse association is weaker for Latino than non-Latino youth. The diminished return of parental educational attainment on perceived tobacco use norms may be due to environmental and structural inequalities at family, school, or neighborhood due to the segregation of ethnic minority communities. Future research should test why and how the same MDRs could not be found for Black youth.

Author Contributions: Conceptualization, E.A., B.N., and A.Y.-B.; Formal analysis, B.N.; Investigation, A.Y.-B.; Software, E.A.; Writing—original draft, E.A., and B.N.; Writing—review and editing, E.A., and B.N. All authors have read and agreed to the published version of the manuscript.

Funding: As a scholar of the Clinical Research Education and Career Development (CRECD) program at Charles R. Drew University of Medicine and Science (CDU), Dr. Adinkrah's research-related activities were supported by the NIMHD/NIH Award # R25 MD007610. A.Y.-B. is funded and supported by the Tobacco-Related Disease Research Program (TRDRP) grant R00RG2347.

Institutional Review Board Statement: This study used publicly available PATH data. All data are fully de-identified. Thus, the study was not human subject research and exempt from full IRB review.

Informed Consent Statement: All youth provided assent. All parents provided consent.

Data Availability Statement: PATH data are publicly available here: https://www.icpsr.umich.edu/web/NAHDAP/series/606 (accessed 12 October 2022).

Conflicts of Interest: The authors declare no conflict of interest.

References

1. Asma, S. *The GATS Atlas: Global Adult Tobacco Survey*; CDC: Atlanta, GA, USA, 2015.
2. Hiscock, R.; Bauld, L.; Amos, A.; Fidler, J.A.; Munafò, M. Socioeconomic status and smoking: A review. *Ann. N. Y. Acad. Sci.* **2012**, *1248*, 107–123. [CrossRef]
3. Gecková, A.M.; Stewart, R.; van Dijk, J.P.; Orosová, O.g.; Groothoff, J.W.; Post, D. Influence of socio-economic status, parents and peers on smoking behaviour of adolescents. *Eur. Addict. Res.* **2005**, *11*, 204–209. [CrossRef]
4. Glendinning, A.; Shucksmith, J.; Hendry, L. Family life and smoking in adolescence. *Soc. Sci. Med.* **1997**, *44*, 93–101. [CrossRef]
5. Jessor, R.; Jessor, S.L. *Problem Behavior and Psychosocial Development: A Longitudinal Study of Youth*; Academic Press: New York, NY, USA, 1977.
6. Pezzella, F.S.; Thornberry, T.P.; Smith, C.A. Race socialization and parenting styles: Links to delinquency for African American and White adolescents. *Youth Violence Juv. Justice* **2016**, *14*, 448–467. [CrossRef]

7. Assari, S. Parental Educational Attainment and Mental Well-Being of College Students; Diminished Returns of Blacks. *Brain Sci.* **2018**, *8*, 193. [CrossRef]
8. Assari, S. Blacks' Diminished Return of Education Attainment on Subjective Health; Mediating Effect of Income. *Brain Sci.* **2018**, *8*, 176. [CrossRef] [PubMed]
9. Assari, S. Socioeconomic Status and Self-Rated Oral Health; Diminished Return among Hispanic Whites. *Dent. J.* **2018**, *6*, 11. [CrossRef]
10. Assari, S. Health Disparities due to Diminished Return among Black Americans: Public Policy Solutions. *Soc. Issues Policy Rev.* **2018**, *12*, 112–145. [CrossRef]
11. Assari, S. Diminished Economic Return of Socioeconomic Status for Black Families. *Soc. Sci.* **2018**, *7*, 74. [CrossRef]
12. Assari, S.; Caldwell, C.H.; Mincy, R. Family Socioeconomic Status at Birth and Youth Impulsivity at Age 15; Blacks' Diminished Return. *Children* **2018**, *5*, 58. [CrossRef]
13. Assari, S.; Caldwell, C.H.; Zimmerman, M.A. Family Structure and Subsequent Anxiety Symptoms; Minorities' Diminished Return. *Brain Sci.* **2018**, *8*, 97. [CrossRef] [PubMed]
14. Assari, S.; Hani, N. Household Income and Children's Unmet Dental Care Need; Blacks' Diminished Return. *Dent. J.* **2018**, *6*, 17. [CrossRef]
15. Assari, S.; Lapeyrouse, L.M.; Neighbors, H.W. Income and Self-Rated Mental Health: Diminished Returns for High Income Black Americans. *Behav. Sci.* **2018**, *8*, 50. [CrossRef] [PubMed]
16. Assari, S.; Mistry, R. Educational Attainment and Smoking Status in a National Sample of American Adults; Evidence for the Blacks' Diminished Return. *Int. J. Environ. Res. Public Health* **2018**, *15*, 763. [CrossRef] [PubMed]
17. Assari, S. Unequal Gain of Equal Resources across Racial Groups. *Int. J. Health Policy Manag.* **2018**, *7*, 1–9. [CrossRef] [PubMed]
18. Assari, S. Understanding America: Unequal Economic Returns of Years of Schooling in Whites and Blacks. *World J. Educ. Res.* **2020**, *7*, 78–92. [CrossRef]
19. Darvishi, M.; Saqib, M.; Assari, S. Diminished Association between Parental Education and Parahippocampal Cortical Thickness in Pre-Adolescents in the US. *Stud. Soc. Sci. Res.* **2021**, *2*, 34–63. [CrossRef]
20. Assari, S. Diminished Returns of Income Against Cigarette Smoking Among Chinese Americans. *J. Health Econ. Dev.* **2019**, *1*, 1–8.
21. Assari, S.; Bazargan, M. Education Level and Cigarette Smoking: Diminished Returns of Lesbian, Gay and Bisexual Individuals. *Behav. Sci.* **2019**, *9*, 103. [CrossRef]
22. Assari, S.; Bazargan, M. Protective Effects of Educational Attainment Against Cigarette Smoking; Diminished Returns of American Indians and Alaska Natives in the National Health Interview Survey. *Int. J. Travel Med. Glob. Health* **2019**, *7*, 105. [CrossRef]
23. Assari, S.; Mistry, R. Diminished Return of Employment on Ever Smoking Among Hispanic Whites in Los Angeles. *Health Equity* **2019**, *3*, 138–144. [CrossRef] [PubMed]
24. Assari, S.; Smith, J.L.; Zimmerman, M.A.; Bazargan, M. Cigarette Smoking among Economically Disadvantaged African-American Older Adults in South Los Angeles: Gender Differences. *Int. J. Environ. Res. Public Health* **2019**, *16*, 1208. [CrossRef] [PubMed]
25. Darvishi, M.; Saqib, M.; Assari, S. Parental Education and Functional Connectivity between Nucleus Accumbens (NAcc) and Frontoparietal Network (FPN). *J. Educ. Cult. Stud.* **2021**, *5*, 61–83. [CrossRef]
26. Assari, S. Socioeconomic Status and Current Cigarette Smoking Status: Immigrants' Diminished Returns. *Int. J. Travel Med. Glob. Health* **2020**, *8*, 66–72. [CrossRef] [PubMed]
27. Assari, S.; Boyce, S.; Caldwell, C.H.; Bazargan, M. Parent Education and Future Transition to Cigarette Smoking: Latinos' Diminished Returns. *Front. Pediatr.* **2020**, *8*, 457. [CrossRef]
28. Assari, S.; Mistry, R.; Caldwell, C.H.; Bazargan, M. Protective Effects of Parental Education Against Youth Cigarette Smoking: Diminished Returns of Blacks and Hispanics. *Adolesc. Health Med. Ther.* **2020**, *11*, 63–71. [CrossRef]
29. Assari, S.B.M.; Chalian, M. Social Determinants of Hookah Smoking in the United States. *J. Ment. Health Clin. Psychol.* **2020**, *4*, 21. [CrossRef]
30. Fuller-Rowell, T.E.; Cogburn, C.D.; Brodish, A.B.; Peck, S.C.; Malanchuk, O.; Eccles, J.S. Racial discrimination and substance use: Longitudinal associations and identity moderators. *J. Behav. Med.* **2012**, *35*, 581–590. [CrossRef]
31. Fuller-Rowell, T.E.; Curtis, D.S.; Doan, S.N.; Coe, C.L. Racial disparities in the health benefits of educational attainment: A study of inflammatory trajectories among African American and white adults. *Psychosom. Med.* **2015**, *77*, 33–40. [CrossRef]
32. Fuller-Rowell, T.E.; Doan, S.N. The social costs of academic success across ethnic groups. *Child Dev.* **2010**, *81*, 1696–1713. [CrossRef]
33. Assari, S. Original Paper Are Teachers Biased against Black Children? A Study of Race, Amygdala Volume, and Problem Behaviors. *J. Educ. Teach. Soc. Stud.* **2021**, 3. [CrossRef]
34. Assari, S.; Caldwell, C.H. Teacher Discrimination Reduces School Performance of African American Youth: Role of Gender. *Brain Sci.* **2018**, *8*, 183. [CrossRef] [PubMed]
35. Boyce, S.; Bazargan, M.; Caldwell, C.H.; Zimmerman, M.A.; Assari, S. Parental Educational Attainment and Social Environment of Urban Public Schools in the U.S.: Blacks' Diminished Returns. *Children* **2020**, *7*, 44. [CrossRef] [PubMed]
36. Assari, S.; Caldwell, C.; Bazargan, M. Parental educational attainment and relatives' substance use of American youth: Hispanics Diminished Returns. *J. Biosci. Med.* **2020**, *8*, 122–134. [CrossRef]
37. Assari, S. Does School Racial Composition Explain Why High Income Black Youth Perceive More Discrimination? *A Gender Analysis. Brain Sci.* **2018**, *8*, 140. [CrossRef]

38. Assari, S.; Moghani Lankarani, M. Workplace Racial Composition Explains High Perceived Discrimination of High Socioeconomic Status African American Men. *Brain Sci.* **2018**, *8*, 139. [CrossRef]
39. Assari, S.; Preiser, B.; Lankarani, M.M.; Caldwell, C.H. Subjective Socioeconomic Status Moderates the Association between Discrimination and Depression in African American Youth. *Brain Sci.* **2018**, *8*, 71. [CrossRef]
40. Dantzler, K.; Altamirano, M.; Anomo, T.; Carrillo, E.; Hall, M.; Hildreth, K.; Nwabuzor, J.; Opong, N.; Okbu, H.; Perez, M.; et al. Learning While Black: A Qualitative Analysis of the Impact of Race in a U. S. High School. *World J. Educ. Res.* **2022**, *9*. [CrossRef]
41. Halliwell, H.A.; IBCLC; King, E.; Gonzalez-Matute, M.; Kirksey, J.A.; Martinez, C.; Pratts, M.; Ybarra, S. It's Like the Elephant in the Room" A Qualitative Analysis of Racism in a U.S. High School. *World J. Educ. Res.* **2022**, *9*. [CrossRef]
42. Assari, S.; Najand, B.; Young-Brinn, A. Minorities' Diminished Returns of Family Socioeconomic Status on Youth Peers' Tobacco Use. *Int. J. Travel Med. Glob. Health* **2022**, *10*, 159–165. [CrossRef]
43. Bazargan, M.; Cobb, S.; Castro Sandoval, J.; Assari, S. Smoking Status and Well-Being of Underserved African American Older Adults. *Behav. Sci.* **2020**, *10*, 78. [CrossRef] [PubMed]
44. Harris, J.C.; Mereish, E.H.; Faulkner, M.L.; Assari, S.; Choi, K.; Leggio, L.; Farokhnia, M. Racial Differences in the Association Between Alcohol Drinking and Cigarette Smoking: Preliminary Findings From an Alcohol Research Program. *Alcohol Alcohol.* **2022**, *57*, 330–339. [CrossRef] [PubMed]
45. Assari, S. General Self-Efficacy and Mortality in the USA; Racial Differences. *J. Racial Ethn. Health Disparities* **2017**, *4*, 746–757. [CrossRef] [PubMed]
46. Assari, S.; Lankarani, M.M. Chronic Medical Conditions and Negative Affect; Racial Variation in Reciprocal Associations Over Time. *Front. Psychiatry* **2016**, *7*, 140. [CrossRef]
47. Lankarani, M.M.; Assari, S. Positive and Negative Affect More Concurrent among Blacks than Whites. *Behav. Sci.* **2017**, *7*, 48. [CrossRef]
48. Assari, S. Race, Education Attainment, and Happiness in the United States. *Int. J. Epidemiol. Res.* **2019**, *6*, 76. [CrossRef]
49. Cobb, S.; Javanbakht, A.; Khalifeh Soltani, E.; Bazargan, M.; Assari, S. Racial Difference in the Relationship Between Health and Happiness in the United States. *Psychol. Res. Behav. Manag.* **2020**, *13*, 481–490. [CrossRef]
50. Maharlouei, N.; Cobb, S.; Bazargan, M.; Assari, S. Subjective Health and Happiness in the United States: Gender Differences in the Effects of Socioeconomic Status Indicators. *J. Ment. Health Clin. Psychol.* **2020**, *4*, 8–17. [CrossRef]
51. Assari, S. Race, sense of control over life, and short-term risk of mortality among older adults in the United States. *Arch. Med. Sci.* **2017**, *13*, 1233–1240. [CrossRef]
52. Topa, G.; Moriano, J.A. Theory of planned behavior and smoking: Meta-analysis and SEM model. *Subst. Abus. Rehabil.* **2010**, *1*, 23–33. [CrossRef]
53. Guo, Q.; Johnson, C.A.; Unger, J.B.; Lee, L.; Xie, B.; Chou, C.-P.; Palmer, P.H.; Sun, P.; Gallaher, P.; Pentz, M. Utility of the theory of reasoned action and theory of planned behavior for predicting Chinese adolescent smoking. *Addict. Behav.* **2007**, *32*, 1066–1081. [CrossRef] [PubMed]
54. Perkins, J.M.; Perkins, H.W.; Jurinsky, J.; Craig, D.W. Adolescent tobacco use and misperceptions of social norms across schools in the United States. *J. Stud. Alcohol Drugs* **2019**, *80*, 659–668. [CrossRef]
55. Buu, A.; Nam, J.K.; Yang, M.; Su, W.-C.; Lin, H.-C. Home e-cigarette rules and youth's vulnerability to initiate and sustain e-cigarette use. *Prev. Med.* **2022**, *164*, 107334. [CrossRef] [PubMed]
56. Unger, J.B.; Rohrbach, L.A.; Howard-Pitney, B.; Ritt-Olson, A.; Mouttapa, M. Peer influences and susceptibility to smoking among California adolescents. *Subst. Use Misuse* **2001**, *36*, 551–571. [CrossRef] [PubMed]
57. Assari, S.; Lankarani, M.M. Education and Alcohol Consumption among Older Americans; Black-White Differences. *Front. Public Health* **2016**, *4*, 67. [CrossRef]
58. Assari, S.; Farokhnia, M.; Mistry, R. Education Attainment and Alcohol Binge Drinking: Diminished Returns of Hispanics in Los Angeles. *Behav. Sci.* **2019**, *9*, 9. [CrossRef]
59. Williams, D.R. Race, socioeconomic status, and health the added effects of racism and discrimination. *Ann. N. Y. Acad. Sci.* **1999**, *896*, 173–188. [CrossRef]
60. Williams, D.R. Miles to go before we sleep: Racial inequities in health. *J. Health Soc. Behav.* **2012**, *53*, 279–295. [CrossRef]
61. Williams, D.R.; Cooper, L.A. Reducing racial inequities in health: Using what we already know to take action. *Int. J. Environ. Res. Public Health* **2019**, *16*, 606. [CrossRef]
62. Williams, D.R.; Lawrence, J.A.; Davis, B.A. Racism and health: Evidence and needed research. *Annu. Rev. Public Health* **2019**, *40*, 105–125. [CrossRef]
63. Hibbs, R.; Rankin, K.M.; David, R.J.; Collins, J.W., Jr. The Relation of Neighborhood Income to the Age-Related Patterns of Preterm Birth Among White and African-American Women: The Effect of Cigarette Smoking. *Matern. Child Health J.* **2016**, *20*, 1432–1440. [CrossRef] [PubMed]
64. Martins, S.S.; Lee, G.P.; Kim, J.H.; Letourneau, E.J.; Storr, C.L. Gambling and sexual behaviors in African-American adolescents. *Addict. Behav.* **2014**, *39*, 854–860. [CrossRef] [PubMed]
65. Assari, S.; Mistry, R. Erratum: Assari, S.; Mistry, R. Educational Attainment and Smoking Status in a National Sample of American Adults; Evidence for the Blacks' Diminished Return. *Int. J. Environ. Res. Public Health* **2018**, *15*, 2084. [CrossRef] [PubMed]
66. Boyce, S.; Darvishi, M.; Marandi, R.; Rahmanian, R.; Akhtar, S.; Patterson, J.; Assari, S. Racism-Related Diminished Returns of Socioeconomic Status on Adolescent Brain and Cognitive Development. *Res. Health Sci.* **2021**, *6*, 1–22. [CrossRef]

67. Assari, S.; Lankarani, M.M.; Burgard, S. Black-white difference in long-term predictive power of self-rated health on all-cause mortality in United States. *Ann. Epidemiol.* **2016**, *26*, 106–114. [CrossRef] [PubMed]
68. Assari, S. Self-rated Health and Mortality due to Kidney Diseases: Racial Differences in the United States. *Adv. Biomed. Res.* **2018**, *7*, 4. [CrossRef] [PubMed]
69. James, S.A.; Hartnett, S.A.; Kalsbeek, W.D. John Henryism and blood pressure differences among black men. *J. Behav. Med.* **1983**, *6*, 259–278. [CrossRef]
70. Duijkers, T.J.; Drijver, M.; Kromhout, D.; James, S.A. "John Henryism" and blood pressure in a Dutch population. *Psychosom. Med.* **1988**, *50*, 353–359. [CrossRef]
71. James, S.A. John Henryism and the health of African-Americans. *Cult. Med. Psychiatry* **1994**, *18*, 163–182. [CrossRef]
72. Clark, R.; Adams, J.H. Moderating effects of perceived racism on John Henryism and blood pressure reactivity in Black female college students. *Ann. Behav. Med.* **2004**, *28*, 126–131. [CrossRef]
73. Subramanyam, M.A.; James, S.A.; Diez-Roux, A.V.; Hickson, D.A.; Sarpong, D.; Sims, M.; Taylor, H.A., Jr.; Wyatt, S.B. Socioeconomic status, John Henryism and blood pressure among African-Americans in the Jackson Heart Study. *Soc. Sci. Med.* **2013**, *93*, 139–146. [CrossRef] [PubMed]
74. Hudson, D.; Sacks, T.; Irani, K.; Asher, A. The Price of the Ticket: Health Costs of Upward Mobility among African Americans. *Int. J. Environ. Res. Public Health* **2020**, *17*, 1179. [CrossRef] [PubMed]
75. Zahodne, L.B.; Meyer, O.L.; Choi, E.; Thomas, M.L.; Willis, S.L.; Marsiske, M.; Gross, A.L.; Rebok, G.W.; Parisi, J.M. External locus of control contributes to racial disparities in memory and reasoning training gains in ACTIVE. *Psychol. Aging* **2015**, *30*, 561. [CrossRef]
76. Assari, S.; Bazargan, M. Educational Attainment and Tobacco Harm Knowledge Among American Adults: Diminished Returns of African Americans and Hispanics. *Int. J. Epidemiol. Res.* **2020**, *7*, 6–11. [CrossRef]

Disclaimer/Publisher's Note: The statements, opinions and data contained in all publications are solely those of the individual author(s) and contributor(s) and not of MDPI and/or the editor(s). MDPI and/or the editor(s) disclaim responsibility for any injury to people or property resulting from any ideas, methods, instructions or products referred to in the content.

MDPI
St. Alban-Anlage 66
4052 Basel
Switzerland
Tel. +41 61 683 77 34
Fax +41 61 302 89 18
www.mdpi.com

International Journal of Environmental Research and Public Health Editorial Office
E-mail: ijerph@mdpi.com
www.mdpi.com/journal/ijerph

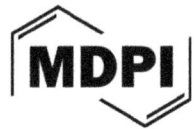

www.ingramcontent.com/pod-product-compliance
Lightning Source LLC
LaVergne TN
LVHW070206100526
838202LV00015B/2008

9 7 8 3 0 3 6 5 6 9 7 8 9